Transcatheter Valve Therapies

Transcatheter Valve Therapies

Christoph Huber

University Clinic for Cardiovascular Surgery
Swiss Heart Center–Bern University Hospital–Inselspital
Bern, Switzerland

Ted Feldman

Evanston Hospital
Evanston, Illinois, USA

with a contribution by Jack D. Lemmon

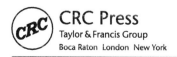

CRC Press
Taylor & Francis Group
Boca Raton London New York

CRC Press is an imprint of the
Taylor & Francis Group, an **informa** business

CRC Press
Taylor & Francis Group
6000 Broken Sound Parkway NW, Suite 300
Boca Raton, FL 33487-2742

First issued in paperback 2017

© 2010 by Taylor & Francis Group, LLC
CRC Press is an imprint of Taylor & Francis Group, an Informa business

No claim to original U.S. Government works

ISBN-13: 978-1-4398-1078-1 (hbk)
ISBN-13: 978-1-138-11610-8 (pbk)

A CIP record for this book is available from the British Library.

Library of Congress Cataloging-in-Publication Data available on application

Visit the Taylor & Francis Web site at
http://www.taylorandfrancis.com

and the CRC Press Web site at
http://www.crcpress.com

To my wife Ann,
and my two daughters Chloé and Sophie

Foreword

Transcatheter valve therapy (TCVT) is a uniquely modern, up-to-date, and integrated scientific work on a new era of heart valve therapy. What is most interesting about this work on percutaneous valve therapy is that the editor is a cardiac surgeon who is espousing interventional techniques for a select patient population requiring valve repair or replacement. Dr. Huber comes with unique qualifications having worked in cardiac surgery as well as having extensive experience with clinical and experimental interventional procedures, thus well-suited to have a precise and scientific overview of this burgeoning field. It is clear that within 10 years many of the devices shown in this book will be available to clinicians to use in a variety of clinical settings. These, along with the increasing numbers of elderly patients who will require valve surgery in one form or another, were important stimuli to produce such a book. Dr. Huber is to be congratulated for putting forth in one concise volume a current overview of transcatheter valve therapy—past, present, and future.

These will be important therapies as the numbers of elderly patients grow and require minimally invasive valve therapy. Another important population that may benefit from these therapies is those with other infirmities or comorbidities in whom traditional open heart surgery for valve therapy would be a very high-risk procedure. Such conditions would include additional systemic diseases such as liver, hepatic cirrhosis, or a previous therapy, such as chest radiation or prior coronary bypass.

Dr. Huber has concisely and completely included prior experimental data on these valve therapies that are important to understand how these devices will work. In addition, he has also provided us with the methods individual practitioners should use to learn how to use these techniques, namely, simulation technology and other models, including animal surgery, where not only insertion of the device is demonstrated, but coordination of teamwork to implant the device can be replicated to obtain a successful result.

The concept of teamwork and an integrative philosophy to make medical disciplines work synchronal is key for this entire area going forward and Dr. Huber has summarized it beautifully. This effort will require experts in imaging, cardiac anesthesia, cardiology, cardiac surgery, and certainly interventionalists. As editor of the *Journal of Thoracic and Cardiovascular Surgery*, I have stated many times that the integrative approach to the medical specialty or a service line concept is clearly the wave of the future and the future is now.

   Dr. Huber's book should be read and studied carefully with a sense toward the future. TCVT stands as an important milestone in our compilation of knowledge and expertise about a field that will be growing exponentially in the next decades.

Lawrence H. Cohn, M.D.
Boston, Massachusetts, U.S.A.

Foreword

Dr. Huber has put together an up to date textbook on catheter therapy with a focus on aortic valve disease. The text is timely, and takes a careful look at where we came from, where we are, and where we are going with aortic valve replacement therapies. The development of catheter based aortic valve replacement rests on a long history of surgical valve replacement, and also as much so on a long history of development of percutaneous, catheter based methods. The expertise that has drawn on both of these antecedent pathways to come together as a means for valve replacement using almost completely noninvasive methods has required true partnership in its development.

Most of the inventors of catheter valve therapies have been cardiac surgeons. Most of the first in-man experience has been generated by interventional cardiologists, always working in conjunction with a team that includes cardiothoracic and vascular surgeons, cardiac anesthesiologists, imaging cardiologists, and a variety of other support staff. The future evolution of this partnership might be modeled after what has developed in the area of vascular surgery. Vascular surgeons adopted catheter based methods over the last decade, and transformed the field of vascular surgery. Similarly, interventional cardiologists have looked to a variety of structural heart interventions that have previously been entirely within the realm of surgery, and adapted a whole host of new procedures including mitral valve repair, atrial septal defect and patent foramen ovale closure, left atrial appendage occlusion, and paravalvular prosthetic leak closure.

The training pathway to acquire all of the necessary skills for catheter based valve therapies is not clear. The traditional case volume model is not easily applicable. In the interventional world, in the United States there are 1 million coronary stent procedures a year. This provides a huge population for volume based training standards. The magic number of PCI procedures required in one year, accredited Interventional training programs, is 250 cases. The volume of valve interventions is orders of magnitude lower, and in addition the interventions are more complicated. Thus, volume driven criteria are not adequate for training. This textbook gives a clear picture of the value of simulation training for the development of skills in this new area of therapy. The importance of participation and trials during the early development of percutaneous valve therapies cannot be emphasized enough. Ultimately, it is experienced gained over a long period of time that will be necessary for the hybrid cardiac physician.

This textbook may soon be followed by textbooks on mitral valve repair and other structural interventions. The field is in an explosive growth mode, with almost all of these new therapies still in the Phase I trial experience. Aortic valve replacement therapy has emerged as the most developed procedure in this field, and this greatly enhances the value of this textbook.

What does the future of this therapy and of the melding of traditional surgical and catheter based interventional skills hold? The appearance of this book is a first step in the roadmap for the future of the partnership and of the field.

Ted Feldman, M.D.
Director, Cardiac Catheterization Laboratory
Evanston Hospital, Evanston, Illinois, U.S.A.

Preface

Transcatheter Valve Therapies not only chronicle the astonishing advances that have taken place in the field but also prepares the reader in a contemporary and unique fashion for the challenging future of cardiac valve therapies. The landscape of cardiac surgery is changing and so is the field of interventional cardiology.

The idea of accessing and replacing a failing valve through the patients vasculature might have been mistakenly dismissed as being an illusionary idea, but has since become the most rapidly expanding therapy of choice in cardiovascular disease. This book is designed to meet the growing needs of the cardiologist, cardiac surgeons, anesthetists and general practitioners—all jointly working towards a better quality of life for patients with heart valve disease.

The aim of the book is to provide a comprehensive overview of transcatheter valve therapies and the necessary understanding for a successful clinical introduction at individual institutions. All aspects from the logistic needs to the clinical outcomes the new therapies are covered in an unique fashion to allow the reader a constructive approach to transcatheter therapies independent of their specialist background. The author's expertise as cardiac surgeon with an extensive interventional background, having been involved in transcatheter techniques since its beginning provide a innovative patient and enduser oriented textbook.

The scope of the book is to provide the reader with handy expertise from both the surgical and interventional experience. By inventing the trans-apical procedure for treating structural heart disease, the author joined fundamental surgical and interventional strategies that are provided to the reader in the following chapters.

In such a rapidly expanding field precise description of devices might only be of limited value. The timeless quality of this book is provided by integrating fundamental development steps leading up to the successful market introduction and clinical implementation. Providing the necessary pathways illustrated by the author's own experience results in a comprehensive resource presenting in similar fashion the past, the present, and the future of transcatheter valve therapies.

All essential topics are represented in this book written for clinicians as well as for researchers in the field of transcatheter valve therapies for structural heart disease. Following a concise chronological chapter order, epidemiologic considerations emphasize the unmet needs of patients suffering from heart valve disease and provide insights into the excepted grow of a patient population at risk. But within the exciting adoption of novel therapy care should be taken to stay unbiased and ready for further changes. Ted Feldman's expertise highlights the complementing aspects of balloon aortic valvuloplasty. As a stand-alone procedure or as part of the transcatheter valve replacement. His chapter presents many technical insights into balloon aortic valvuloplasty. Introduction of a new technology requires a multilevel approach to reach successful acceptance. Many hurdles needed to be taken and the introduction of the technology chapter provides the reader with valuable hints of how transcatheter valve therapies were implemented into the surgical practice and why the introduction of the transapical approach became a strategic technique to merge interventional and surgical advantages for a given patient's best benefits. New imaging modalities as well as outlines and necessities of the hybrid environment in the context of a team-based collaboration are conveniently summarized in the same chapter.

An essential resource is found in the section highlighting the particularities of transcatheter access. Understanding the unique and demanding aortic root anatomy provides the necessary ground for most accurate device delivery and future device development. Emerging technologies require constant improvements and the author's own step-wise development might serve as a guide for future design improvements. Innovation paired with strikingly easy technical construction can provide promising solutions to complex tasks as described in the experimental work chapter, featuring not only development steps of aortic devices but also potential solutions for transcatheter tricuspid, mitral and pulmonary valve replacement. Jack Lemmon summarizes the rigorous testing requirements for endovascular medical devices in his chapter Preclinical Valved Stent Device Testing.

The clinical overview in chapter 12 Clinical Results of Aortic Transcatheter Valve Therapies provides the most recent data of the worldwide transcatheter aortic valve experience with detailed outcomes and complications in easy accessible text and table formats.

The author's personal vision of the future on transcatheter valve therapies is outlined in the Conclusion and will prepare the reader to embark into the fascinating future of endoluminal cardiac therapies.

SUMMARY

The book represents one of the earliest attempts to provide the reader in a comprehensive fashion with all key features of transcatheter valve therapies. In a remarkable overview all essential topics are discussed based on the author's own clinical and experimental experience in the field. The book is a must read for everyone planning to get involved into transcatheter valve implantation, a most useful resource for experienced clinicians wishing to become more involved in improving transcatheter valve therapies further and finally the book provides the fundament for researchers and for the industry to build and create new medical technologies for shaping the cardiovascular landscape of the future.

Christoph Huber

Acknowledgments

I would like to thank the many people I had the pleasure to work with. It is a rare opportunity to contribute to what might be one of the most promising steps into a new era of cardiovascular medicine. The inspiration and perseverance to write the first book on aortic transcatheter valve therapies came from all the patients to profit from these exciting new techniques as well as from all the open-minded, encouraging, and visionary colleagues and friends I had the honor to meet and work with. I would like to mention Ludwig K. von Segesser and the whole team of the surgical experimental laboratory at the University Hospital of Lausanne, in particular Iker Mallabiabarena and Monique Augstburger for their early support of my animal work. I also thank my dear colleagues; we shared many late hours at the lab, which include Piergiorgio Tozzi, Bettina Marty, Jun Quing Zhou and Liang Ma.

Great thanks go to Larry Cohn, possibly my most important surgical mentor, whose visionary spirit and belief in my research helped ignite the worldwide interest as expressed in his foreword to this book. My thanks extend to Ted Feldman for his valuable contribution to the present textbook expressing the view of the cardiologist and emphasizing the need for a close interdisciplinary collaboration as well as for his insight into balloon aortic valvuloplasty. I also thank Jack Lemmon for contributing the chapter on valve testing. Thanks go to the publisher Informa Healthcare for their so helpful editorial presence and prompt response.

Finally, I thank my wife Ann and my two adorable daughters Sophie and Chloé for their support, understanding, and patience for the many nights and after-work hours I spent writing this book and I thank my parents and my sister, Laurence, for their encouraging spirit.

Contents

List of Abbreviations

AAA	Abdominal aortic aneurysms
AVD	Aortic valve disease
AVR	Aortic valve replacement
CABG	Coronary artery bypass grafting
CBF	Coronary blood flow
CCS	Canadian Cardiovascular Society
CK	Creatinin kinase
CKMB	Creatinin kinase MB fraction
CPB	Cardiopulmonary bypass
DAVR	Direct access valve replacement
EACTS	European Association of Cardiothoracic Surgery
EF	Ejection fraction
EVAR	Endovascular aortic repair
FOV	Field of view
GI	Gastrointestinal
HLM	Heart-lung machine
ICE	Intracardiac echo
IVUS	Intravascular ultrasound
LA	Left atrium
LAD	Left anterior descending
LCA	Left coronary artery
LV	Left ventricle
LVDD	Left ventricle end-diastolic diameter
LVOT	Left ventricular outflow tract
MI	Myocardial infarction
MRI	Magnetic resonance imaging
MSCT	Multislice computer tomography
MVSDO	Muscular ventricular septum defect occluder
PAVR	Percutaneous aortic valve replacement
PTCA	Percutaneous transluminal coronary angioplasty
RCA	Right coronary artery
RCSSI	Residual coronary sinus stent index
RV	Right ventricle
RVOT	Right ventricular outflow tract
SAVR	Surgical aortic valve replacement
SHD	Structural heart disease
SPAP	Systolic pulmonary artery pressure
STJ	Sinotubular junction

TAP	Transapical procedure
TCV	Transcatheter valve
TCVT	Transcatheter valve therapies
TEE	Transesophageal echo
TIA	Transient ischemic attack
TTE	Transthoracic echo

Disclosure

The book *Transcatheter Valve Therapies* was in part supported by the Swiss National Research Grant No 3200B0-113437 titled "Direct Access Valve Replacement (DAVR) for aortic valves via the Trans Apical Procedure (TAP)" Bern, Switzerland, and by the Fond CardioMet of the Centre for Cardiovascular And Metabolic Research, titled: "Direct Access Aortic Valve Replacement," University Hospital Lausanne, CHUV, Switzerland.

This book has kindly been sponsored by Edwards Lifesciences and CoreValve.

Christoph Huber is founder and stockholder of EndoHeart AG, a Winterthur, Switzerland-based company, active in the development of new transcatheter therapies.

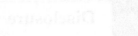

1   Introduction

RESHAPING THE TREATMENT LANDSCAPE OF STRUCTURAL HEART DISEASE

Treating structural heart disease (SHD) has been the driving force behind the development of what is nowadays known as open heart surgery. Since the first successful attempt of repairing a failing mitral valve by Eliott Cutler and Samuel Levine (1), performed at the former Peter Bent Brigham Hospital in Boston, on a 12-year-old girl using a valvulotome, several technical developments have allowed gaining safe access to the inner heart. The probably most important contribution to modern open heart surgery was John Gibbon's heart-lung machine (2). Ever since, heart valve surgery is performed with the heart-lung machine.

Nevertheless, very little progress has been made since. Indeed, new longer-lasting heart valves have been designed, sizes of apparatus used in the operation rooms have decreased drastically, and handling has become easier. Several new approaches to the diseased valve were experienced, and it is certainly worth mentioning that outcome and patient safety improved significantly in all risk classes and age ranges (3). But despite of all progress, no new breakthroughs were achieved.

Nonsurgical techniques, for example, balloon aortic valvuloplasty, initially thought to become the most promising percutaneous alternative, was widely popularized in the 1980s and initially showed satisfying acute results. But poor mid- and long-term outcomes led to the large abandonment of this technique for adult aortic valve stenosis (4–7).

The early days of coronary balloon angioplasty followed a similar pattern after initial enthusiasm. Important drawbacks followed as experienced first by Andreas Roland Grüntzig in 1978 (8). Despite improvements in technical equipment and growing experience of the operators, two major limitations of balloon angioplasty remained unchanged. Vessel wall dissection and abrupt postangioplasty closure complicated 5% of procedures (9), and restenosis occurred in 30% to 40% of patients (10–12).

Only by combining a novel technology aiming toward supporting the vessel wall with a scaffolding device, balloon angioplasty eventually spread to become the most frequently performed cardiac intervention. A self-expanding mesh stent as proposed and first in-man implantation by Ulrich Sigwart in 1986 (13) became the precursors of nowadays routinely implanted coronary stents.

Getting back to the treatment of the aortic valve stenosis, a very similar development can be observed today. Balloon dilatation alone was insufficient as a standalone procedure for coronary interventions as was balloon aortic valvuloplasty. Only the introduction of stents consolidated the former technique. A lesson learned and applied currently with the introduction of valved supporting elements into the aortic root after aortic balloon valvuloplasty for aortic stenosis. The valved anchoring scaffold called valved stent is gaining wider popularity as transcatheter valve therapies (TCVT) for SHD and has ignited an accelerated enthusiasm adopted by cardiac surgeons and interventional cardiologists (14).

Henning Rud Andersen was the first to describe the concept of valved stent in 1990 (15, 16). In his new concept, he combined a tissue valve with a balloon-expandable and self-anchoring scaffold. The obtained device was suitable for a collapsed insertion via a femoral artery and endoluminal expansion and delivery over the native aortic valve. In a porcine model, he implanted five valved stents into the descending aorta, two into the ascending aorta, and another three into a subcoronary position of the aortic root. Andersen also filed the earliest patent application dating back to May 18, 1990 (17).

The same year, Dusan Pavcnik described a prosthetic caged-ball aortic valve for transcatheter implantation performed in 12 adult mongrel dogs (18). Both studies clearly proved feasibility of a remote aortic valve insertion without the need for cardiopulmonary support. Even though the results were very encouraging, valved stents were far-off from becoming a clinical alternative to surgical aortic valve replacement. It took several other experimental feasibility studies and a full decade for the first in-man implantation of a remotely inserted heart valve performed by Philipp Bonhoeffer in 2000 (19). A 12-year-old boy with stenosis and insufficiency of a prosthetic conduit from the right ventricle to the pulmonary artery underwent the first percutaneous implantation of a bovine jugular valve in his conduit.

The excellent postinterventional result encouraged further development of TCVT. Two years later, in a French town called Rouen, Alain Cribier implanted the first percutaneous heart valve in a 57-year-old man in cardiogenic shock with highly calcified aortic stenosis as last-resort therapy (20). The early clinical experience identified important limitations of the novel technique.

From 2001 onward, the author has aimed toward improving and further developing TCVT to what might become one of the most promising new therapies for SHD. Introducing the direct access valve replacement technique via the transapical procedure, first publicly disclosed by the author in 2004 (21), created ideal conditions to improve and further spread popularity and support for this new line of treatment for SHD.

Leading the path through aortic TCVT to allow better and safer patient care is the main topic of the present work.

REFERENCES

1. Cutler EC, Levine SA. Cardiotomy and valvulotomy for mitral stenosis: Experimental observations and clinical notes concerning an operated case with recovery. Boston Med Surg J 1923; 188:1023–1027.
2. Gibbon JH Jr. Application of a mechanical heart and lung apparatus in cardiac surgery. Minn Med 1954; 37:171.
3. Huber CH, Göber V, Berdat P, et al. Benefits of cardiac surgery in octogenarians—A postoperative quality of life assessment. Eur J Cardiothorac Surg 2007; 31:1099–1105.
4. NHLBI Balloon Valvuloplasty Registry Participants. Percutaneous balloon aortic valvuloplasty. Acute and 30-day follow-up results in 674 patients from the NHLBI Balloon Valvuloplasty Registry. Circulation 1991; 84(6):2383–2397.
5. O'Neill WW. Predictors of long-term survival after percutaneous aortic valvuloplasty: Report of the Mansfield Scientific Balloon Aortic Valvuloplasty Registry. J Am Coll Cardiol 1991; 17(1):193–198.

6. Lieberman EB, Bashore TM, Hermiller JB, et al. Balloon aortic valvuloplasty in adults: Failure of procedure to improve long-term survival. J Am Coll Cardiol 1995; 26(6):1522–1528.
7. Kuntz RE, Tosteson AN, Berman AD, et al. Predictors of event-free survival after balloon aortic valvuloplasty. N Engl J Med 1991; 325(1):17–23.
8. Gruntzig A. Transluminal dilatation of coronary-artery stenosis. Lancet 1978; 1(8058):263.
9. Ellis SG, Roubin GS, King SB III, et al. In-hospital cardiac mortality after acute closure after coronary angioplasty: Analysis of risk factors from 8,207 procedures. J Am Coll Cardiol 1988; 11(2):211–216.
10. Leimgruber PP, Roubin GS, Hollman J, et al. Restenosis after successful coronary angioplasty in patients with single-vessel disease. Circulation 1986; 73(4):710–717.
11. Anderson HV, Roubin GS, Leimgruber PP, et al. Primary angiographic success rates of percutaneous transluminal coronary angioplasty. Am J Cardiol 1985; 56(12):712–717.
12. Urban P, Meier B, Finci L, et al. Coronary wedge pressure: A predictor of restenosis after coronary balloon angioplasty. J Am Coll Cardiol 1987; 10(3):504–509.
13. Sigwart U, Puel J, Mirkovitch V, et al. Intravascular stents to prevent occlusion and restenosis after transluminal angioplasty. N Engl J Med 1987; 316(12):701–706.
14. Vassiliades TA, Block PC, Cohn LH, et al. The clinical development of percutaneous heart valve technology. A position statement of the Society of Thoracic Surgeons (STS), the American Association for Thoracic Surgery (AATS), and the Society for Cardiovascular Angiography and Interventions (SCAI). J Am Coll Cardiol 2005; 45:1554–1560.
15. Andersen HR, Knudsen LL, Hasenkam JM. Transluminal catheter implantation of a new expandable artificial cardiac valve in the aorta and the beating heart of closed chest pigs [abstract]. Eur Heart J 1990; 11(suppl):224a.
16. Andersen HR, Knudsen LL, Hasenkam JM. Transluminal implantation of artificial heart valves. Description of a new expandable aortic valve and initial results with implantation by catheter technique in closed chest pigs. Eur Heart J 1992; 13(5):704–708.
17. Andersen HR, Hasenkam JM, Knudsen, LL. Valve prosthesis for implantation in the body and a catheter for implanting such valve prosthesis. No 1246/90, May 18, 1990, Denmark.
18. Pavcnik D, Wright KC, Wallace S. Development and initial experimental evaluation of a prosthetic aortic valve for transcatheter placement. Work in progress. Radiology 1992; 183(1):151–154.
19. Bonhoeffer P, Boudjemline Y, Saliba Z, et al. Percutaneous replacement of pulmonary valve in a right-ventricle to pulmonary-artery prosthetic conduit with valve dysfunction. Lancet 2000; 356(9239):1403–1405.
20. Cribier A, Eltchaninoff H, Bash A, et al. Percutaneous transcatheter implantation of an aortic valve prosthesis for calcific aortic stenosis: First human case description. Circulation 2002; 106(24):3006–3008.
21. Huber CH, Nasratulla M, Augstburger M, et al. Ultrasound navigation through the heart for off-pump aortic valved stent implantation: New tools for new goals. J Endovasc Ther 2004; 11:503–510.

Historical Background

"There are three stages in the history of every medical discovery. When it is first announced, people say that it is not true. Then, a little later, when truth has been borne in on them, so that it can no longer be denied, they say it is not important. After that, if its importance becomes sufficiently obvious, they say that anyhow it is not new." (1)

Drawing back what led to the transcatheter techniques for structural heart disease requires following down two pathways. The first recreates the story of heart surgery and the second the advances of catheter techniques. Both originated separately, joined a first time, separated again, and currently got back together to unite synergies into transcatheter valve therapies.

THE EARLY DAYS OF HEART VALVE SURGERY

Knowledge and understanding of the aortic valve started with the exceptional work of Leonardo da Vinci (Fig. 1) (2,3) and Andreas Vesalius (4) (Fig. 2), in the 15th and 16th centuries. Courageous, secret dissections of mortal bodies resulted not only in beautiful *oeuvres d'art* and detailed anatomical drawings of the heart and its structures, but also in functional understanding of biological valves and even in name giving. It is said that da Vinci compared the left-sided atrioventricular valve as resembling a "bishop's miter" and gave the "mitral valve" its name. Several centuries and discoveries followed until wider understanding of the heart and blood circulation was obtained. In 1628, experiments by William Harvey (5) established the concept of the blood circulation and marked the beginning of modern cardiology (Fig. 3).

At the end of the 19th century, a warning and discouraging ban was expressed by leading surgeons.

"Any surgeon who wishes to preserve the respect of his colleagues would never attempt to suture the heart" (6).

Stephan Paget little later published a personal point of view: "Surgery of the heart has probably reached the limits set by nature, no new methods and no new discovery can overcome the natural difficulties that attend a wound of the heart." (7) On the Continent, Professor Theodor Billroth joined in: "A surgeon who tries to suture a heart wound deserves to lose the esteem of his colleagues." Paget and Billroth's pessimism not withstanding, Ludwig Rehn of Frankfurt— a former German hussar turned surgeon—made the first successful suture of a human heart wound in September of the same year, 1896 (8).

Very fortunately, the pioneers and founders of modern cardiac surgery bravely faced the foreseen challenges in the 20th century.

CLOSED HEART VALVE SURGERY IN THE YEAR BEFORE
THE HEART-LUNG MACHINE

On July 13, 1912, Theodore Tuffier successfully digitally dilated a stenotic aortic valve in a 26-year-old Belgian patient by pushing the invaginated aortic wall

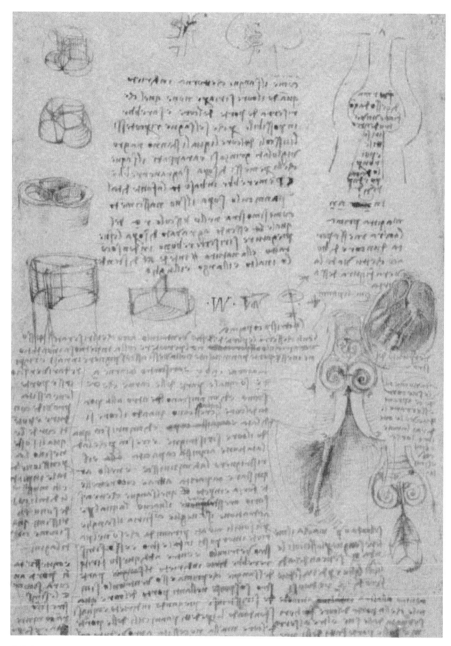

FIGURE 1 Leonardo da Vinci's notes on the valve of the heart and flow of blood within it, with illustrative drawings, ca 1513. Downloaded from www.universalleonardo.org (The Royal Collection).

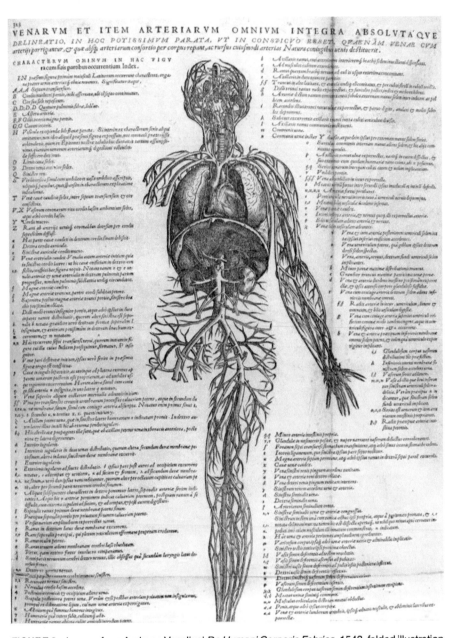

FIGURE 2 Images from Andreas Vesalius' *De Humani Corporis Fabrica*, 1543, folded illustration on the arteries and the heart, p. 313 (i.e., p. 314). Downloaded from www.quod.lib.umich.edu.

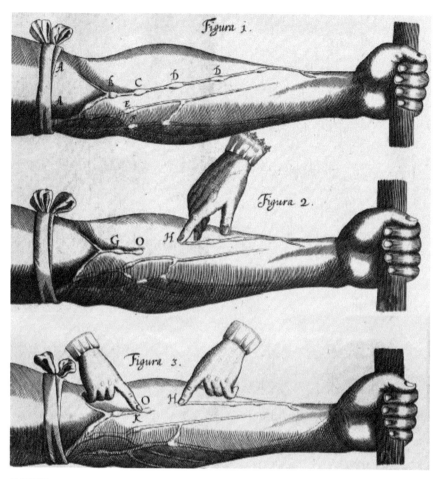

FIGURE 3 Illustration from William Harvey's *De Motu Cordis*, 1628. *Figura 1* shows distended veins in the forearm and position of valves. *Figura 2* shows that if a vein has been "milked" centrally and the peripheral end compressed, it does not fill until the finger is released. *Figura 3* shows that blood cannot be forced in the "wrong" direction. (*Source*: From Wellcome Institute Library, London.)

trough the disease valve (9). Without doubt, this excellent result has to be considered with great care. Russel Brock, more than 30 years later, in the 1940s, attempted instrumental aortic valved dilatation via an endovascular approach, but his results lacked Tuffier's success. In the following years, different tools to dilate the pulmonary and aortic valve were invented, for example, the Brock and the Bailey dilatator (Fig. 4), and new access route to the disease aortic valve explored (10,11). Despite ingenious new therapies, results remained poor with high mortality and finally the procedures got abandoned.

In parallel, intense development for the treatment of mitral valve disease succeeded. For the first time in the history of cardiovascular disease, a collaborative effort between Elliot Cutler, a young cardiac surgeon, and Samuel Levine, a cardiologist, led to the earliest successful mitral valvulotomy in a 12-year-old girl with a failing mitral valve at the former Peter Bent Brigham Hospital,

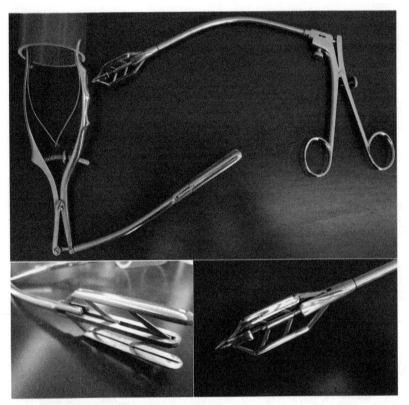

FIGURE 4 The Bailey aortic (*right*) and mitral valve (*left*) dilatator with the respective detailed view lower part. (*Source*: From Div. Cardiac Surgery, Brigham and Women's Hospital Collection of prosthetic cardiac valves.)

today's Brigham and Women's Hospital in Boston, MA. Unfortunately, subsequent patients suffered and frequently died from postoperative mitral regurgitation because of too generous mitral valvulotomy (12). Once more, the technique was abandoned.

Two years later, an English surgeon, Henry Souttar, reported the first successful digital mitral commissurotomy (13), an isolated intervention he did not repeat because of misunderstanding and peer pressure as pointed out in a written correspondence with Dwight Harken in 1961, "... it is of no use to be ahead of one's time ..." (14).

Following Brock's and Charles Bailey's pioneering works on the pulmonary and aortic valves, respectively, an artificial heart valve was developed and implanted in the descending aorta of a dog by Charles Hufnagel in Washington, DC. The early concept of the caged ball valve might have originated from an improved bottle stopper patented by Jeremiah Williams on February 9, 1858 (Fig. 5).

Hufnagel reported an initial clinical experience of 23 patients with aortic regurgitation in 1952 with a 26% mortality greatly caused by the steep learning curve of the new procedure (15). The implantation technique consisted in fixing a methacrylate tube caged ball valve into the descending aorta by two

UNITED STATES PATENT OFFICE.

J. B. WILLIAMS, OF NEW YORK, N. Y.

IMPROVED BOTTLE-STOPPER.

Specification forming part of Letters Patent No. **19,323,** dated February 9, 1858.

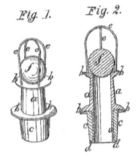

Fig. 1.   *Fig. 2.*

To all whom it may concern:

Be it known that I, JEREMIAH B. WILLIAMS, of the city and county of New York, in the State of New York, have invented a new and useful Improvement in the Manufacture of Bottle-Stoppers; and I do hereby declare the following to be a full, clear, and exact description of the construction of the same, reference being had to the accompanying drawings, making a part of this specification, in which—

Figure 1 represents a perspective view of the article in question; and Fig. 2 represents a central vertical section through the same.

Similar letters of reference where they occur in the separate figures denote like parts of the stoppers in both of them.

and use my invention, I will proceed to describe the same with reference to the drawings.

a represents a tube of metal, either cast, struck up, or made in any of the usual well-known ways, and furnished with the accustomed flanges, *b b*—one to rest on the top of the neck of the bottle and the other to form a lip over which the liquid flows. The lower end of the tube is incased by a conical cork cylinder or belt, *c*, which, when slipped on, is retained in its place by turning a flange, *d*, against it on the lower end of the tube *a*. To the top flange *b* are fastened two or more wires, *e*, so as to form a guide or frame in which a loose ball, *f*, may freely roll when the bottle is canted, so as to leave a free passage through the tube *a*. When the bottle is

FIGURE 5 U.S. Patent 19323, Improved bottle-stopper, dated February 9, 1858, by Jeremiah B. Williams as a possible precursor of the first ball-and-cage valve designs.

multiple-point fixation rings (16) (Fig. 6). The intrinsic design allowed rapid and sutureless implantation without the heart-lung machine (17)—a brilliant anchoring concept, again much in advance of its time.

OPEN HEART SURGERY AFTER INTRODUCTION OF THE HEART-LUNG MACHINE

A pivotal point was reached for modern open heart surgery with the development of the heart-lung machine.

One of the first and most successful reports on tissue perfusion has been published as cover story of *Time* of the June 13, 1938 issue (Fig. 7). The cover page

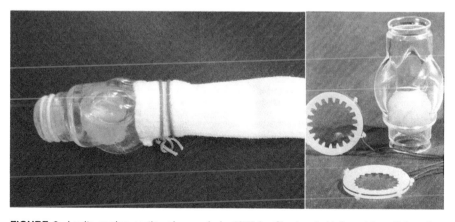

FIGURE 6 Lucite canine aortic valve made in 1950 by Charles A. Hufnagel in collaboration with Carl Hewson. It was made of methacrylate (Plexiglas), was available in four sizes, with a diameter of 0.75–1.25 in. The flared ends and the joining groove allowed extravascular anchoring. (*Source:* From Div. Cardiac Surgery, Brigham and Women's Hospital Collection of prosthetic cardiac valves.)

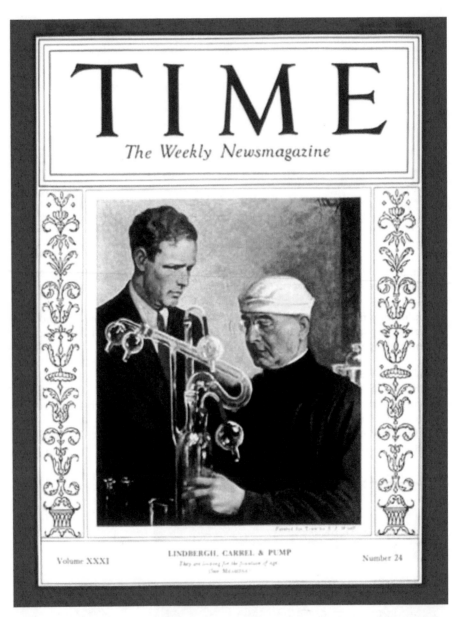

FIGURE 7 Time magazine cover from June 13, 1938, displaying Charles A. Lindbergh & Dr. Alexis Carrel.

presents Charles A. Lindbergh and Alexis Carrel standing next to their tissue perfusion apparatus that served to perfuse a cat thyroid gland for 18 days.

> "From this moment [we are] opening to experimental investigation a forbidden field: the living human body. . . . Organs removed from the human

body, in the course of an operation or soon after death, could be revived in the Lindbergh pump, and made to function again when perfused with an artificial fluid. . . . When larger apparatus are built, entire human organs, such as pancreas, suprarenal, thyroid, and other glands . . . would manufacture in vitro the substances supplied today to patients by horses or rabbits" (18).

Organs were kept alive for several days but eventually degenerated.

It was Jay McLean's major research work on phospholipids and his discovery of heparin that solved one of the greatest drawback of tissue perfusion— clotting. Anticoagulation allowed using blood-based perfusion solution in artificial circuits (19).

In the 1930s, John Gibbon, a doctor in Boston, became fascinated by the idea of supporting the body with an artificial perfusion system to temporarily replace the heart and lung function. His fascination turned into a lifetime achievement. Over the following 20 years, Gibbon's road to success was fought with setbacks, delays, and technical difficulties, yet Gibbon, with his perseverance, was able to pursue his dream to its end. He describes his first success as an "event that I hardly dreamed of in 1931," the year he was first inspired by the idea of extracorporeal circulation (Fig. 8). On May 6, 1953, Gibbon performed the first successful open heart operation with the use of the heart-lung machine by closing an atrial septal defect in an 18-year-old girl (20). At the same time, Charles Walton Lillehei and colleagues of the University of Minnesota introduced the concept of controlled cross-circulation. This method was based on the principle of connecting the patient's circulation with the donor patient; usually the patient's parent or a close relative provided the cardiopulmonary support. Both circulations were connected via a motor pump controlling and equalizing the reciprocal blood exchange.

On March 26, 1954, a 12-month-old infant was connected to his anesthetized father serving as the oxygenator. The patient's blood flow was routed from his caval system to the father's femoral vein and lungs, where it was

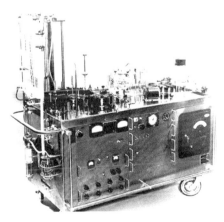 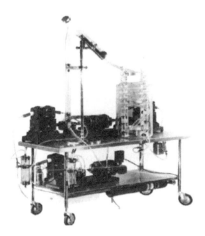

FIGURE 8 The John Gibbon heart-lung machine (*left*) and the DeWall bubble oxygenator (*right*).

oxygenated, and then returned to the patient's carotid artery. The ventricular septal defect was repaired with a total pump time of 19 minutes. Over the following year, Lillehei operated on 45 patients (21), with otherwise irreparable complex interventricular defects, using a modified setup integrating a bubble oxygenator engineered by Richard DeWall (Fig. 8). Even though cross-circulation was a breakthrough, it was not widely adopted because it posed a serious risk to the "donor." Nevertheless, this method opened the door to modern heart surgery.

The same year in 1955, John W. Kirklin at the Mayo Clinic, less than 150 km from the University of Minnesota, started open heart surgery using a modified Gibbon heart-lung machine. The race was on, and from 1955 to 1957 both surgeons intermittently produced extraordinary surgical achievements in the domain of congenital cardiac surgery (22).

DEVELOPMENT OF PROSTHETIC HEART VALVES

The Mechanical Heart Valve

The early clinical work on prosthetic heart valves by Hufnagel and J.M. Campbell might have been inspired by a bottle stopper patent published in 1858 (Fig. 5). Both independently designed and built a prosthetic heart valve consisting of a cage and a mobile spherical poppet. Hufnagel's valve was composed from a lucent methacrylate (Plexiglas) cage surrounding a silicon-coated nylon poppet. Hufnagel performed the first implantation of his caged ball valve in September 1952, but no reports on implantation of Campbell's valve have been found. Lefrak and Starr described the first human implantation of the Hufnagel valve as "igniting the fire of prosthetic valve implantation (23). Regardless of Hufnagel's encouraging results in the first 23 patients, no other heart valve implantation were performed until 1955, the year of the first reported mitral valve replacement performed by Judson T. Chesterman (24). The caged ball valve was made of Perspex and consisted of an outer cage, a poppet, and two buttons used for fixation to the outer surface of the heart, designed by Clifford Lambourne. On July 22, 1955, at the City General Hospital in Sheffield, England, Chesterman implanted the first mitral valve. The patient survived surgery for 14 hours but died when the poppet twisted out of position.

After that, several groups of researchers attempted to implant various designs of prosthetic heart valves but with poor results, often because thrombotic events presented a major drawback (25,26).

The development of the first successful artificial heart valve started in 1958, the year in which Lowell Edwards, a semiretired electrical engineer, at age 65, stepped into Starr's office. Their collaborative effort prompted in the first human mitral valve replacement on August 25, 1960 (27). The valve was based on an earlier design concept from Ellis and Bulbulian of the Mayo Clinic published in 1958 (28). A silicone rubber ball was placed within a methyl methacrylate cage composed of four thick struts. The ball was trapped and the cage closed by acetone welding of the ring to the cage. Another interesting caged ball prosthetic valve concept was developed in the 1960s by Edward A. Smeloff and Cutter (Cutter Laboratories, Berkeley, CA) featuring an open cage at the upper and lower ends (Fig. 9).

Starr and Edwards, unlike Ellis and Bulbulian, did not abandon their attempts to develop the ball valve design, because they saw the ball valve design as a solution to thrombus formation at the hinge points of the previous artificial

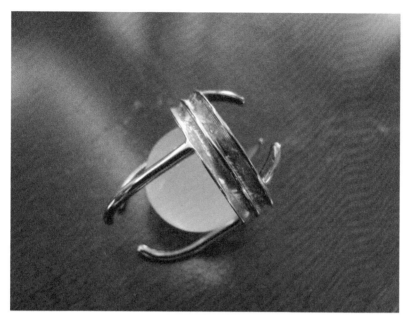

FIGURE 9 Smeloff-Cutter aortic ball valve, with the Teflon cloth seat removed, used in the mid-1960s. (*Source:* From Div. Cardiac Surgery, Brigham and Women's Hospital Collection of prosthetic cardiac valves.)

valve designs because the constant motion of the ball might remove the thrombus as it formed. An important barrier was overcome and development of a medical device moved away from coping nature to construct adapted functionality. This might have led to the famous quote of Starr "Let's make a valve that works and not worry about its looks." What followed was a success story of multiple design modifications and succeeding clinical mitral valve replacements (Fig. 10). Just one year after the first successful digital mitral commisurotomy (13), Edwards Laboratories issued a 9–key-items charta for the development of artificial heart valves. Since 1968, this charta has not lost any of its initial validity:

1. Embolism prevention (free-floating ball, no hinge points)
2. Durability (introduction of stainless steel struts)
3. Ease and security of attachment (modification of the sewing ring)
4. Improved preservation of surrounding tissue (less traumatic cage covering)
5. Minimizing turbulence (increasing the orifice/ball ratio)
6. Reduction of hemolysis (improved neoendothelialization)
7. Noise suppression (silicon ball)
8. Increased biocompatibility of all components (stellite, stainless steel, methyl methacrylate, Teflon cloth and sutures, silicone rubber)
9. Improved methods of storage and sterilization

The Starr-Edwards ball valve prosthesis functioned well, and became one of the most successfully and widely used prosthetic valves with continued clinical use today.

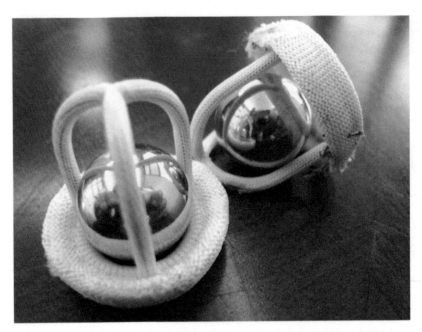

FIGURE 10 The Starr-Edwards 2310 series was a small cloth-covered aortic valve used in the late 1960s. (*Source:* From Div. Cardiac Surgery, Brigham and Women's Hospital Collection of prosthetic cardiac valves.)

Following Hufnagel's pioneering work on ectopic sutureless valve implantation, in the mid-1960s the concept of sutureless aortic valve implantation gained new popularity. The Magovern-Cromie aortic prosthesis was designed for orthotopic aortic implantation (Fig. 11). The prosthesis features a double-barbed anchoring ring with a snap-on mechanism to sandwich the native annular tissue for valve anchoring. The top part of the cage is open and the annular ring traps the ball in the diastolic position.

The physiological disadvantages of ball valve prostheses were soon recognized. There was an inevitable low-grade but tolerable hemolysis from the serial impact of the ball on the cage. In addition, the effective cross-sectional area of the valve orifice was not ideal because the poppet occupied a significant percentage of the orifice area. These considerations led to the development of disk prostheses.

Viking Bjork, at the Karolinska Institute in Stockholm, Sweden, working in conjunction with the Shiley Corporation in California reported in 1969 about what was to become the Bjork-Shiley tilting disk prosthesis (29) (Fig. 12). Other disk prostheses were developed around the same time, including the Lillehei-Cruz-Kaster tilting disk valve (1963) and Wada-Cutter tilting disk heart valve (1966) (Fig. 13), but the Bjork valve quickly became the disk valve of choice and was widely used for many years.

In 1977, the St. Jude pyrolytic carbon disk bileaflet heart valve became the first mechanical valve to achieve a major success. Twenty years later, it remains

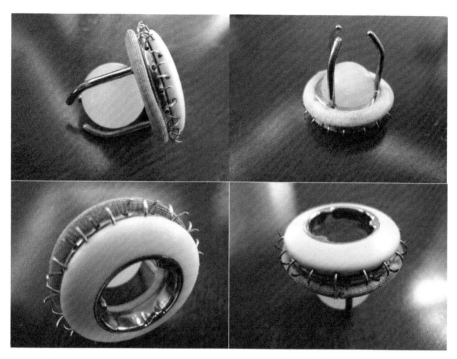

FIGURE 11 The Magovern-Cromie sutureless valve was a large aortic valve design for suture-less anchoring. (*Source:* From Div. Cardiac Surgery, Brigham and Women's Hospital Collection of prosthetic cardiac valves.)

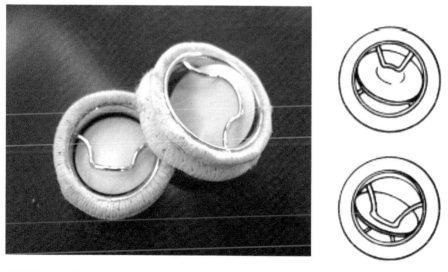

FIGURE 12 Two original Bjork-Shiley tilting disk valve prostheses with white single leaflet Delrin disk from the 1970s. (*Source:* From Div. Cardiac Surgery, Brigham and Women's Hospital Collection of prosthetic cardiac valves.)

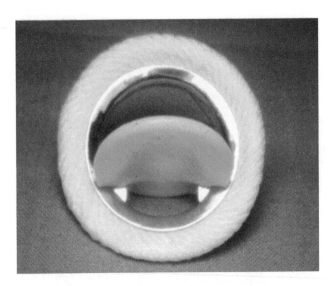

FIGURE 13 Wada-Cutter tilting disk valve prosthesis.

one of the most popular and durable prostheses (30) [Fig. 14(A)]. The same year, Demetre Nicoloff, coinventor and cardiovascular surgeon at the University of Minnesota, reported the first clinical implant on October 3. Currently, diverse bileaflet mechanical valves are in clinical use, including the Medtronic-Hall (1977) [Fig. 14(B)], Omniscience (1978), Carbomedics (1986), and ATS valves (1992). Mechanical heart valve prosthesis underwent numerous cycles of design engineering as expressed in the great variety of models. However, only a few remain clinically important today (Figs. 15 and 16).

BIOPROSTHETIC HEART VALVES
The Achilles' heel of mechanical prostheses leading to frequent thromboembolic complications seemed insolvable. New investigations into biological tissue prostheses were initiated. Various autogenous materials underwent experimental usability testing with a strong emphasis on the pericardium, dura mater, and fascia lata. Ake Senning's groups in Zurich, Switzerland, revealed a significant reduction of thromboembolic complication (31) using fascia lata compared to mechanical prosthesis. In the 1960s, Jean-Paul Binet's group in Paris, France, also began developing tissue valves (32).

Successful aortic valve replacement using aortic homografts were reported as early as 1962 by Donald Ross in (33) London, United Kingdom, and in 1964 by Sir Brian Gerald Barratt-Boyes, Auckland, New Zealand (34). The encouraging results of Mark O'Brien's work (35), Brisbane, Australia, in 1987 on long-term experiences with cryopreservation showed viable homograft tissue even after 10 years of preservation. Cryopreservation is currently generally accepted as the homograft preservation technique of choice. However, the limited availability of homograft valves, the technically challenging operation, and the excellent results of the current bioprosthetic valves has restricted its widespread use.

In 1967, Donald Ross (36), London, United Kingdom, reported the ingenious concept of replacing the failing aortic valve with the patient's own

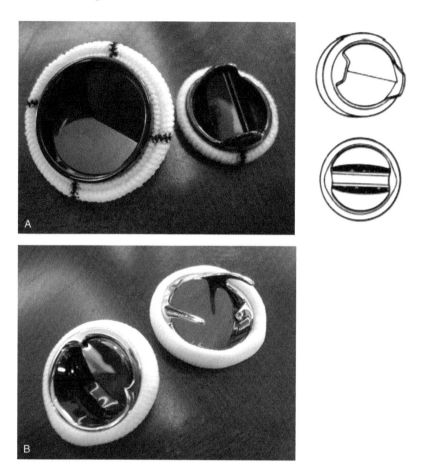

FIGURE 14 (**A**) St. Jude disk valve of pyrolytic carbon is the prototype bileaflet valve from the 1980s and remains the current industrial leader. (**B**) Medtronic-Hall tilting disk valves with a black disk of pyrolytic carbon (90% Pyrolite) from the 1990s till today. (*Source*: From Div. Cardiac Surgery, Brigham and Women's Hospital Collection of prosthetic cardiac valves.)

pulmonary valve (autologous tissue valve), and then replacing the absent pulmonary valve with a pulmonary valve homograft. The rationale to make a double valve disease from a single valve disease, as the Ross procedure was criticized, comes from the homograft's durability in the low pressure system of the right heart being longer than in the aortic position and the autologous pulmonary valve showed very promising results when placed in the aortic position. Freedom from anticoagulation and good valve durability made the operation become increasingly popular throughout the United States and Europe. The aortic valve replacement with a pulmonary autologous graft still is considered one of the prime choices for aortic valve replacement up into the young adulthood. The availability of cryopreserved grafts for the mandatory pulmonary valve replacement has further expanded the acceptance of the Ross operation.

After the low frequency of thromboembolic event from tissue valves was recognized, the search for a heterograft valve began because of the limited

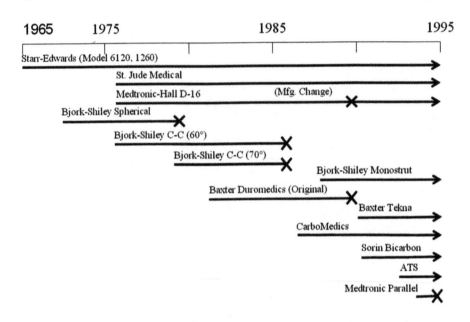

FIGURE 15 Time-related development of some selected mechanical heart valve prosthesis.

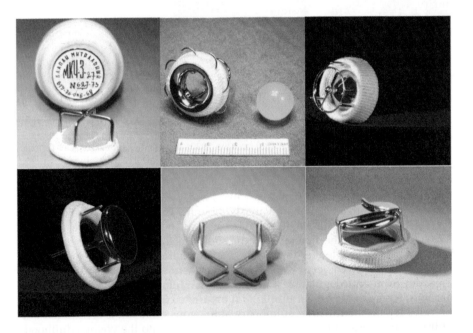

FIGURE 16 Overview of the large variety of mechanical heart valve designs.

availability of homograft valves. Formaldehyde-preserved heterogenic valves showed good acute outcome data, but failed within two to three years because of tissue degeneration and calcification (37). Fortunately, a few years later, it was discovered that glutaraldehyde was an excellent tissue preservative. This inspired Alain Carpentier (38), Paris, France, in the mid-1960s to explore the functionality and durability of glutaraldehyde-preserved porcine aortic valves. In contrast to all other experiences with different forms of heterograft preservation, the durability of glutaraldehyde-preserved prostheses was dramatically better—more than 90% functioned satisfactorily 5 years after implantation, and 75% to 85% after 10 years. This result revived the interest in xenograft valves by fixating porcine valves with glutaraldehyde. In 1966, Carpentier started to mount his valves on a stent facilitating handling and suturing. The first stented valve xenograft implant took place in 1967 in collaboration with Charles Dubost. From then onward, bioprosthetic tissue valves became a permanent feature of valvular heart surgery landscape, and the early work resulted in the widespread use of the Carpentier-Edwards porcine valves and the implantation of Hancock and Angell-Shiley bioprostheses in a large number of patients (39, 40).

CARDIAC CATHETERIZATION: A HISTORICAL GLIMPSE
  "...Cardiac Catheter was ... the Key in the Lock" (41)

Accessing the inside of the human heart safely has inspired numerous researchers and clinicians to undertake formidable journeys and achieve extraordinary discoveries.

From the ancient Egyptian bladder catheterizations in 3000 BC with metallic pipes to Hippocrates of Kos in 400 BC using hollow reeds and brass pipes to push water and air into cadaver vasculature to Harvey's inferior vena cava catheterization in 1651, all have contributed to the development of catheter-based techniques.

Intracardiac measurements were first reported by Stephen Hales in 1711 (42). His realization was followed by the French physiologist Claude Bernard in 1844 inserting a long mercury thermometer via the carotid artery of horses into the left ventricle. Less than 30 years later, the German physicist Adolph Fick in 1870 described a most brilliant method to calculate blood flow (43). A new era began with the German surgical resident Werner Forssmann's electrifying experiments in July 1929. After realizing from cadaver studies how simple it was to advance a urologic catheter from the brachial vein into the right atrium, Forssmann was facing enormous resistance from his superiors to support his work. Forssmann went on to do self-experimentation, and inserted a 65-cm bladder catheter into his right heart (44). He was fired the same day and never went back into cardiology. Forssmann together with André Cournand and Dickinson Richards shared the Nobel Prize in Medicine in 1956 for their outstanding contributions to cardiac catheterization. The key to the door started to turn with the improved radiology equipment, the intravascular technique for left heart catheterization by Henry A. Zimmerman in 1950 (45), and Sven-Ivar Seldinger's catheter-over-a-needle technique in 1953 (46).

Mason Sones, a pediatric cardiologist, set the standard of selective coronary angiography in October 1958 by accidental injection of contrast into the right coronary. Soon after his surprisingly positive incident, he set out to design a specific rigid body catheter with a tapered tip (47). Later, Melvin Judkins, an associate of Charles Dotter, challenged the first Sones coronary catheters with new designs accounting for various aortic root sizes (48). The same duo in 1964 performed the first intensional transluminal dilatation of a stenosed popliteal artery by inserting a guidewire over the lesion and dilating it with double polyethylene catheters, a technique already known from dilatation of urethral strictures.

The key definitively turned and the door opened when Andreas Grüntzig spent time as guest fellow in a radiology laboratory in Engelskirchen, Germany. After having learned Dotter's technique of transluminal angioplasty, he moved to Zurich, Switzerland, in 1970, where he began to conceive angioplasty balloons to refine the quite crude procedure. In May 1977, at the St. Mary's Hospital in San Francisco, Grüntzig performed the first coronary angioplasty during coronary artery bypass surgery (49).

The door swung open completely with the introduction of intravascular scaffolding devices providing firm support to the vessel wall. Dotter's initial experiments in 1969 with plastic tubing and stainless steel coil spring prosthesis for peripheral vascular disease identified the stainless steel devices as the only viable device when heparin was administered during the first four days. In contrast, all the plastic tubes grafts clotted within the first 24 hours (50). In 1983, aortic stent design was brought further by Dierk Maass from the Zurich group, experimenting with self-expanding stent designs based on the coil spring principle, but only the double helix structure (51) proved to be free of migration or thrombotic complications. Unfortunately, deployment required a bulky delivery system making it unsuitable for small arteries as the coronaries.

The final breakthrough was achieved by Ulrich Sigwart in 1987 by reporting the first human coronary stent implantation (52). He replaced the coil structure with a mesh configuration composed of interwoven stainless steel strands from vessel wall supporting constructs to anchoring and sealing devices.

All the above-mentioned pioneers, and in particular Maass and Sigwart's work, built the key concept of transcatheter valve therapies. Using the stents secondary characteristics to carry and anchor a valve anywhere in a vessel allowed the future Valved Stent development (see Development of Transcatheter Valve Therapies).

RISE, FALL, AND RENAISSANCE OF BALLOON AORTIC VALVULOPLASTY

William Rashkind might have been the first to introduce therapeutic balloon dilatation in an attempt to increase oxygen saturation in a patient with a cyanotic heart defect in 1966 (53). In line with the congenital cardiac population, Jean Kan in 1982 applied balloon dilatation to the stenosed pulmonary valve (54) and James Lock (55) to aortic coarctations. Early reports on mitral and congenital aortic balloon valvuloplasties followed in 1984 by Kanji Inoue (56) and by Zuhdi Lababidi (57), respectively. Encouraged by the highly successful valvuloplasty results, a novel less-invasive therapy promising to cure aortic valve stenosis emerged. In 1985, Alain Cribier performed the first adult balloon aortic valvuloplasty (58). The early enthusiasm of this reasonably safe procedure became somewhat tempered by the fact that the increment in aortic valve area was far smaller than expected compared to the surgical results. The quote "the procedure starts with aortic stenosis and ends with aortic stenosis" might best reproduce the essential limitations of the intervention (59). The hospital mortality might reach 14%, and in close to one-third periprocedural complications are experienced. Indication for balloon aortic valvuloplasty became very restricted to nonoperable patients or as a bridge to surgical aortic valve replacement. Most currently, a new debate ignited about the use of balloon aortic valvuloplasty as stand-alone procedure. A greater role might be attributed to balloon aortic valvuloplasty beyond its use for valve predilatation during percutaneous trans-catheter aortic valve therapies. The technique might be of substantial benefit to the expanding very elderly population in regards of midterm quality-of-life gain (see Chap. 4).

DEVELOPMENT OF TRANSCATHETER VALVE THERAPIES

The era of sutureless heart valves dates back to September 11, 1952, when Hufnagel inserted a sutureless ball cage valve into the descending aorta for aortic regurgitation (16). A little over a decade later in 1965, Davies reported about a catheter-mounted unicuspid valve that was deployed above the aortic valve position for the temporary relief of aortic insufficiency (60). In the 1970s, Moulopoulos (61) and Phillips (62) designed catheter-mounted aortic valves for experimental use. However all those devices did miss the one essential feature—the capability of endovascular anchoring, and therefore remained limited to only temporary use. The next milestone leading to development of the valved stents was reached in 1986, when Sigwart developed and successfully implanted the first coronary stent (52).

One year later, at Arizona Heart Institute in Phoenix, in a vast and crowded auditorium, cardiac specialists from all over the world were listening to the groundbreaking news. Among them sat a 39-year-old Danish cardiology registrar, Henning-Rud Andersen, who was to become the inventor of the valved stent, watching the metal mesh being placed around a crimped balloon catheter, and in a later step inserted into the target coronary and reexpanded in situ. Andersen became inspired by what he first called a ridiculous idea—a similar scaffold allowing anchoring of a valve within the heart. On his flight back to Aarhus, Denmark, he decided to focus his research on this topic. One of his first actions back in Aarhus was to rush down to the local butcher shop and buy pig hearts. He opened them, cut the heart valve free, and placed the valve on a hand folded latticed metal tube,which then squeezed around a balloon.

The valved stent was born (Fig. 17). The idea was both simple and brilliant—to introduce the catheter-mounted valved stent through an artery into the heart, place it over the native aortic valve, and then anchor the stent-supported valve by balloon expansion of the stainless steal scaffold, thus resulting in a new valve, but no scar.

It is said that because of lack of equipment and poor working conditions in the basement animal research laboratory, the pigs were moved upstairs into the regular operating rooms after terminating the scheduled operating room program. Despite the simplest self-made technical equipment, Andersen reported the first successful implantation on May 1, 1989.

Everyone was much excited, and a publication in a formidable high-impact journal became within range. Surprisingly enough, the paper was at first rejected—too crazy the idea that might be worth being patented but not published in a scientific journal. Eventually the work was printed in the *European Heart Journal* in May 1992 (63,64), and finally the Andersen patent was sold for a lump sum of $10,000 to an American company. The initial Anderson device measured 32 mm in outer diameter in the expanded state and 12 mm in the

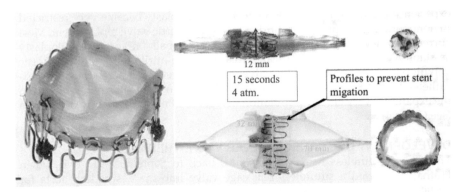

FIGURE 17 The original H. Andersen valved stent made from a manually folded stainless steel stent and a porcine native aortic valve in the expanded and the crimped stage. (*Source*: Modified in part from Ref. 64.)

crimped state. A bulky 41F delivery device was necessary to insert the valved stent. The access vessels were chosen accordingly—only the ascending and the descending aortas allowed direct insertion. As a matter of fact, at the time the transapical access was not even considered an option, most likely because nobody had thought about it until the author introduced the transapical procedure (65, 66). This third access option (Chap. 6. Access to the Aortic Valves) for TCV implantation was first publicly disclosed by the author in February 2004 at the annual International Society of Endovascular Surgery meeting in Scottsdale, AZ (65). Anecdotally, the presentation took place in the same auditorium where Sigwart's presentation inspired Andersen to invent the valved stent concept 16 years earlier. Experimental results in nine pigs were excellent with nine successfully placed devices and only trivial regurgitation in two animals and unchanged end-diastolic pressure in all.

However, the device race was started, Andersen being the first to patent. He was not the only one working on transcatheter valve devices. The same year, the radiologist Dusan Pavcnik, Prague, Czech Republic, demonstrated the feasibility of transcatheter implantation of a caged ball valve (Fig. 18) in the aortic position of mongrel dogs (67). The proposed device consisted of a modified barbed Gianturco-Rösch self-expanding stainless steel Z-stent scaffold creating a doming cage at the upper or distal end to house an expandable latex balloon ball and a springlike coiled stainless steel wire creating the annular or proximal end. The future ball valve was seated on the tip of a 60-cm-long 5F catheter.

In a second step, after delivery of the stent, the balloon-ball was to be positioned within the cage and expanded with either air, contrast medium, or a polymerizing silicon substrate. Successful implantation is reported via an 11 or 12F PTFE delivery sheath in the infracoronary position in 12 dogs. Excellent valve function is reported from the early postinterventional phase, but within three hours the ball valve escaped into the aorta. Four years later, in 1996, Nader Moazami, St. Louis, described acceptable hemodynamic performance in a porcine feasibility study with transluminal aortic valve insertion using a self-design trileaflet bovine pericardial valve mounted in a collapsible stent (68).

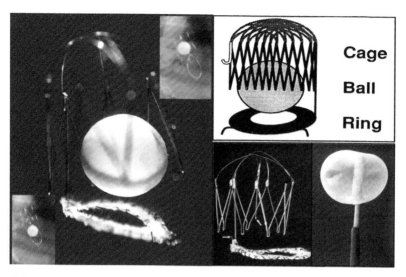

FIGURE 18 Caged ball design as proposed by D. Pavcnik for percutaneous insertion and in situ device construction. (*Source*: Modified in part from Ref. 64.)

Another four years later, Jan Sochman of the same group as Pavcnik, Prague, Czech Republic, published the successful percutaneous transcatheter aortic flexible tilting disk valve prosthesis implantation in mongrel dogs.

A mechanical but flexible oval tilting disk made of a 0.010-in nitinol-braided PTFE membrane of 0.1 mm thickness was captured within a Z-stent build scaffold. The two-step delivery process via a 10 to 12F delivery device consisted of first stent deployment followed by the disk valve implantation. In a later communication, Jan Sochman presented a one-step approach using an SX-braided stent carrier and a locking flexible disk membrane (69).

In parallel to the aortic valve, the pulmonary valve was addressed in an experimental setting by Philipp Bonhoeffer and Younes Boudjemline in 2000, reporting of a valved stent transcatheter implantation in pulmonary position in lambs (70), Hôpital Necker pour Enfants Malades, Paris, France. The device consisting of a biological bovine jugular vein conduit of approximately 2.5 cm length sutured into platinum-iridium alloy stent. Bonhoeffer made valved stents a reality by his major clinical breakthrough. He reported the first human valved stent implantation on October 21, 2000, in a failing right ventricle to pulmonary artery prosthetic conduit (71). The same group also investigated on aortic devices by a modification of the pulmonary-valved stent implanted in the descending aorta (72,73). All heterotopic implants in the animal aortic insufficiency model functioned well but none of the animals were alive after 24 hours. Most likely the death was related to the acute onset of a severe aortic insufficiency of iatrogenic origin rather than to a gradually progression of aortic regurgitation. A latter attempt implanting the devices in native aortic valve position failed because of repeated coronary obstructions, and led to the construction of a two-layered stent with an outer layer made from three nitinol hooks protruding like little arms and ensuring orientation by landing within the three commissures and by the previously described inner stent. The follow-up controls at two months showed most satisfying results with good valve function, no migration, and no coronary obstruction (74).

In 2002, Georg Lutter, a cardiac surgeon working in Fribourg, Germany, at the time successfully deployed a valved stent (Chap. 13) in the porcine aorta (75). Six of these valved stents were implanted in the descending aorta and eight in the ascending aorta of anaesthetized pigs, eleven of which successfully implanted and demonstrated low transvalvular gradients (mean end-systolic gradient 5.4 ± 3.3 mm Hg) and mild leakage. The device made from a porcine aortic valve sutured into a 21-mm-long nitinol stent with anchoring barbs was delivered via a 22F sheath. The coronary orifice, however, remained one of the most difficult problems to overcome. The stent was later elongated to 28 mm of height to overcome the problem of twisting (Chap. 7 Device-Related Insights into the Aortic Root Anatomy).

A year later, the author's research group presented their initial work on vena cava valved stent to treat tricuspid regurgitation (76), and a year later the author published the landmark paper about valved stent and coronary flow patterns (77).

The nest milestone was definitively achieved by Alain Cribier, Rouen, France, one of the pioneers of balloon aortic valvuloplasty. He successfully implanted the first in-man aortic valved stent on April 16, 2002, as a lifesaving last-resort option (78). The patient survived for 17 weeks and died of noncardiac cause.

Encouraged by those positive and most promising developments, numerous groups worldwide started to become involved into transcatheter valve therapies research and engineering targeting to improve the clinical outcome of those novel treatment strategies.

REFERENCES

1. Wilson RM. The Beloved Physician: Sir James Mackenzie. New York: Macmillan, 1926:177.
2. Da Vinci L. Studies of a Three-Cusp Valve and Schema for a Model of the Neck of the Aorta. Windsor Castle, The Royal Collection, 19082r, 1516.
3. Nicholl C. Leonardo da Vinci. Flights of the Mind. New York: Viking-Penguin, 2004.
4. Vesalius A. De Humani Corporis Fabrica Libri Septem [Title page: Andreae Vesalii Bruxellensis, Scholae Medicorum Patauinae Professoris De Humani Corporis Fabrica Libri Septem]. Basileae [Basel]: Ex Officina Joannis Oporini, 1543.
5. Snellen HA. History of Cardiology: A Brief Outline of the 350 Years' Prelude to an Explosive Growth. Netherlands: Donker Academic Publications, 1984:19–26.
6. Bilroth CAT. Speech at the Vienna Medical Society Meeting. 1880.
7. Paget S. The Surgery of the Chest. Illustrated. Bristol: John Wright & Co., London: Simpkin, Marshall, Hamilton, Kent, & Co., Ltd. 10s. 6d. net., 1896.
8. Rehn L. Ueber penetrierende Herzwunden und Herznaht. Archiv Für Klinische Chirurgie 1897; 55:315–329.
9. Tuffier T. Etat actuel de la chirurgie intrathoracique. Trans Int Congr Med 1913 (London 1914); 7. Surgery 1914; 2:249.
10. Brock R. Aortic subvalvular stenosis: Surgical treatment. Guys Hosp Rep 1957; 106:221.
11. Bailey CP, Bolton HE, Nichols HT, et al. Commissurotomy for rheumatic aortic stenosis. Circulation 1954; 9:22.

12. Cutler EC, Levine SA. Cardiotomy and valvulotomy for mitral stenosis: Experimental observations and clinical notes concerning an operated case with recovery. Boston Med Surg J 1923; 188:1023–1027.
13. Souttar HS. Surgical treatment of mitral stenosis. Br Med J 1925; 2:603.
14. Acierno LJ. The History of Cardiology. New York: Parthenon Publishing Group, 1994:633.
15. Hufnagel CA, Harvey WP, Rabil PJ, et al. Surgical correction of aortic insufficiency. Surgery 1954; 35:673.
16. Hufnagel CA. Aortic plastic valvular prostheses. Bull Georgetown Univ Med Cent 1951; 4:128.
17. Campbell JM. Artificial aortic valve. J Thorac Cardiovasc Surg 1958; 19:312.
18. Men in black—Charles A. Lindbergh & Dr. Alexis Carrel. Time 1938;13.
19. McLean J. The discovery of heparin. Circulation 1959; 19:78.
20. Gibbon JH Jr. Application of a mechanical heart and lung apparatus in cardiac surgery. Minn Med 1954; 37:171.
21. Lillehei CW, Cohen M, Warden HE, et al. The direct-vision intracardiac correction of congenital anomalies by controlled cross circulation. Surgery 1955; 38:11–29.
22. Kirklin JW. The middle 1950s and C. Walton Lillehei. J Thorac Cardiovasc Surg 1989; 98:822.
23. Lefrak EA, Starr A. Historic aspects of cardiac valve replacement. In: Lefrak EA, Starr A. eds. Cardiac Valve Prostheses. New York: Appleton-Century-Crofts, 1979: 3–37.
24. Norman AF. The first mitral valve replacement [letter]. Ann Thorac Surg 1991; 51:525–526.
25. Kay EB. Early years in artificial valve development. Ann Thorac Surg 1989; 48:S24–S25.
26. Braunwald NS, Cooper T, Morrow AG. Complete replacement of the mitral valve: Successful clinical application of a flexible polyurethane prosthesis. J Thorac Cardiovasc Surg 1960; 40:1–11.
27. Starr A, Edwards ML. Mitral replacement: Clinical experience with a ball-valve prosthesis. Ann Surg 1961; 154:726–740.
28. Ellis FH Jr, Bulbulian AH. Prosthetic replacement of the mitral valve. I. Preliminary experimental observations. Mayo Clin Proc 1958; 33:532–534.
29. Bjork VO. A new tilting disc valve prosthesis. Scand J Thorac Cardiovasc Surg 1969; 3:1–10.
30. Emery RW, Mettler E, Nicoloff DM. A new cardiac prosthesis: The St. Jude Medical cardiac valve: In vivo results. Circulation 1979; 60:48–54.
31. Senning A, Rothlin M. The late fate of autologous fascia lata valve grafts in the aortic position. Isr J Med Sci 1975; 11:179–84.
32. Binet JP, Carpentier A, Langlois J, et al. Implantation de valves heterogenes dans le traitment des cardiopathies aortiques. C R Acad Sci Paris 1965; 261:5733.
33. Ross DN. Homograft replacement of the aortic valve. Lancet 1962; 2:487.
34. Barratt-Boyes BG. Homograft aortic valve replacement in aortic incompetence and stenosis. Thorax 1964; 19:131–50.
35. O'Brien MF, Stafford EG, Gardner MA, et al. The viable cryopreserved allograft valve. J Cardiac Surg 1987; 2(suppl):153–167.
36. Ross DN. Replacement of aortic and mitral valves with a pulmonary autograft. Lancet 1967; 2:956–958.
37. Binet JP, Planche C, Weiss M. Heterograft replacement of the aortic valve. In: Ionescu MI, Ross DN, Wooler GH, eds. Biological Tissue in Heart Valve Replacement. London: Butterworth, 1971:409.
38. Carpentier A, Deloche A, Relland J, et al. Six-year follow-up of glutaraldehyde-preserved heterografts. With particular reference to the treatment of congenital valve malformations. J Thorac Cardiovasc Surg 1974; 68:771–782.
39. Carpentier A. Principles of tissue valve transplantation. In: Ionescu MI, Ross DN, Wooler GH, eds. Biological Tissue in Heart Valve Replacement. London: Butterworth, 1971:49.

40. Kaiser GA, Hancock WD, Lukban SB, et al. Clinical use of a new design stented xenograft heart valve prosthesis. Surg Forum 1969; 20:137.
41. Cournand AF. Control of the pulmonary circulation in man with some remarks on methodology. Nobel Lecture, 1956.
42. Hales S. Statistical essays. In: Innys W, Manby R, Woodwards T, eds. Containing Heamostaticks, Vol. 2. London: 1733.
43. Fick A. Über die Messung des Blutquantums in den Herzventrikeln. In: Sitzungs-berichte der Phys. Med. Ges. zu Würzburg. XIV. Sitzung am 9 Juli, 1870:16.
44. Forssmann W. Experiments on Myself: Memories of a Surgeon in Germany. New York: St. Martin's Press, 1974:84–85.
45. Zimmerman HA, Scott RW, Becker NO. Catheterization of the left side of the heart in man. Circulation 1950; 357–359.
46. Seldinger SI. Catheter replacement of the needle in percutaneous arteriography: A new technique. Acta Radiol 1953; 39:368–376.
47. Sones FM Jr, Shirey EK, Proudfit WL, et al. Cine-coronary arteriography [Abstract]. Circulation 1959; 20:773.
48. Dotter CT, Judkins MP, Frische LH. Safety guidesprings for percutaneous cardiovas-cular catheterization. Am J Roentgenol Radium Ther Nucl Med 1966; 9:957–60.
49. Grüntzig AR, Myler RK, Hanna ES, et al. Coronary transluminal angioplasty [abstract]. Circulation 1977; 84:55–56.
50. Dotter CT. Transluminally placed coil-spring endarterial tube grafts: Long-term patency in canine popliteal artery. Invest Radiol 1969; 4:329–332.
51. Maass D. Transluminal implantation of self-adjusting expandable prosthesis: Princi-ples, techniques, and results. Prog Artif Org 1983; 2:979–987.
52. Sigwart U, Puel J, Mirkovitch V, et al. Intravascular stents to prevent occlusion and restenosis after transluminal angioplasty. N Engl J Med 1987; 316:701–706.
53. Rashkind WJ, Miller WW. Creation of an atrial septal defect without thoracotomy. A palliative approach to complete transposition of the great arteries. JAMA 1966; 196(11):991–992.
54. Kan JS, White RI Jr, Mitchell SE, et al. Percutaneous balloon valvuloplasty: A new method for treating congenital pulmonary stenosis. N Engl J Med. 1982; 307(9):540–542.
55. Lock JE, Bass JL, Amplatz K, et al. Balloon dilatation angioplasty of aortic coarctations in infants and children. Circulation 1983; 68(1):109–116.
56. Inoue K, Owaki T, Nakamura F, et al. Clinical application of transvenous mitral com-missurotomy by a new balloon catheter. J Thorac Cardiovasc Surg 1984; 87(3):394–402.
57. Labaibidi Z, Wu JR, Walls JT. Percutaneous balloon aortic valvuloplasty: Results in 23 patients. Am J Cardiol 1984; 53(1):194–197.
58. Cribier A, Savin T, Saudi N, et al. Percutaneous transluminal valvuloplasty of acquired aortic stenosis in elderly patients: An alternative to valve replacement? Lancet 1986; 1(8472):63–67.
59. NHLBI Balloon Valvuloplasty Registry Participants. Percutaneous balloon aortic valvuloplasty. Acute and 30-day follow-up results in 674 patients from NHLBI Bal-loon Valvuloplasty Registry. Circulation 1991; 84:2383–2397.
60. Davies H. Catheter-mounted valve for temporary relief of aortic insufficiency. Lancet 1965; 1:250.
61. Moulopoulos SD, Anthopoulos L, Stamatelopoulos S, et al. Catheter mounted aortic valves. Ann Thorac Surg 1971; 11:423–430.
62. Phillips SJ, Ciborski M, Freed PS, et al. A temporary catheter-tip aortic valve: Hemo-dynamic effects on experimental acute aortic insufficiency. Ann Thorac Surg. 1976; 21:134–137.
63. Andersen HR, Knudsen LL, Hasenkam JM. Transluminal catheter implantation of a new expandable artificial cardiac valve in the aorta and the beating heart of closed chest pigs (abstract). Eur Heart J 1990; 11(suppl):224a.
64. Andersen HR, Knudsen LL, Hasenkam JM. Transluminal implantation of artificial heart valves. Description of a new expandable aortic valve and initial results with

implantation by catheter technique in closed chest pigs. Eur Heart J 1992; 13(5):704–708.

65. Huber CH, Nasratulla M, Augstburger M, et al. Ultrasound navigation through the heart for off-pump aortic valved stent implantation: New tools for new goals. J Endovasc Ther 2004; 11(4):503–510.

66. Huber CH, inventor. United States published patent application. US patent 2006/0074484 A1. 2004.

67. Pavcnik D, Wright KC, Wallace S. Development and initial experimental evaluation of a prosthetic aortic valve for transcatheter placement. Work in progress. Radiology 1992; 183(1):151–154.

68. Moazami N, Bessler M, Argenziano M, et al. Transluminal aortic valve placement. A feasibility study with a newly designed collapsible aortic valve. ASAIO J 1996; 42(5):M381–M385.

69. Sochman J, Peregrin JH, Rocek M, et al. Related articles, links percutaneous transcatheter one-step mechanical aortic disc valve prosthesis implantation: A preliminary feasibility study in swine. Cardiovasc Intervent Radiol 2006; 29(1):114–119.

70. Bonhoeffer P, Boudjemline Y, Saliba Z, et al. Transcatheter implantation of a bovine valve in pulmonary position: A lamb study. Circulation 2000; 102(7):813–816.

71. Bonhoeffer P, Boudjemline Y, Saliba Z, et al. Percutaneous replacement of pulmonary valve in a right-ventricle to pulmonary-artery prosthetic conduit with valve dysfunction. Lancet 2000; 356(9239):1403–1405.

72. Boudjemline Y, Bonhoeffer P. Percutaneous implantation of a valve in the descending aorta in lambs. Eur Heart J 2002; 23(13):1045–1049.

73. Boudjemline Y, Bonhoeffer P. Steps toward percutaneous aortic valve replacement. Circulation 2002; 105(6):775–778.

74. Boudjemline Y, Bonhoeffer P. Percutaneous aortic valve replacement: Will we get there? Heart 2001; 86(6):705–706.

75. Lutter G, Kuklinski D, Berg G, et al. Percutaneous aortic valve replacement: An experimental study. I. Studies on implantation. J Thorac Cardiovasc Surg 2002; 123:768–776.

76. Zhou JQ, Corno AF, Huber CH, et al. Self-expandable valved stent of large size: Off-bypass implantation in pulmonary position. Eur J Cardiothorac Surg 2003; 24(2):212–216.

77. Huber CH, Tozzi P, Corno AF, et al. Do valved stents compromise coronary flow? Eur J Cardiothorac Surg. 2004; 25(5):754–759.

78. Cribier A, Eltchaninoff H, Bash A, et al. Percutaneous transcatheter implantation of an aortic valve prosthesis for calcific aortic stenosis: First human case description. Circulation 2002; 106(24):3006–3008.

Epidemiologic Consideration on Transcatheter Therapies for Structural Heart Disease—An Unmet Clinical Need

INTRODUCTION

In the United States alone, more than 50,000 open heart surgical aortic valve replacements (SAVRs) are performed every year (Annex 1), but the patient population with aortic valve disease (AVD) is far larger. Results presented at the 27th Cowen Healthcare Conference in Boston, March 2005, estimate that in the U.S. aortic valve replacement (AVR) market alone 45% of patients meeting treatment criteria and being eligible for surgical AVR are not referred to surgical therapy, another 22% of patients meeting treatment criteria are not eligible because of age or important risk profile, and finally, only 33% of the patients requiring aortic valve therapy undergo SAVR.

The invasiveness of surgical valve replacement, the operative risk, and the prolonged and costly recovery preclude large numbers of sick patients from having the operation performed. To that effect, two major limitations are associated with SAVR:

1. Significant mortality and morbidity and lengthy postoperative recovery period due to the routine use of the heart-lung machine and the necessity for a midline sternotomy. A large proportion of patients requiring AVR from a clinical perspective are denied surgery because of unacceptable high surgical risk (so-called inoperable or high-risk patients). Another large group of patients, being offered aortic valve surgery, themselves do not wish to assume the risk and/or undergo a lengthy and strenuous recovery after the operation (so-called low-risk patients).
2. Between the two choices of implantable aortic valves, mechanical and bioprosthetic (tissue) valves, bioprosthetic valves are increasingly recommended and used. The lifespan of bioprosthetic valves is 12 to 15 years and after this time period the patient must typically undergo aortic valve reoperation. Reoperation is technically more challenging and confers an even higher rate of complication, mortality, and morbidity compared to the initial open heart surgical operation.

AVD POPULATION—A MARKET PERSPECTIVE

The following epidemiologic assessment by Richard Harbaugh reflects on future developments and trends of AVD population from a market perspective. (Summarized and excerpted with client permission from copyrighted proprietary market research executed by CONSILIUM Associates LLC, Irvine, CA. Original study dated December 15, 2005, and updated July 30, 2006. Courtesy of CoreValve Inc., Irvine, CA.)

The incidence of AVD is increasing in developed countries and is contributing to the worldwide rise in cardiovascular-related morbidity and mortality.

AVD can affect patients of all ages, but it primarily affects the elderly. In the early 1960s, the advent of open heart surgery provided AVD patients with the opportunity to undergo AVR. Today, after dramatic technology and surgical technique improvements, a large percentage of patients are candidates for SAVR. New less invasive procedures are also being developed in an effort to offer treatment to patients less suitable for surgery. Questions arise concerning the number of people who could benefit from AVR technologies during the next few decades. The objective of this AVD patient population assessment is to

- Determine the current prevalence and incidence of AVD in developed countries.
- Estimate the prevalence of AVD in 2025.
- Estimate the patient population that could benefit from AVR in 2025.

Population Shifts
This analysis focuses on countries where AVR treatment is expected to be readily available to a majority of the population during the study time frame. These include the United States, Canada, Japan, and the 27 European countries referred to as the EU27 (new members Bulgaria and Romania are included). Less developed nations are specifically excluded from this analysis.

Table 1 shows that by the end of 2004, only 15.4% of the people in the 30 countries included in this assessment were older than 65 years. By 2025, this percentage will have grown to 21.6%. In 2005, there were 145 million people older than 65 years, and by 2025 this number will have grown to 218 million. In contrast, the total population in the target countries will grow only 7%—from approximately 938 million to just more than 1 billion. In 2005, the U.S. population aged 65 and older (the most populated country in the group) represented 25% of the total, and in 2025 would represent 30% of the total population. In all countries combined, the net increase in the age 65+ population will be 52% over the 20 years of the assessment period (includes attrition within the population).

Table 2 provides estimates on the cohort changes within the elderly population between 2004 and 2025 for all 30 countries. Not only will the age 65+ population increase, but the segment of the population older than 85 years in the target countries will nearly double from 16.5 million in 2005 to 31.6 million in 2025. This factor will be a major contributor to a predicted increase in the prevalence of symptomatic AVD over the time period.

Incidence of AVD
Despite the significant number of people being treated for AVD, neither the Center for Disease Control nor U.S. insurance payers specifically include AVD in their statistics. In addition, few other countries maintain statistics for the number of people who have been diagnosed or are being treated. The shortage of reliable data is partially explained by the absence of standardized diagnostic and treatment standards.

In the United States, the incidence and prevalence of AVD has been studied extensively. Stewart et al. performed echocardiography on 5201 people older than 65 years who were enrolled in the cardiovascular health study. AVD was identified in 26% of this random population of seniors and significant stenosis was found in 2% (1). In this study, the incidence of AVD in 75- to 84-year-olds

TABLE 1   Estimates for Population Growth from 2004 to 2025

	Total population		Percentage 65+		Population 65+	
	2004	2025	2004	2025	2004	2025
Austria	8,114	8,501	15.50%	22.10%	1,258	1,879
Belgium	10,396	10,898	17.10%	22.50%	1,778	2,452
Bulgaria	7,801	6,465	17.10%	23.80%	1,334	1,539
Cyprus	730	897	11.90%	19.20%	87	172
Czech Republic	10,212	9,812	14.00%	22.40%	1,430	2,198
Denmark	5,398	5,557	14.90%	21.20%	804	1,178
Estonia	1,351	1,224	16.10%	19.90%	218	244
Finland	5,220	5,439	15.60%	24.60%	814	1,338
France	59,901	64,392	16.30%	22.40%	9,764	14,424
Germany	82,532	82,108	18.00%	24.60%	14,856	20,199
Greece	11,041	11,394	17.80%	22.80%	1,965	2,598
Hungary	10,117	9,588	15.50%	22.00%	1,568	2,109
Ireland	4,028	4,922	11.10%	16.50%	447	812
Italy	57,888	57,751	19.20%	25.00%	11,114	14,438
Latvia	2,319	2,068	16.20%	19.70%	376	407
Lithuania	3,446	3,134	15.00%	19.20%	517	602
Luxembourg	452	544	14.10%	18.00%	64	98
Malta	400	468	13.10%	21.30%	52	100
Netherlands	16,258	17,429	13.90%	20.60%	2,260	3,590
Poland	38,191	36,836	13.00%	21.10%	4,965	7,772
Portugal	10,475	10,730	16.90%	22.10%	1,770	2,371
Romania	21,711	19,746	14.50%	19.00%	3,148	3,752
Slovakia	5,380	5,237	11.50%	18.90%	619	990
Slovenia	1,996	2,014	15.00%	22.80%	299	459
Spain	42,345	45,556	16.90%	22.00%	7,156	10,022
Sweden	8,976	9,769	17.20%	22.20%	1,544	2,169
United Kingdom	59,652	63,792	16.00%	20.90%	9,544	13,333
EU27	486,330	496,271	16.40%	22.60%	79,758	112,245
Japan	127,687	121,612	19.50%	27.30%	24,899	33,200
Canada	31,714	36,105	12.80%	22.30%	4,059	8,046
United States	292,801	353,120	12.30%	18.20%	35,919	64,268
Total	**938,532**	**1,007,108**	**15.41%**	**21.62%**	**144,635**	**217,759**

Source: U.S. Bureau of the Census – 30 countries – and International Data Base (http://www.census.gov/ipc/www/idb/).

TABLE 2   Segmented Estimates for Age >65 Population Growth from 2004 to 2025

Age →	65–74		75–84		85+	
	2004	2025	2004	2025	2004	2025
EU27	44,282	56,726	28,782	35,865	8,271	16,450
US	18,623	35,688	12,952	19,825	5,120	8,010
Canada	2,247	4,456	1,506	2,397	330	950
Japan	13,736	14,372	8,344	13,054	2,738	6,233
Total	**78,888**	**111,242**	**51,584**	**71,141**	**16,459**	**31,643**

Source: U.S. Bureau of the Census – 30 countries – and International Data Base (http://www.census.gov/ipc/www/idb/).

increased to 37% and among those older than 85 the percentage was 52%. These data support the conclusion that symptoms of AVD increase with age, as does the percentage of these patients who require valve replacement.

A study by Otto et al. assessed the aortic valve of a random sample of 5621 people older than 65. As assessed by echocardiogram, 29% showed stenosis without outflow obstruction versus restrictive stenosis in 2% (2). Other (smaller) studies of random populations of seniors have shown a prevalence of symptomatic aortic valve stenosis as high as 9% (3).

Prevalence Trends in AVD

It is anticipated that several factors other than age will contribute to an increase in AVD prevalence over the next two decades. Another significant factor that is contributing to an increase in AVD is obesity and its associated conditions including hypertension, coronary artery disease (CAD), and diabetes (4–6).

The best available indication of the extent to which obesity may affect the number of AVD patients can be seen in the estimates of obese population shown in Table 3. It is important to note that these data represent only the change that is expected in this patient population over a five-year period. The World Health Organization expects to see the percentage of people who are obese increase significantly in 23 of the countries included in this assessment. How the effects of obesity will influence the long-term incidence of AVD is difficult to predict until large cohort tracking research is carried out, but this observation supports the premise that the overall prevalence percentage of AVD will be larger in 2025 than it is in 2005.

Research indicating other contributors to AVD is ongoing. In a 2006 study by the American Heart Association Kidney and Cardiovascular Disease Council, the Councils on High Blood Pressure Research, Cardiovascular Disease in the Young, and Epidemiology and Prevention, it was shown that kidney and cardiovascular diseases accelerate the symptoms and severity of each other (6).

The Contribution of Bicuspid Aortic Valves

Clinical evidence shows a higher incidence of AVD in people with bicuspid valves. Studies have reported that between 1% and 2% of the overall population has a bicuspid aortic valve, and that 46% of these people will develop AVD if they live past 50 years (7).

The Contribution of CAD

CAD is the most common form of heart disease and a leading cause of death in all countries studied. Although more often closely allied with other factors, there are a number of studies indicating a correlation between aortic valve sclerosis and CAD. The most recent article by Soydinc et al. showed "aortic valve sclerosis is strongly interrelated with the coronary angiographic Gensini score" (8).

The Contribution of Diabetes

Diabetes has been shown to be a factor in the early onset of AVD. While the studies on the effects of obesity are rarely focused on an AVD correlation, Katz et al. have conducted research that assessed aortic valve calcium on 6780 participants in the Multi-Ethnic Study of Arthrosclerosis (MESA) (9). This study cohort included 1016 patients with diabetes mellitus, the most common type in adults,

TABLE 3 Prevalence of Population with a Body Mass Index Greater than 25 kg/m^2 (in 30 Countries) Between 2005 and 2010

Country/Region	2005		2010	
	Men	Women	Men	Women
Austria	61.0%	53.2%	62.9%	55.2%
Belgium	51.9%	40.7%	54.1%	42.9%
Bulgaria	62.8%	45.5%	62.8%	45.5%
Canada	65.1%	57.1%	66.9%	59.5%
Czech Republic	58.1%	47.8%	60.1%	49.3%
Cyprus	51.7%	60.6%	53.8%	63.0%
Denmark	52.5%	39.1%	55.0%	41.4%
Estonia	50.7%	33.8%	50.7%	33.8%
Finland	64.9%	52.4%	67.1%	54.5%
France	45.6%	34.7%	48.0%	36.9%
Germany	65.1%	55.1%	67.2%	57.1%
Greece	75.7%	61.3%	77.5%	63.2%
Hungary	55.9%	47.4%	55.9%	47.4%
Ireland	51.5%	41.7%	53.9%	43.9%
Italy	52.7%	38.3%	55.0%	40.0%
Japan	27.0%	18.1%	29.8%	16.2%
Latvia	49.9%	44.7%	49.9%	44.7%
Lithuania	62.3%	43.9%	62.3%	43.9%
Luxembourg	54.4%	54.0%	56.9%	56.2%
Malta	71.4%	66.1%	73.3%	67.6%
Netherlands	48.0%	44.0%	50.2%	46.1%
Poland	50.7%	44.3%	50.7%	44.3%
Portugal	58.5%	49.2%	60.9%	51.2%
Romania	37.7%	40.6%	37.7%	40.6%
Slovakia	52.0%	60.6%	54.0%	62.9%
Slovenia	56.0%	63.5%	57.9%	65.7%
Spain	55.8%	47.7%	57.9%	49.8%
Sweden	54.5%	44.9%	57.0%	47.2%
United Kingdom	65.7%	61.9%	67.8%	63.8%
United States	75.6%	72.6%	80.5%	76.7%

whose aortic valve was assessed via computer tomography. Among women and men with diabetes mellitus, respectively 17% and 24% had aortic valve calcium. These percentages can be compared to a population of 4024 included in the study that had neither diabetes mellitus nor metabolic syndrome. The diabetes-free women and men had a prevalence of only 8% and 14% respectively. Another controlled study of the ICD-9 codes was completed by the Veterans Health Administration hospitals. This study analyzed in-patient treatment of 845,747 patients from all Veterans Health Administration hospitals and found that people with type 2 diabetes mellitus were 25% more likely to have AVD than those who did not have diabetes (10). Currently, there are approximately 200 million people with type 2 diabetes in the world. This figure is expected to increase to 333 million by 2025, with a high prevalence rate in the developed countries (11). As shown in Table 4, in the 30 countries studied, there are approximately 47 million diabetic patients in 2005. It is estimated that this number will grow to 70 million (12) by 2025. This finding supports the premise that the overall prevalence percentage of AVD will be larger in 2025 than it is in 2005.

TABLE 4 Current and Projected Prevalence of Diabetes (in 30 Countries) Between 2005 and 2010

Country/Region	2005	2025
Austria	239,000	366,000
Belgium	317,000	461,000
Bulgaria	472,000	458,000
Canada	2,006,000	3,543,000
Czech Republic	336,000	441,000
Cyprus	50,000	87,000
Denmark	157,000	232,000
Estonia	46,000	43,000
Finland	157,000	239,000
France	171,0000	2,645,000
Germany	2,627,000	3,771,000
Greece	853,000	1,077,000
Hungary	333,000	376,000
Ireland	86,000	157,000
Italy	4,252,000	5,374,000
Japan	6,765,000	8,914,000
Latvia	82,000	90,000
Lithuania	114,000	146,000
Luxembourg	12,000	21,000
Malta	39,000	57,000
Netherlands	426,000	720,000
Poland	1,134,000	1,541,000
Portugal	662,000	882,000
Romania	1,092,000	1,395,000
Slovakia	153,000	220,000
Slovenia	66,000	87,000
Spain	2,717,000	3,752,000
Sweden	292,000	404,000
United Kingdom	1,765,000	2,668,000
United States	17,702,000	30,312,000
Total	**15,753**	**17,612**

The Contribution of Dialysis

The calcium accumulation associated with dialysis can contribute to aortic valve calcification. Several studies have shown a high incidence of AVD in this population. Reported percentages range from 28% to 55% of ESRD patients who become AVD symptomatic 10 to 20 years earlier than the general population (13–16). In one study of 135 chronic hemodialysis patients, 105 (78%) presented with aortic valve calcification (17). The population of ESRD patients is of particular interest to the groups working on percutaneous aortic valve replacement procedures. Currently, most of these patients do not receive prosthetic valves, as they tend to be a poor surgical risk. In most cases, their general hemodynamic health is poor, they have a high potential for renal failure to be caused by anesthesia during and after surgery. In addition, it can be difficult to manage their hypertension and hyperkalemia as well as their arteriovenous fistula. Nearly 21% of the patients identified as dialysis subjects undergoing AVR experience mortality/morbidity in hospital (18).

TABLE 5 Estimated Deaths owing to Rheumatic Heart Disease in 2000 by WHO Region

	Deaths N ($\times 10^3$)	Rate (per 100,000 population)
Africa	29	4.5
The Americas	15	1.8
Eastern Mediterranean	21	4.4
Europe	38	4.3
South-East Asia	117	7.6
Western Pacific	115	6.8
World	**332**	**5.5**

Currently, there are approximately 1.5 million people worldwide on dialysis with approximately two-thirds (1 million) of these in the 30 countries studied (19). This number is expected to double by 2025 (20). This finding supports the premise that the overall prevalence percentage of AVD will be larger in 2025 than it is in 2005.

It would be easy to discount the *contribution of rheumatic fever*, since it has largely been eradicated from developed nations. Worldwide, however, rheumatic disease is a significant cause of morbidity and mortality, and in 1998 it was the 14th leading cause of death in people aged 15 to 44 years in less developed nations (Table 5).

The treatment burden from rheumatic fever is shifted to the nations studied through the mechanism of immigration. It is anticipated that immigration will contribute to the prevalence of AVD in the studied countries. This observation contributes to the premise that the prevalence percentage of AVD will be larger in 2025 than it is in 2005.

The *contribution of changing attitudes toward AVR* may play a role. It was anticipated that patients would remain in the pool of those requiring a heart valve replacement for a relatively short period of time as they were expected to either undergo surgery or expire. Most AVD patients do exit the pool within one to three years. Surprisingly, however, it was found that some patients remain in the pool for several years (21). Reasons for this are numerous and include clinical cardiologists' attitudes concerning the surgical risk versus potential improvement in quality of life (QoL). One of the most recent clinical studies indicates that approximately one-third of the patients who present within the health care system, and could benefit from AVR, never undergo the surgery (22). Changing patient and physician attitudes may lead not only to more, but also to earlier intervention, and thus larger numbers of patients for AVR.

Finally, there *may be a contribution* from the large number of people who utilized the combination of fenfluramine and phentermine for weight loss in the United States during the late 1990s. Between 1995 and the time the FDA disallowed sale of these drugs, an estimated 14 million prescriptions were written for either fenfluramine or phentermine (fen/phen) (23). The user population was typically young adults, and their use of the drug combination is expected to have two effects on the prevalence of AVD, specifically in the United States. The first effect is that patients who are predisposed to AVD will not only have a much higher risk of becoming AVD symptomatic, but also that this will occur at an earlier age. In addition, longer life expectancy is likely to contribute some patients who previously would have expired prior to their AVD becoming symptomatic. Typically, this indication would not be included in this type of analysis; however, the large number of prescriptions written mean that an estimated more than five million people took the combination of drugs for more than six months, which is long enough to have caused permanent damage to their aortic valve (23). It is difficult to predict an actuarial on this population, but it is undeniable that there will be an effect during the study period.

The combination of all factors can support the hypothesis that the incidence of AVD and the prevalence of need for AVR will increase from 26% to 35%, and 2% to 3% respectively of the age 65+ population. By either measure, current studied incidence or extrapolated future incidence estimates, the patient population requiring AVR over the next two decades will grow very dramatically. In addition, addressing their disease state will require further improvement in treatment methods and techniques.

In conclusion, as demonstrated in Table 6, the number of people with symptomatic AVD requiring AVR treatment is expected to rise dramatically between 2005 and 2025 for the following reasons:

1. Symptomatic AVD is largely age related and the world population is aging. Today there is already a higher percentage of people older than 65 years than ever before, and this percentage will continue to grow over the period assessed.
2. People are living longer. While previous generations of patients with AVD often died of other causes prior to their condition aggravating, today and in the future, they will live long enough to require AVR.
3. The incidence of AVD and the prevailing need for AVR increases with each age segment above 65. The relative age group distribution will change dramatically over the next two decades as 80-, 85-, and 90-year-olds become larger cohorts.
4. Comorbidities that cause people to experience AVD symptoms earlier, such as diabetes, obesity, and cardiovascular disease, continue to be very prevalent.

TABLE 6 Population with AVD That Requires Valve Replacement Target Countries in 2005 and 2025

	2005	2025
Total population in the target countries	938,532,000	1,007,108,000
Percentage of people older than age 65	15.41%	21.62%
Number of people older than age 65	144,635,000	217,759,000
Percentage with AVD by current incidence	26%	26%
Number with AVD by current incidence	37,605,000	56,617,000
Percent with symptomatic AVD by current incidence	2%	2%
Number with symptomatic AVD by current incidence	2,890,000	4,355,000
Age and comorbidity-adjusted percent with AVD	Not applicable	35%
Age and comorbidity-adjusted number with AVD	Not applicable	76,216,000
Age and comorbidity-adjusted percent with symptomatic AVD	Not applicable	3%
Age and comorbidity-adjusted number with symptomatic AVD	Not applicable	6,533,000

5. The population requiring dialysis is growing dramatically, and a high percentage of such patients acquire AVD. In addition, the life expectancy of patients requiring dialysis is increasing and more are expected to live long enough to require AVR.

BENEFITS OF CARDIAC SURGERY IN THE OLDER PATIENT

Transcatheter aortic valve therapies are targeting two populations. First, the so-called inoperable or not-eligible aortic valve patient, and second, the eligible but not referred patient. Unfortunately, it is a widespread and common misbelief that the older patients should be classified as inoperable as they might not survive or at least not benefit from SAVR.

In the following study, the author has studied mortality, morbidity, and QoL in patients older than 80 years undergoing valvular, coronary, or combined heart surgery. The results are extremely satisfying and should always be kept in mind when withholding older patients from surgery or selecting them for transcatheter aortic valve implantation.

The following study is in part reproduced from Huber CH, et al. Benefits of cardiac surgery in octogenarians—a postoperative quality of life assessment. Eur J Cardiothorac Surg 2007; 31:1099–1105.

Epidemiologic Considerations of a Progressively Older Growing Population

Life expectancy has increased during recent decades leading to an older growing population. In 1982, life expectancy at birth for the overall population in Switzerland, the United Kingdom, and the United States was 76.3, 75.7, and 75.5 years, respectively. Ten years later, life expectancy has been increased to 79.9 years for Switzerland, 77.9 years for the United Kingdom, and >77 years for the United States. By 2022, life expectancy will reach 82.0 years for Switzerland, 80.8 years for the United Kingdom, and 80.2 for the United States. An 80-year-old Swiss man or woman will live another 6.6 or 7.8 years, respectively. Sixteen percent of the Western European population is over 65 years of age, 13% in the USA and 15% in Switzerland. In contrast only about half (7%) of the world's population falls into the same age group. Five percent of the Swiss population is aged 80 years and above, and this age group continues to rise. It is estimated that the U.S. population will include more than 25 million persons aged at least 80 years by 2050 (24).

Considering that heart diseases are the leading cause of death in industrialized nations, and the prevalence of CAD is 18% in the United States, it is estimated the number of patients seeking treatment will further increase. Despite maximum medical therapy, many patients of this age group remain severely symptomatic of their cardiovascular disease. Cardiovascular diseases are functionally limiting more than 25% of the population aged 80 years and above (25).

Continuous advances in operative techniques, myocardial protection, and perioperative care have led to a steady decline in operative mortality, and cardiac surgery can be performed safely in patients aged 80 years and older with good midterm results.

QoL is becoming an increasingly important aspect of assessing the outcome of any therapeutic intervention as well as a personal perception of health, physical well-being, and mental state. Elkington in 1966 (26) described QoL as "not just the absence of death but life with the vibrant quality that was associate with the vigor of youth."

Methodical Assessment
Introducing a new technology should entirely focus on the intended patient benefits. The older patient fall by virtue of their age into a higher surgical risk group, and are therefore more likely to be treated by transcatheter technologies. But the simple fact of being old is not sufficient to withhold surgery. The following work illustrates good surgical outcomes in patients older than 80 years.

Of 161 octogenarians with consecutive heart operations between January 1999 and December 2003 at a single Swiss institution, all patients with isolated coronary artery bypass grafting (CABG), isolated AVR, or combined CABG/AVR were selected ($n = 136$).

Data were extracted from retrospective review of patient's records. Information on QoL of the 120 surviving patients and causes of deaths were obtained via telephone interviews during a two-month period by the same investigator. The surviving patient was questioned in the first line, relatives, patient's general practitioners or cardiologists, and hospital autopsy records served to acquire additional information.

The postoperative QoL assessment is based on the modified Seattle Angina Questionnaire and is 100% complete. The mean follow-up was 890 days (max 1853, min 69 days).

Preoperative Patient's Characteristics
The mean age of the 136 patients at operation was 82.3 ± 2.1 years, ranging from 80 to 91 years. More than 13% of the patients were 85 years or older. Eighty (59%) were male patients. Two-thirds presented with symptoms of NYHA class III or IV, respectively Canadian Cardiovascular Society angina grade (CCS) class III or more. Body mass index was 25.5 ± 3.8 kg/m^2. The preoperative variables are summarized in Table 7.

Isolated CABG (n = 61 Patients)
Unstable angina pectoris was the most common symptom. Forty-two (69%) patients had a CCS of III or more. Twenty-seven (44%) patients had a history of myocardial infarction, in eleven patients less than 14 days before, and in sixteen patients more than 2 weeks before surgery. The left ventricular ejection fraction (LVEF) was $59 \pm 13\%$, and only five (8.2%) patients presented with an LVEF of equal or less than 35%.

In 53 (87%) patients three-vessel and in 7 (11%) patients two-vessel disease was present. Left main stem disease was diagnosed in 25 (41%) patients.

Quintuple CABG was performed in 7 (11%) patients, quadruple in 25 (41%) patients, triple in 23 (38%) patients, while two-vessel revascularization was performed six times (10%). In 47 (77%) patients, a left internal mammary artery was harvested, and 47 (77%) patients got one or more arterial conduits. Eight (13%) radial arteries were harvested and implanted. The operation time was 168 ± 40 minutes and the bypass time was 77 ± 29 minutes. Mean aortic cross-clamp time was 46 ± 18 minutes. Nine (15%) patients needed inotropic support during weaning from cardiopulmonary bypass (CPB) and one (1.6%) patient required support via an intra-aortic balloon pump (IABP).

TABLE 7 Preoperative Patient Characteristics

Variables	No. of patients (%)			
	All (n = 136)	CABG (n = 61)	AVR (n = 34)	CABG/AVR (n = 41)
Males	80 (59)	39 (64)	15 (44)	26 (63)
Age	82.3 ± 2.1	82.0 ± 1.8	82.6 ± 2.0	82.5 ± 2.6
NYHA or CCS ≥III	90 (66)	43 (70)	21 (62)	26 (63)
Hypertension	83 (61)	38 (62)	15 (44)	30 (73)
Dyslipidemia	70 (51)	33 (54)	14 (41)	23 (56)
Pos. family history	34 (25)	14 (23)	6 (18)	14 (34)
NIDDM/IDDM	14 (10)/2 (1.5)	6 (10)/2 (3.3)	3 (9)/0	5 (13)/0
Creatinine ≥120 μmol/L	26 (19)	10 (16)	7 (21)	9 (22)
COPD	21 (15)	7 (11)	7 (21)	7 (17)
Tobacco abuse	33 (24)	23 (38)	4 (12)	6 (15)
PAD	19 (14)	10 (16)	4 (12)	5 (12)
Atrial fibrillation	26 (19)	7 (11)	10 (29)	9 (22)
Previous MI	35 (26)	27 (44)	2 (6)	6 (15)
Anticoagulation	14 (10)	8 (13)	5 (15)	1 (2.4)

Abbreviations: BMI, body mass index; CAD, coronary artery disease; CCS, Canadian Cardiovascular Society; COPD, chronic obstructive airway disease; MI, myocardial infarction; IDDM, insulin-dependent diabetes mellitus; NIDDM, non–insulin-dependent diabetes mellitus; LVEF, left ventricular ejection fraction; NYHA, New York Hear Association; PAD, peripheral arterial disease.

Aortic Valve Replacement (n = 34 Patients)

Twenty-one (62%) operated patients were in NHYA ≥III and LVEF was 60.4 ± 14%.

Severe aortic stenosis was the leading pathology in all 34 (100%) patients. In 16 (47%) patients, concomitant aortic insufficiency grade I or II was noted. Nineteen (29%) patients showed slight to moderate mitral valve insufficiency.

Stented bioprosthesis was implanted in 25 (74%) patients, stentless in 1 (3%) patient, and a mechanical valve in 8 (24%) patients. Mean CPB time was 76 ± 28 minutes and mean aortic cross-clamp time was 53 ± 14 minutes. The overall operation time was 152 ± 37 minutes.

Inotropic support for CPB weaning was necessary in 10 (29%) patients, but no patient required IABP support.

CABG in Combination with AVR (n = 41 Patients)

Six (15%) patients had left main disease, ten (24%) patients presented with triple-vessel, and thirty-five (87%) patients had either double- or single-vessel CAD. Twenty (48%) patients had single, fourteen (34%) patients had double, and eleven (27%) patients had triple or more vessel revascularization. Thirteen (31%) left internal mammary arteries and three (7.3%) radial arteries were harvested.

Stented bioprosthesis was implanted in 34 (83%) patients, stentless bioprosthesis in 1 (2.4%) patient, and a mechanical valve in 13 (31%) patients. Mean CPB time for combined AVR and CABG was 90 ± 35 minutes and mean aortic cross-clamp time was 62 ± 19 was minutes. The overall operative time was 169 ± 41 minutes.

Nineteen (46%) patients required inotropic drugs for CPB weaning, but IABP was never necessary in the perioperative phase.

Early Postoperative Outcomes

Table 8 lists early complications (<30 days) in relation to the type of surgery.

The most frequent postoperative complication in all groups was arrhythmias with atrial fibrillation in 29 (21%) patients. A permanent pacemaker became necessary in two (1.5%) patients only.

Four (3%) patients suffered perioperative myocardial infarction after combined AVR/CABG, but none required IABP support in this group. Twenty-seven (20%) patients needed inotropic drugs to wean from CPB, and in twenty-one (15%) patients, inotropes had to be continued for more than 24 hours. Prolonged mechanical ventilation (>2 days) was necessary in eight (5.9%) patients. The average length of stay in the intensive care unit (ICU) was 2.7 ± 1.6 days, and five (3.7%) patients stayed more than 1 week. Temporary dialysis was required in two (1.5%) patients, but in both the renal function recovered completely. Eight (5.9%)

TABLE 8   Early Complications (<30 d) in Relation to the Type of Surgery and Additionally Assessed Postoperative Variables

	No. of patients (%)			
Variable	All ($n = 136$)	CABG ($n = 61$)	AVR ($n = 34$)	CABG/AVR ($n = 41$)
Inotropic drug support required	27 (19.9)	9 (14.8)	9 (26.4)	9 (22.0)
IABP	1 (0.7)	1 (1.6)	0	0
ICU (d)	2.7 ± 1.6	2.8 ± 1.5	2.6 ± 1.2	2.7 ± 2.1
Prolonged ventilation (>24 h)	8 (5.9)	4 (6.6)	3 (8.8)	3 (7.3)
Duration of inotropes (h)	13.5 ± 29.0	8.3 ± 22.3	17.6 ± 33.0	0.75 ± 1.4
No. of intraoperative EC	1.5 ± 2.0	1.4 ± 1.8	1.8 ± 2.2	1.5 ± 2.0
No. of postoperative EC	1.0 ± 5.1	1.4 ± 7.4	0.9 ± 2.0	0.5 ± 1.2
Transient neurological impairment	3 (2.2)	1 (1.6)	0	2 (4.9)
Permanent neurological impairment	5 (3.7)	4 (6.6)	1 (2.9)	0
Myocardial infarction	4 (2.9)	0	0	4 (9.8)
Temporary dialysis	3 (2.2)	1 (1.6)	1 (2.9)	1 (2.4)
Antibiotic treatment (>48 h)	26 (19.1)	5 (8.2%)	11 (32.4%)	10 (24.4)
Deep sternal infections needing reoperation	2 (1.5%)	0	2 (5.9%)	0
Reoperation for bleeding	6 (4.4%)	2 (3.3%)	2 (5.9%)	2 (4.8)
Atrial fibrillation	29 (21.3%)	8 (13.2%)	10 (29.4%)	11 (26.8)
Permanent pacemaker	2 (1.5%)	0	2 (5.9%)	0
Hospital stay mean time (d)	14.2 ± 10.1	14.1 ± 13.5	13.8 ± 5.9	14.8 ± 6.2
No. of drugs at discharge	5	5	5	5

Abbreviations: EC, erythrocyte concentrate; IABP, intra-aortic balloon pump; ICU, intensive care unit.

patients underwent reintervention, in six (4.4%) patients for persistent bleeding, and in two (1.5%) patients because of deep sternal wound infection.

Five (3.7%) patients suffered from permanent neurological impairment and three (2.2%) patients recovered fully from a transient neurological impairment.

Hospital stay was 14.2 ± 10.1 days, including six (4.4%) patients with a stay longer than 25 days (range 5–110).

Mortality (Cumulative Survival in Brackets)

In-hospital death occurred in six (4.4%) patients. One month after surgery, 130 (95%) patients were alive. Survival at one, three, and five years was 93%, 90%, and 73%, respectively. The highest midterm survival rate was recorded in the isolated AVR with 31 (75%) patients alive. In contrast, combined operations with CABG/AVR showed the lowest five-year survival with 35 (65%) patients alive. The CABG group survival positioned itself between AVR and CABG/AVR groups with 54 patients alive corresponding to a cumulative five-year survival of 70% (Fig. 1).

Causes of the 16 deaths over five years were mostly of noncardiac origin. Fatal pneumonia caused death in five (31.3%) patients. In two (12.5%) patients cerebrovascular accidents, in three (18.8%) patients septicemia, in one (6.3%) patient mesenterial infarction, in one (6.3%) patient cerebral hemorrhage, and in one female (6.3%) patient euthanasia led to death. In five (31.3%) patients, a cardiac cause has been found to be at the origin of death. Table 9 shows a comparison of intervention-linked cumulative survival in octogenarians after cardiac surgery.

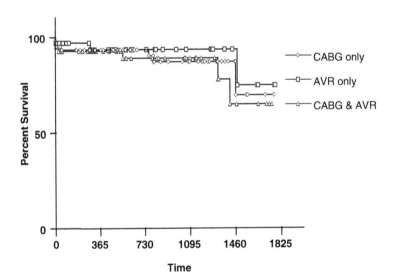

FIGURE 1 Kaplan-Meyer survival curves, comparing CABG, AVR, and combined procedures in patients older than 80 years. The unit on the time axis is expressed in days and the unit on the survival axis is expressed in percentage.

TABLE 9 Comparison of Intervention-Linked Cumulative Survival in Octogenarians After Cardiac Surgery[a]

Operation	30-day Survival	1-year Survival	3-year Survival	5-year Survival
All operations ($n = 136$)	95% ± 1.7 (7)	93% ± 2.0 (9)	90% ± 2.1 (12)	73% ± 7.9 (16)
Isolated CABG ($n = 61$)	95% ± 2.7 (3)	93% ± 3.2 (4)	87% ± 5.3 (6)	70% ± 16.1 (7)
Isolated AVR ($n = 34$)	97% ± 2.8 (1)	94% ± 4.3 (2)	94% ± 4.3 (2)	75% ± 17.1 (3)
AVR and CABG ($n = 41$)	92% ± 4.0 (3)	92% ± 4.0 (3)	88% ± 5.3 (4)	65% ± 15.2 (6)

[a]Cumulative absolute numbers of occurred death within every survival interval given in brackets.

Midterm Results

Quality of life

The mean follow-up length was 890 days (range from 69 to 1853). Information was collected by telephone interviews.

One hundred thirty patients left the hospital, and at follow-up one hundred twenty patients were alive. A validated Seattle Angina Questionnaire including two additional questions regarding dyspnea was used to assess the QoL [Fig. 4(A)]. This 11-item multiple-choice instrument examines mobility and activity, cardiac symptoms perception, disease perception, treatment satisfaction, as well as emotional well-being and enjoyment of life. In terms to assess also valve pathologies, dyspnea as an additional symptom was added to the questions regarding chest pain.

QoL improved considerably after cardiac surgery. Overall, 97 (81%) patients were not or little disabled in their daily activities (Fig. 2). Physical exercise was not or little limited in 84 (70%) patients. Symptoms decreased post cardiac surgery in 112 (93%) patients; only 2 (1.7%) patients felt worse than before operation and 6 (5%) patients described unchanged symptoms (Fig. 3). Eighty-six (72%) patients were free of angina or dyspnea, while eight (6.6%) patients

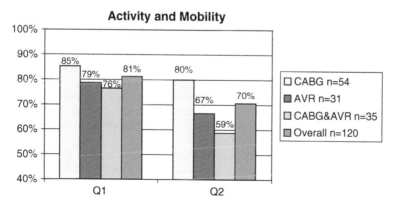

FIGURE 2 Percentage and absolute numbers of patients having answered questions 1 and 2 with no or little limitations in their daily activities.

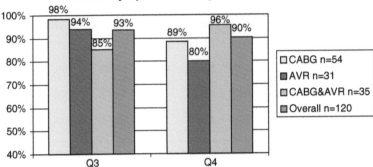

FIGURE 3 Percentage and absolute numbers of patients having answered question 3 with much less or less angina or dyspnea and question 4 with angina or dyspnea less than once a week or never in the last 4 wk.

remained moderately to severely symptomatic. In the CABG group, 42 (77.7%) patients did not have to take nitroglycerin anymore. Overall, 93 (77%) patients were very satisfied, and another 21 (17.4%) patients were satisfied by the previous treatment. Only six (5%) patients felt not satisfied to take their prescribed medication. Furthermore, 112 (93.4%) patients were very reassured to have continuous full access to medical treatments [Fig. 4(A)].

Interference of cardiac disease with daily enjoyment of life was described by only 9 (7.5%) patients, while 111 (92.5%) patients had no reduction in their QoL. Sixty-nine (58%) patients were very optimistic to conserve their present activity of life. Thirty-three (27.7%) patients did think about recurrence of their heart disease from time to time, but only seventeen (14.2%) patients were anxious about having a heart attack more frequently or dying suddenly [Fig. 4(B)]. In contrast, 30 (45%) patients undergoing AVR, with or without concomitant CABG, worried at least once a day of dying versus 6 (11.1%) patients after isolated coronary artery bypass surgery.

Finally, 116 (97%) patients at follow-up lived in their own homes and preserved a high degree of self-care.

Discussion
Since the mid-1980s, the peri- and postoperative survival in octogenarians, after cardiac surgery, has steadily increased to become highly acceptable nowadays (27). Patients 80 years and older represent a very distinct population from younger cardiac patients (28). Measurement of morbidity and mortality provide only a small amount of information about the patient's postoperative physical, functional, emotional, and mental well-being.

Little is known about the postoperative symptom perception in patients 80 years and older after cardiac surgery. This study analyses the postoperative QoL in 120 consecutive octogenarians post CABG, AVR, or a combination of both procedures. Mean follow-up was approximately 2.5 years, and none of the surviving patients was lost at follow-up. Information on QoL was obtained from close family members in the three patients with permanent neurological

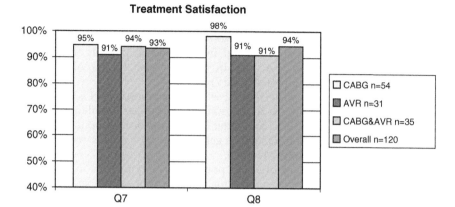

(A)

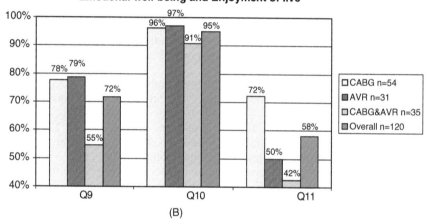

(B)

FIGURE 4   (**A**) Percentage and absolute numbers of patients having answered questions 7 and 8 and satisfied or very satisfied with their treatment. (**B**) Percentage and absolute numbers of patients having answered questions 9 and 10 with little or no interference and satisfied or very satisfied about their emotional well-being, question 8 and satisfied or very satisfied with their treatment, and question 11 and rarely or never worrying about a heart attack or sudden death event.

impairment. No one refused to answer the questionnaire. The QoL of 54 patients after CABG surgery, of 31 patients after AVR, and 35 patients after combined procedures was compared.

The initial assessment was based on the two main cardiac functional symptoms: chest pain and dyspnea. As older patients are known to have advanced symptoms at presentation for surgery, NYHA classes III and IV are more common findings in octogenarians as they are in younger patients. Alexander et al. (27) described NYHA classes III to IV heart failure being present in 16.6% compared to 9.8% in patients younger than 80 years. Fruitman and coworkers (28) have also shown a significant higher presence of NYHA IV in octogenarians.

Questions 1 to 5 of the Seattle Angina Questionnaire all address either one or both symptoms. In CABG patients, unstable angina pectoris was the presenting symptom with more than two-thirds of the patients being in CCS ≥III. Near-equal distribution was found for dyspnea in patients undergoing AVR with 62% being in NYHA ≥III. In the combined CABG/AVR group, dyspnea was the leading symptom (Table 7).

The gender difference is decreasing with age progression: 41% of patients were women opposed to 20% to 30% described in younger population (27,29). We did not identify either a trend for higher female or male in-hospital mortality as described by others. Therefore, female gender may be a weaker risk factor in the elderly compared to younger women.

The higher difference of pre- and postoperative symptoms in this older patient subgroup is a further argument for the benefit of early operative treatment in patients older than 80 years.

In 42%, left main disease was present, and CAD showed to be more extensive in older patients at the time of surgery. In contrast, LVEF did not differ from values in younger collectives, and preoperative COPD or diabetes mellitus was less likely to be found in octogenarians.

Compared to the literature (30), we used the left thoracic artery more often (78%) for revascularization of the left artery descending territory. In our opinion the principle of the thoracic artery as the graft of choice in CABG is valid in patients 80 years as well.

Peripheral vascular disease was more commonly present in CABG patients (17%) compared to patients undergoing AVR with or without concomitant CABG (12%).

Three years after surgery, 124 (90%) patients were alive, and 120 (73%) patients five years after their operation (Table 9). These survival rates are comparable or slightly higher than the ones described in other studies (27,29,31,32) and show good early and midterm postoperative results justifying not withholding cardiac surgery from the increasing elderly and very old population.

Longevity is not the primary goal in patients older than 80 years—good operative outcomes imply safety and survival and also the gain of comfort in daily life. The marked improvement of the NYHA functional class as well as improvement of the CCS class we found (72% free of angina or dyspnea) has been reported previously (28,33,34). Nevertheless, only marginal attention had been paid in most studies to the improvement of emotional well-being, treatment satisfaction, and disease perception. The results of the present study demonstrate a remarkable QoL and an important improvement in the patient's functional status after cardiac surgery in octogenarians.

Activity and mobility improved in ischemic and valvular diseases, with nearly 80% of the patients feeling no or only little limitation in their daily activity (Fig. 2). The improvement in exercise tolerance is less homogenously distributed, reporting 80% of CABG patients being virtually free of limitation and only 59% of the patients in the combined procedures group. This difference in exercise tolerance is reflected again in the patient symptom perception. Ninety-eight percent of the CABG patients compared to eighty-five percent of CABG and AVR patients felt important improvement of their angina or dyspnea compared to their preoperative clinical condition. The vast majority (93%) of all the octogenarians felt much better after surgery (Fig. 3). Toward all types of operations, more than 90% of the patients were at least satisfied or very satisfied with the overall treatment of their heart disease. And it is noteworthy that nearly 100% of the CABG patients as well as 91% of the AVR or CABG and AVR patients felt pleased to have access to full medical treatment, despite their advanced age [Fig. 4(A)]. More than 95% of the patients at follow-up lived in their own homes and enjoyed a high degree of autonomy. Similar results have been found by Fruitman et al. (28), Heijmeriks et al. (35), Rumsfeld et al. (36), Kumar et al. (33), and Yun et al. (37).

Looking at an economical scale, hospital costs have been reported to be 20% to 27% higher in the older population (38). Avery et al. attributed the increase of total direct hospital costs for octogenarians to a more severe risk profile and to longer consecutive ICU and hospital stay (29). However, emphasis on early extubation and timely aggressive mobilization after surgery also in this elderly patient population has successfully decreased the overall intubation time and length of stay in ICU to 2.8 days (Table 8). This is between the previously reported 6.8 (27) or 5.1 days (31) and the 1.7 to 1.1 days of Dalrymple-Hay et al. (39). Prolonged ventilation (>24 hours) was required in only 8.7% summarizing all cardiac procedures in our study population. Our hospital stay of 14.5 days is in the range of previous publications (34). The excellent postoperative recovery and QoL gave back the potential of self-care and reduced consecutive disease-associated costs compared to medical treatments with repeated hospitalization for repetitive heart failure (40).

In summary, selected patients aged 80 years and older after cardiac surgery show a remarkable QoL and a considerable increase in their emotional well-being [Fig. 4(B)] as well as an important increase in their functional status with a satisfactory medium-term five-year survival (Fig. 1) at a reasonably low risk. The stunning recovery from being a bedridden patient to a self-caring patient is further a very important advantage after cardiac surgery in this challenging age group. Therefore in selected octogenarians, early operative treatment should not be withheld, and adoption of an early referral practice might further increase the postoperative patients benefits.

Limitations
The present study has several limitations. The use of a modified Seattle Angina Questionnaire instead of the SF-36 questionnaire (41,42) was motivated by the increased age, the specific disease, and treatment characteristics of the analyzed patient population. SF-36 is a multipurpose short-form health survey with 36 questions. It yields an eight-scale profile of functional health and well-being scores as well as psychometrically based physical and mental health summary. It is known to be a generic measure, as opposed to one that targets a specific age, disease, or treatment group. The Seattle Angina Questionnaire (43,44) as opposed to the SF-36 is a shorter 11-item questionnaire measuring five dimensions including physical limitation, anginal stability, anginal frequency, treatment satisfaction, and disease perception targeting a specific disease and treatment group. The lower number of questions and the nature of the questions were found to be more adequate to the very old patient population. All questions investigating angina-related outcomes had to be supplemented with the symptom of dyspnea to address AVD as well (Table 10). This modification is by itself not validated, but does not interfere with the angina assessment and provides a simple tool to measure valve-related QoL perception.

Further, the 136 patients represent a selective subgroup of the entire population. CAD as well as valve pathologies might follow a different disease

TABLE 10 Questionnaire used for Quality of Life Assessment via Telephone Interview[a]

No	Question (Q)/Answer options (A)
1.	Q: How limited are you in your daily activities inside your flat/house? A: Severely limited/moderately limited/limited/little limited/not limited
2.	Q: How limited are you moving upstairs or walk up a little hill? A: Severely limited/moderately limited/limited/little limited/not limited
3.	Q: Compare your angina or dyspnea today and before the operation? A: Lot more/somewhat more/unchanged/less/much less
4.	Q: Over the past 4 wk, on average, how many times have you had angina or dyspnea? A: 4 times or more a day/1–3 times day/3 or more times a week/less than once a week/never in the last 4 wk
5.	Q: Over the past 4 wk, on average, how many times have you taken nitroglycerin? A: 4 times or more a day/1–3 times day/3 or more times a week/less than once a week/never in the last 4 wk
6.	Q: How bothersome is it for you to take your pills as prescribed? A: Very/moderately/little/not at all/no drugs prescribed
7.	Q: How satisfied are you that everything possible is being done to treat your heart? A: Not satisfied/somewhat satisfied/satisfied/very satisfied
8.	Q: How satisfied are you with the overall treatment of your heart disease? A: Very dissatisfied/somewhat dissatisfied/little dissatisfied/satisfied/very satisfied
9.	Q: Over the last 4 wk, how much has your angina or dyspnea interfered with your enjoyment of life? A: Strongly interfered/somewhat interfered/little interfered/not interfered
10.	Q: If you had to spend the rest of your life with your actual discomfort, how would you feel about this? A: Very dissatisfied/somewhat dissatisfied/little dissatisfied/satisfied/very satisfied
11.	
(a)	Q: (a) How often do you worry that you may have a heart attack or die suddenly? A: Can't stop/often/from time to time/rarely/never
(b)	Q: (b) Where do you live? A: At home/with my family/with friends/at a nursery home

[a]Translated from German.

progression in these older patients and certainly show a delayed onset. A further limitation is the relatively small sample size decreasing the ability to detect factors influencing the outcome. However, the number of patients in the present series was similar to previous studies assessing cardiac surgery in octogenarians. Although we extracted retrospective data, no patient was lost in the follow-up.

This study reports postoperative results of a single centre, which may introduce institutional bias. Despite those possible limitations, postoperative survival and overall QoL in patients 80 years and older was very good.

REFERENCES

1. Stewart BF, Siscovick D, Lind BK, et al; for the Cardiovascular Health Study. Clinical factors associated with calcific aortic valve disease. J Am Coll Cardiol 1997; 29:630–634.
2. Otto CM, Lind BK, Kitzman DW, et al; for the Cardiovascular Health Study. Association of Aortic Valve Sclerosis with Cardiovascular Mortality and Morbidity in the Elderly. N Engl J Med 1999; 341(3):142–147.
3. Lindoroos M, Kupari M, Heikkila J, et al. Prevalence of aortic valve abnormalities in the elderly: An echocardiographic study of a random population sample. J Am Coll Cardiol 1993; 21:1220–1225.

4. Exadactylos N, Sugrue DD, Oakley CM. Prevalence of coronary artery disease in patients with isolated aortic valve stenosis. Br Heart J 1984; 51(2):121–124.
5. Peter M, Hoffmann A, Parker C, et al. Progression of aortic stenosis. Role of age and concomitant coronary artery disease. Chest 1993; 103:1715–1719.
6. Detection of kidney disease in patients with or at increased risk of cardiovascular disease American Heart Association Kidney and Cardiovascular Disease Council; The Councils on High Blood Pressure Research, Cardiovascular Disease in the Young, and Epidemiology and Prevention; and the Quality of Care and Outcomes Research Interdisciplinary Working Group; In Collaboration With the National Kidney Foundation Date: September 5, 2006. Circulation 2006; 114:1083–1087.
7. Fenoglio JJ Jr, McAllister HA Jr, DeCastro CM, et al. Congenital bicuspid aortic valve after age 20. Am J Cardiol 1977; 39(2):164–169.
8. Soydinc S, Davutoglu V, Dundar A, et al. Relationship between aortic valve sclerosis and the extent of coronary artery disease in patients undergoing diagnostic coronary angiography [published online ahead of print May 29, 2006]. Cardiology 2006; 106(4): 277–282.
9. Katz R, Wong ND, Kronmal R, et al. Features of the metabolic syndrome and diabetes mellitus as predictors of aortic valve calcification in the Multi-Ethnic Study of Arthrosclerosis. [Published online ahead of print April 24, 2006.] Circulation 2006; 113:2113–2119.
10. Movahed MR, Hashemzadeh M, Hamal MM. Type II diabetes mellitus is independently associated with non-rheumatic aortic valve stenosis or regurgitation. Chest 2005.
11. Celebrating World Health Day 2002, Welcare Hospital in Dubai. Community Action, December 9, 2002, COPYRIGHT 2002 Community Action Publishers. This material is published under license from the publisher through the Gale Group, Farmington Hills, Michigan.
12. World Health Organization (WHO), 2006. The world health report 2006—working together for health. http://www.who.int/whr/2006/en/.
13. Braun J, Oldendorf M, Moshage W, et al. Electron beam computed tomography in the evaluation of cardiac calcifications in chronic dialysis patients. Am J Kidney Dis 1996; 27:394–401.
14. Baglin A, Hanslik T, Vaillant JN, et al. Severe valvular heart disease in patients on chronic dialysis. Ann Med Interne (Paris) 1997; 148:521–526.
15. Urenã P, Malergue MC, Goldfarb B, et al. Evolutive aortic stenosis in hemodialysis patients: Analysis of risk factors. Nephrologie 1999; 20:217–225.
16. Maher ER, Pazianas M, Curtis JR. Calcific aortic stenosis: A complication of chronic uremia. Nephron 1987; 47:119–122.
17. Ventura JE, Tavella N, Romero C, et al. Aortic valve calcification is an independent factor of left ventricular hypertrophy in patients on maintenance haemodialysis. Nephrol Dial Transplant 2002; 17:1795–1801.
18. Herzog CA, Ma JZ, Collins AJ. Long-Term Survival of Dialysis Patients in the United States with Prosthetic Heart Valves. Should ACC/AHA Practice Guidelines on Valve Selection Be Modified? From the Cardiovascular Special Studies Center, US Renal Data System (C.A.H., J.Z.M., A.J.C.), and Department of Internal Medicine, Divisions of Cardiology (C.A.H.) and Nephrology (A.J.C.), Hennepin County Medical Center, University of Minnesota, Minneapolis, and the Department of Preventive Medicine, University of Tennessee, Memphis (J.Z.M.). Circulation 2002; 105:1336–1341.
19. Lysaght MJ. Maintenance dialysis population dynamics: Current trends and long-term implications. J Am Soc Nephrol 2002; 13:S37–S40.
20. Prüss-Üstün A, Corvalán C. Preventing disease through healthy environments: Towards an estimate of the environmental burden of disease. World Health Organization 2006.
21. Carabello BA, Crawford FA. Valvular heart disease. NEJM 1997; 337(1):32–41.
22. Iung B, Baron G, Butchart EG, et al. A prospective survey of patients with valvular heart disease in Europe: The Euro Heart Survey on Valvular Heart Disease. Eur Heart J 2003; 24:1231–1243.

23. IMS HEALTH. National Prescription Audit Plus, Therapeutic Category Report Documentation: Confidence Limit Tables—Prescribed and Dispensed Drugs, 1996–2001. Plymouth Meeting, PA: IMS HEALTH, 2001.

24. Spencer G; US Bureau of Census. Projections of the Population of the United States by Age, Sex and Race: 1988 to 2080. Washington, DC: US Government Printing Office, 1989. Current Population Reports, Series P-25, No 1018.

25. U.S. Bureau of the Census. Statistical Abstract of the United States/1994, 114th ed. Washington, DC: Department of Commerce, 1994: 84.

26. Elkington JR. Medicine and quality of life. Ann Inter Med 1966; 64:711–714.

27. Alexander KP, Anstrom KJ, Muhlbaier LH, et al. Outcomes of cardiac surgery in patients > or = 80 years: Results from the National Cardiovascular Network. J Am Coll Cardiol 2000; 35(3):731–738.

28. Fruitman DS, MacDougall CE, Ross DB. Cardiac surgery in octogenarians: Can elderly patients benefit? Quality of life after cardiac surgery. Ann Thorac Surg 1999; 68(6):2129–2135.

29. Avery GJ II, Ley SJ, Hill JD, et al. Cardiac surgery in the octogenarian: Evaluation of risk, cost, and outcome. Ann Thorac Surg 2001; 71(2):591–596.

30. Kolh P, Kerzmann A, Lahaye L, et al. Cardiac surgery in octogenarians: Peri-operative outcome and long-term results. Eur Heart J 2001; 22(14):1235–1243.

31. Akins CW, Daggett WM, Vlahakes GJ, et al. Cardiac operations in patients 80 years old and older. Ann Thorac Surg 1997; 64(3):606–614; discussion 614–615.

32. Rosengart TK, Finnin EB, Kim DY, et al. Open heart surgery in the elderly: Results from a consecutive series of 100 patients aged 85 years or older. Am J Med 2002; 112(2):143–147.

33. Kumar P, Zehr KJ, Chang A, et al. Quality of life in octogenarians after open heart surgery. Chest 1995; 108(4):919–926.

34. Sundt TM, Bailey MS, Moon MR, et al. Quality of life after aortic valve replacement at the age of >80 years. Circulation 2000; 102(19 suppl 3):III70–III74.

35. Heijmeriks JA, Pourrier S, Dassen P, et al. Comparison of quality of life after coronary and/or valvular cardiac surgery in patients > or = 75 years of age with younger patients. Am J Cardiol 1999; 83(7):1129–1132; A9 1999 #64.

36. Rumsfeld JS, Magid DJ, O'Brien M, et al. Department of Veterans Affairs cooperative study in health services: Processes, structures, and outcomes of care in cardiac surgery. Changes in health-related quality of life following coronary artery bypass graft surgery. Ann Thorac Surg 2001; 72(6):2026–2032.

37. Yun KL, Sintek CF, Fletcher AD, et al. Time related quality of life after elective cardiac operation. Ann Thorac Surg 1999; 68(4):1314–1320.

38. Peterson ED, Cowper PA, Jollis JG, et al. Outcomes of coronary artery bypass graft surgery in 24461 patients aged 80 years or older. Circulation 1995; 92(9 suppl):II85–II91.

39. Dalrymple-Hay MJ, Alzetani A, Aboel-Nazar S, et al. Cardiac surgery in the elderly. Eur J Cardiothorac Surg 1999; 15(1):61–66.

40. Sollano JA, Rose EA, Williams DL, et al. Cost-effectiveness of coronary artery bypass surgery in octogenarians. Ann Surg 1998; 228(3):297–306.

41. Immer FF, Althaus SM, Berdat PA, et al. Quality of life and specific problems after cardiac surgery in adolescents and adults with congenital heart diseases. Eur J Cardiovasc Prev Rehabil 2005; 12(2):138–143.

42. Immer FF, Lippeck C, Barmettler H, et al. Improvement of quality of life after surgery on the thoracic aorta: Effect of antegrade cerebral perfusion and short duration of deep hypothermic circulatory arrest. Circulation 2004; 110(11 suppl 1):II250–II255.

43. Spertus JA, Winder JA, Dewhurst TA, et al. Development and evaluation of the Seattle Angina Questionnaire: A new functional status measure for coronary artery disease. J Am Coll Cardiol 1995; 25(2):333–341.

44. Dougherty CM, Dewhurst T, Nichol WP, et al. Comparison of three quality of life instruments in stable angina pectoris: Seattle Angina Questionnaire, Short Form Health Survey (SF-36), and Quality of Life Index-Cardiac Version III. J Clin Epidemiol 1998; 51(7):569–575.

ANNEX 1

U.S. national statistics by HCUPnet provides trend information for the 5-year period from 2000 to 2005. Data formatted and provided by KCI Partners Inc., Oakmont.

Outcomes by Patient and Hospital Characteristics for ICD-9-CM Principal Procedure Code 35.21 Replacement Aortic Valve Tissue

		Total number of discharges		LOS, days (mean)	LOS, days (median)	In-hospital deaths	
All discharges		30,668	100.00%	11.6	8.0	1,343	4.38%
Age group	<1	*	*	*	*	*	*
	1–17	403	1.31%	6.1	5.0	*	*
	18–44	904	2.95%	10.2	6.0	*	*
	45–64	5,300	17.28%	9.6	7.0	112	2.11%
	65–84	21,762	70.96%	11.9	9.0	1,050	4.82%
	85+	2,244	7.32%	14.8	11.0	146	6.51%
	Missing	*	*	*	*	*	*
Sex	Male	18,833	61.41%	11.2	8.0	735	3.90%
	Female	11,814	38.52%	12.3	9.0	608	5.14%
	Missing	*	*	*	*	*	*

*, not significant.
Abbreviation: LOS, length of stay.

ICD-9-CM Principal Procedure Code 35.21, Replace Aortic Valve Tissue

	2000	2001	2002	2003	2004	2005
Total number of discharges	18,591	23,618	25,519	26,308	27,826	30,668
LOS, days (mean)	10.9	11.3	10.9	11.2	11.2	11.6
LOS, days (median)	8.0	8.0	8.0	8.0	8.0	8.0
In-hospital deaths	1,048 (5.64%)	1,310 (5.55%)	1,375 (5.39%)	1,462 (5.56%)	1,352 (4.86%)	1,343 (4.38%)

Abbreviation: LOS, length of stay.

ICD-9-CM Principal Procedure Code 35.22, Replace Aortic Valve Mechanical

	2000	2001	2002	2003	2004	2005
Total number of discharges	31,533	31,541	28,599	29,867	26,574	26,132
LOS, days (mean)	10.6	10.3	10.5	10.7	10.6	10.8
LOS, days (median)	8.0	8.0	8.0	8.0	8.0	8.0
In-hospital deaths	1,696 (5.38%)	1,683 (5.33%)	1,315 (4.60%)	1,372 (4.59%)	1,304 (4.91%)	1,103 (4.22%)

Abbreviation: LOS, length of stay.

Balloon Aortic Valvuloplasty: Current Techniques and Clinical Utility*

BALLOON AORTIC VALVULOPLASTY

After its introduction in 1995 by Cribier, balloon aortic valvuloplasty (BAV) was rapidly adopted and experienced intense interest and explosive growth in 1986 and 1987 (1,2). The rapid recognition of restenosis in the majority of patients, and a clear appreciation for the lack of any improvement in the survival curve in the generally elderly patients targeted for this procedure led to as rapid a decline in its use (3–6). Ultimately, guideline recommendations directed the use of BAV only for high-risk patients for conventional surgery, for use as a bridge to conventional aortic valve replacement (AVR). What has been lost in this process is recognition of the value of BAV as a palliative procedure for patients who otherwise receive no specific therapy (7). There is a large population of patients for whom AVR surgery is extremely high risk. Many of these patients will decline surgery when referred, and many more are never referred because of their advanced age and/or comorbid conditions. There are as many patients in this high-risk category as there are who actually receive operation annually, and there is growing recognition that they may receive significant improvement in symptoms with the use of BAV (8).

The outcome from surgery in this population is not as well documented as many think. High-risk patients who score in the 90th percentile with Society for Thoracic Surgery risk calculator probably do not have improved survival after surgical AVR, experience stroke between 10% and 15%, and have high surgical mortality. More than half of octogenarian patients undergoing AVR recover in a rehabilitation facility. Twenty percent of the Medicare population is rehospitalized within 30 days after AVR for complications, including wound infections, arrhythmias, and failure to thrive (9). The quality of life after AVR in the octogenarian population is not uniformly improved. While many patients have a complete hemodynamic correction of their aortic valve stenosis, a significant proportion never regain any functional capacity, and may never recover from a surgery.

In my own discussions with octogenarian patients, it is common for them to have little concern for procedure mortality, and to be greatly preoccupied with loss of quality of life. They are concerned about prolonged hospitalization, and especially about stroke. Since between 8% and 15% of this population will experience perioperative stroke or transient ischemic attack, and the majority will spend several weeks or longer in a rehabilitation facility, the prospect of a less invasive therapy, which offers relief of symptoms for anywhere between six months and two years, is more attractive to this patient population than many cardiology or cardiovascular surgery practitioners fully appreciate (10,11). Most

---

This chapter contributed by Ted Feldman, Cardiac Catheterization Laboratory, Evanston Hospital, Evanston, Illinois, U.S.A.

patients have 12 to 18 months of clinical improvement after BAV, with improved symptoms and freedom from repeated hospitalizations for heart failure (12). The procedure can be repeated in patients who respond well to the first therapy. The vast majority spends only one to two nights in the hospital, and are ambulatory often on the dame day as the procedure. Although conventional AVR can be performed after several weeks in some patients, the vast majority of BAV patients are not converted into surgical candidates.

BAV has its application in this elderly population. The ideal patient is the ambulatory octogenarian or nonagenarian, who is highly symptomatic with severe aortic stenosis, and typically has some other comorbid conditions.

RETROGRADE BAV

The retrograde technique for BAV has evolved significantly since its introduction in the mid-1980s (13,14). The advent of percutaneous AVR approaches has led to improvements in the basic BAV technique. The importance of femoral arterial access cannot be overemphasized. Fluoroscopy should be used to locate the midfemoral head prior to puncture, such that puncture in the common femoral artery is optimized. The use of a micropuncture set allows introduction of a 21-gauge needle into the femoral artery. A test injection of contrast can demonstrate whether the common femoral has been entered. A high puncture above the lowest course of the inferior epigastric or femoral circumflex vessel, or entry into the superficial femoral or profunda branches, is easily aborted with repuncture adjusted accordingly such that common femoral access is ensured. This is necessary because of the large sheath size needed for BAV.

Once an initial 5 or 6F arterial sheath is in place, and angiography has demonstrated a good position in the common femoral artery and adequate arterial caliber for retrograde BAV, the next step is preclosure with a suture closure device (15,16). A variety of preclosure approaches are commonly used. A 10F Prostar device, a single ProGlide device, or two ProGlide devices placed at 90-degree angles in exchange for a small sheath are ideal. An extra-stiff guidewire is then placed via the suture closure device and used to introduce a 10, 11, or 12F arterial sheath, depending on the balloon size intended for BAV. Left femoral venous 8 and 5F sheaths are placed as well, for Swan and temporary pacemakers respectively. After the sheaths are securely in place, heparin is administered to achieve an activated clotting time between 250 and 300 seconds. Basic hemodynamic assessments are obtained via venous access and a pulmonary artery catheter.

The aortic valve is crossed in typical retrograde fashion using most commonly an Amplatz-shaped catheter or a specifically designed catheter for retrograde aortic valve access (17). A movable-core straight guidewire facilitates directing the catheter, such that the point of wire passage can be controlled. The valve is interrogated with gentle probing until the wire and catheter enter the ventricle. At this point, transaortic valve pressure gradient can be assessed and the valve area determined (18,19).

Rapid ventricular pacing is a key adjunct to BAV. A 5F pacemaker is placed in the right ventricular apex and tested. Once a stable threshold is obtained, burst pacing between rates of 180 to 220 beats/min is tested. The objective is to achieve a phasic peak systolic blood pressure no greater than 50 or 60 mm Hg. This allows balloon inflations to be performed without the balloon being "watermelon seeded" or ejected from the ventricle during balloon inflations. Testing of pacing should be kept to a minimum, since significant left ventricular systolic functional depression is caused by rapid pacing in these patients.

Once pacing is confirmed, a 0.035-in extra-stiff guidewire is placed in the ventricle through the initial diagnostic access catheter. The tip of the wire should be shaped over the end of a scissors or hemostat to create a "ram's horn" configuration, such that the wire may sit in the left ventricular apex without perforating the left ventricular chamber. The wire is used as a rail to deliver a valvuloplasty balloon. Balloon size is determined from preprocedure assessment of an echocardiogram to roughly gauge the annulus diameter. A 1:1 balloon to annulus ratio is the usual first balloon size used.

The balloon is passed across the aortic valve and inflated until a full inflation is clearly achieved (Fig. 1). This involves observing the balloon to lock into

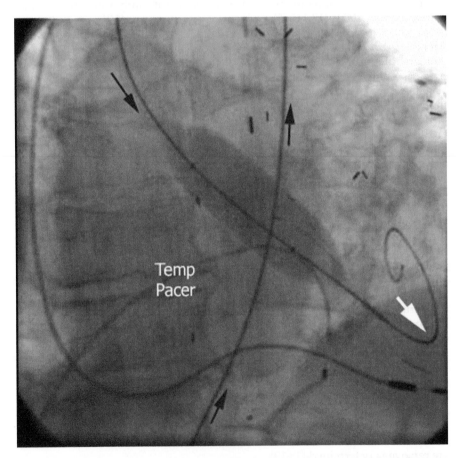

FIGURE 1 Retrograde BAV. A 0.035-in extra-stiff guidewire has been passed retrograde across the aortic valve (*black arrows*). The tip of the wire has been ribboned over the edge of a hemostat to form a large radius curved loop (*white arrow*). Despite the patient having a permanent pacemaker, a temporary right ventricular pacing wire has been placed for rapid ventricular pacing. The inflated balloon is centered in the valve and remains stable because the rapid pacing causes hypotension and precludes ejection of the balloon by left ventricular systolic motion.

the valve during right ventricular rapid pacing, such that full expansion of the waist of the balloon is achieved without the balloon slipping during inflation. Contrast diluted to 9 or 10:1 is used for balloon inflation, such that deflation is as rapid as possible.

In most cases, two or three inflations can be performed. It is less common for current balloons to burst or rupture during the inflation process. If balloon rupture occurs, it is usually in a longitudinal dimension and still allows easy removal from the patient.

After balloon inflations, the balloon is withdrawn over the wire, and pig-tail catheter exchanged for assessment of a final gradient in conjunction with reassessment of the cardiac output. At this point, catheters are removed, and a wire left in place through the femoral sheath, such that suture closure may be accomplished with the wire in place. This allows repassage of a sheath in the event that suture closure is not successful.

ANTEGRADE BAV

Antegrade BAV is much less commonly practiced. The antegrade technique involves delivery of a valvuloplasty balloon via right femoral venous access, utilizing transseptal puncture (20,21). The advantage of the technique is use of the venous system for placement of a large sheath and balloon delivery. This obviates arterial bleeding complications almost entirely. The disadvantage of the approach is the need for transseptal puncture, and the comparatively complex placement of a circulatory wire loop for delivery of the balloon to the aortic valve. A nonrandomized comparison of retrograde and antegrade approaches have shown larger valve areas using the antegrade technique, most probably because larger balloons are used via the antegrade than the retrograde approach.

The procedure setup involves placement of left femoral venous and arterial sheaths for an arterial catheter and pulmonary artery catheter, respectively. Right femoral venous access is achieved with a 14F sheath from the outset of the procedure. Transseptal puncture is performed via the 14F sheath using standard A French Mullins sheath and a transseptal needle. Once the Mullins sheath is in place in the left atrium, a soft-body 7F balloon-tipped catheter is used to cross the mitral valve antegrade, and this allows measurement of left ventricular pressure via the transseptal route, and arterial pressure via the left femoral arterial access. Once the transaortic valve pressure gradient and cardiac output are used for valve area assessment, the single lumen balloon catheter is looped in the left ventricular apex and passed across the aortic valve and into the descending aorta. A 0.032-in guidewire is delivered from the Mullins sheath, through the left ventricular balloon catheter loop, into the aortic arch, and then descending aorta. This wire is snared from the arterial access, and the snare left in place to anchor the wire in the arterial circulation. Thus, a circulatory loop is achieved. This allows a stable rail for passage of a balloon catheter. The single lumen balloon catheter and Mullins sheath are removed.

For the balloon, my own preference is to use an Inoue valvuloplasty balloon for the antegrade approach (Fig. 2). The balloon is delivered through the 14F sheath over the wire rail and tracked around the left ventricular apex into the aortic valve. A single balloon inflation is used. Most male patients do well with a 25- or 26-mm-diameter inflation of a 26-mm Inoue balloon catheter. Female

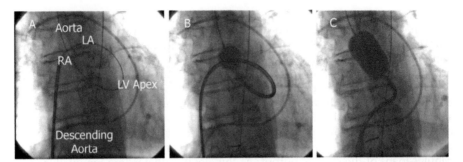

FIGURE 2 Antegrade BAV. Panel A shows the guidewire loop from the inferior vena cava, through the RA, across the atrial septum into the LA, and traversing the LV apex, crossing the valve, and finally being anchored in the descending aorta with a snare. Panel B shows the distal portion of the balloon inflated and pulled back to engage the aortic valve. Panel C shows the fully inflated balloon. *Abbreviations*: LA, left atrium; LV, left ventricular; RA, right atrium.

patients are usually treated with a single inflation of 24 or 25 mm, again with a 26-mm Inoue balloon catheter. After the balloon is inflated and deflated, the balloon catheter is withdrawn over the wire loop. The Mullins sheath is replaced and a 5F pigtail is passed through the Mullins sheath from the venous side, over the wire into the ascending aorta. This is a critical step, since the guidewire must be withdrawn through the protective covering of a diagnostic catheter. Withdrawal of the guidewire without placing a diagnostic catheter first will result in the guidewire acting as a "cheese cutter" on the aortic and/or mitral valves with catastrophic results. Once the guidewire is removed inside the pigtail catheter, the pigtail can be moved back into the left ventricle for final assessment of the transaortic valve pressure gradient.

ECHOCARDIOGRAPHIC ASSESSMENT
Echocardiographic evaluation prior to BAV is essential. The key findings on the echocardiogram include an assessment of left ventricular function, measurement of the aortic annulus diameter, appreciation for associated mitral regurgitation, and in the case of patients for whom antegrade access is planned, interrogation of the left atrial appendage for thrombus. Additionally, transesophageal echocardiography gives valuable information regarding the burden of atheroma in the aortic arch. Mobile atheroma poses substantial risk for these patients during valvuloplasty by any route, or in the event that subsequent aortic valve or coronary surgery might be planned.

COMPLICATIONS OF AORTIC VALVULOPLASTY
The most frequent complications relate to arterial access sheath management (22–25). This highlights the importance of careful attention to good common femoral artery puncture at the beginning of the procedure. An errant puncture merits repuncture or rescheduling of the procedure. In some instances, when sheath angiography demonstrates a puncture above the inguinal ligament, suture closure may be attempted before heparin is given. If a good closure is achieved, it is reasonable to repuncture the artery below the initial site, to gain common femoral arterial access. Use of a micropuncture needle with small

contrast injections prior to introducing a sheath allows ideal sheath placement without committing to punctures that may be too high or too low. Transfusions have been necessary in up to a quarter of patients undergoing this procedure, though suture closure techniques with preclosure have reduced this complication dramatically.

Hypotension during the procedure is ubiquitous. All patients drop their pressure during balloon inflations, with occlusion of the aortic outflow. Pressure recovery is usually rapid, occurring in 10 to 30 seconds, but in some cases pressors are required until the patients are able to generate a blood pressure on their own. Some patients never recover after the balloon is deflated, and this contributes to the 5% to 8% hospital mortality reported in most series. In my practice, patients with systolic pressure less than 110 mm Hg or cardiac output less than 2.5 L/min are usually started on a pressor agent before the balloon is inflated. Neo-Synephrine or dopamine to support blood pressure or dobutamine to augment cardiac output can be used. Coronary ischemia from hypotension during balloon inflations can contribute to slow recovery or collapse after the balloon is deflated, and great care must be taken to minimize the occurrence and duration of ischemia.

Left ventricular apical perforation from the guidewire or tip of the balloon catheter is one of the more important complications. Careful attention to the pulsatility of the cardiac fluoroscopic silhouette is important to help detect perforations before they become hemodynamically catastrophic. Adjuncts to monitoring for this complication include a ubiquitous presence of a right heart catheter, the occasional use of intracardiac echocardiography, and the uniform availability of at least transthoracic echo on short notice when hypotension occurs during BAV procedures. Familiarity and expertise in pericardiocentesis is requisite for BAV performance.

The heavily calcified aortic valve may impinge on a conducting system during BAV. Patients with preexisting left or right bundle branch block require the presence of a temporary pacemaker because transient complete heart block will occur in this subgroup of patients. Occasionally, complete heart block will not resolve within the first several hours after a procedure, and permanent pacing may be necessary. This occurs in 1% or 2% of BAV procedures.

Stroke is remarkably infrequent. Embolization of calcific material from the valve is rarely described. Although asymptomatic embolization occurs in a high proportion of patients even during diagnostic catheterization for aortic valve stenosis, the liberation of large masses of calcium is rare. In my own experience, stroke is more commonly related to thromboemboli from the guidewires used during the procedure. It is possible to displace calcific nodules into the left main orifice, with catastrophic consequences in the unbypassed patient. Immediate recognition of this complication can lead to salvage with left main coronary stenting.

ADVANCES IN TECHNIQUE

The advent of catheter valve replacement has led to a variety of innovations in BAV technique. The most notable is the use of rapid ventricular pacing to keep the balloon from being ejected from the ventricle during balloon inflations. Refinements in the use of suture closure for both arterial and venous access have developed as well. In cases where arterial bleeding is noted prior to sheath removal, contralateral access can be used for placement of an occlusion balloon. In addition, a balloon may be inflated at low pressure at the puncture site via contralateral access, so that suture closure does not result in stricture or deformation of the artery at the site of suture closure. There is preliminary evidence that external proton beam radiation after BAV may extend the durability of the result (26).

SUMMARY

BAV has had a resurgence because of the rapid growth of percutaneous valve replacement (27,28). The procedure has an important role beyond its use for valve predilatation during percutaneous AVR. The application of BAV in clinical practice should be reevaluated. The increasing numbers of poor surgical candidates in the expanding very elderly population suggest a greater role for BAV to improve quality of life. The time has arrived for BAV to be revisited, and a resurgence of this procedure is occurring because of both improved knowledge and improvements in catheter techniques.

REFERENCES

1. Cribier A, Savin T, Saoudi N, et al. Percutaneous transluminal valvuloplasty of acquired aortic stenosis in elderly patients: An alternative to valve replacement? Lancet 1986; 1:63–67.
2. Eltchaninoff H, Cribier A, Tron C, et al. Balloon aortic valvuloplasty in elderly patients at high risk for surgery, or inoperable: Immediate and mid-term results. Eur Heart J 1995; 16:1079–1084.
3. Otto CM, Mickel MC, Kennedy JW, et al. Three-year outcome after balloon aortic valvuloplasty: Insights into prognosis of valvular aortic stenosis. Circulation 1994; 89:642–650.
4. Feldman T, Glagov S, Carroll JD. Restenosis following successful balloon valvuloplasty: Bone formation in aortic valve leaflets. Cathet Cardiovasc Diagn 1993; 29:1–7.
5. Percutaneous balloon aortic valvuloplasty: Acute and 30-day follow-up results in 674 patients from the NHLBI Balloon Valvuloplasty Registry. Circulation 1991; 84:2383–2397.
6. Kuntz RE, Tosteson AN, Berman AD, et al. Predictors of event-free survival after balloon aortic valvuloplasty. N Engl J Med 1991; 325:17–23.
7. Bonow O, Carabello B, Chaterjee K, et al. ACC/AHA 2006 Guidelines for the Management of Patients with Valvular Heart Disease. Executive Summary. Circulation 2006; 114:450–527. American Heart Association Web site. http://www.americanheart.org.
8. Iung B, Baron G, Butchart EG, et al. A prospective survey of patients with valvular heart disease in Europe: The Euro Heart Survey on Valvular Heart Disease. Eur Heart J 2003; 24:1231–1243.
9. Goodney PP, Stukel TA, Lucas FL, et al. Hospital volume, length of stay, and readmission rates in high-risk surgery. Ann Surg 2003; 238:161–167.
10. Kolh P, Kerzmann A, Lahaye L, et al. Cardiac surgery in octogenarians: Peri-operative outcome and long-term results. Eur Heart J 2001; 22:1235–1243.
11. Edwards MB, Taylor KM. Outcomes in nonagenarians after heart valve replacement operation. Ann Thorac Surg 2003; 75:830–834.
12. Agarwal A, Kini AS, Attanti S, et al. Results of repeat balloon valvuloplasty for treatment of aortic stenosis in patients aged 59 to 104 years. Am J Cardiol 2005; 95:43–47.
13. Feldman T. Core curriculum for interventional cardiology: Percutaneous valvuloplasty. Catheter Cardiovasc Interv 2003; 60:48–56.
14. Feldman T, Chiu YC, Carroll JD. Single balloon aortic valvuloplasty: Increased valve areas with improved technique. J Invasive Cardiol 1989; 1:295–300.

15. Solomon LW, Fusman B, Jolly N, et al. Percutaneous suture closure for management of large French size arterial puncture in aortic valvuloplasty. J Invasive Cardiol 2001; 13:592–596.
16. Feldman T. Percutaneous suture closure for management of large French size arterial and venous puncture. J Intervent Cardiol 2000; 13:237–242.
17. Feldman T, Carroll JD, Chiu YC. An improved catheter for crossing stenosed aortic valves. Cathet Cardiovasc Diagn 1989; 16:279–283.
18. Fusman B, Faxon D, Feldman T. Hemodynamic rounds: Transvalvular pressure gradient measurement. Catheter Cardiovasc Interv 2001; 53:553–561.
19. Feldman T, Laskey W. Alchemy in the cath lab: Creating a gold standard for the evaluation of aortic stenosis. Cathet Cardiovasc Diagn 1998; 44:14–15.
20. Feldman T. Transseptal antegrade access for aortic valvuloplasty. Catheter Cardiovasc Interv 2000; 50:492–494.
21. Sakata Y, Sayed Y, Salinger MH, et al. Percutaneous balloon aortic valvuloplasty: Antegrade transseptal vs. conventional retrograde transarterial approach. Catheter Cardiovasc Interv 2005; 64:314–321.
22. Feldman TE. Balloon valvuloplasty. In: Nissen SE, Popma JJ, Kern MJ, et al, eds. CathSAP II. Bethesda, MD: American College of Cardiology, 2001.
23. Feldman T. Chapter 25—Percutaneous therapies for valvular heart disease. In: Baim DS, Grossman W, eds. Grossman's Cardiac Catheterization, Angiography & Intervention, 7th ed. Philadelphia, PA: Lippincott Williams & Wilkins, 2005:543–561.
24. Feldman T, Grossman W. Chapter 28—Profiles in valvular heart disease. In: Baim DS, Grossman W, eds. Grossman's Cardiac Catheterization, Angiography & Intervention, 7th ed. Philadelphia, PA: Lippincott Williams & Wilkins, 2005:637–659.
25. Feldman T. Retrograde percutaneous aortic valvuloplasty. In: Nguyen T, Colombo A, Hu D, et al, eds. Practical Handbook of Advanced Interventional Cardiology, 3rd ed. Blackwell Futura, 2008:489–497.
26. Pedersen WR, Van Tassel RA, Pierce TA, et al. Radiation following percutaneous balloon aortic valvuloplasty to prevent restenosis (RADAR pilot trial). Catheter Cardiovasc Interv 2006; 68:183–192.
27. Hara H, Pedersen WR, Ladich E, et al. Percutaneous balloon aortic valvuloplasty revisited: Time for a renaissance? Circulation 2007; 115:e334–e338.
28. Feldman T, Leon MB. Prospects for percutaneous valve therapies. Circulation 2007; 11:2866–2877.

Introduction of New Technologies

"The Seven Ages in the Evolution of an Idea – with particular reference to the critics"(1).

All treatment modalities thrive toward decreasing invasiveness. Less invasive treatment options are new opportunities (2) to improve patient care and decrease procedure-related morbidity and mortality. Novel approaches also widen treatment indications and increase the patient pool amendable to a curative therapy (Chap. 3).

The current developments in the treatment of heart valve disease are an example of how a medical specialty has to evolve in order to modernize and become less invasive. In a technology-driven field like cardiac surgery, progress is based upon two pillars: surgical skills and device engendering. Both go hand in hand and one cannot exist by itself. Cardiac surgery only fully developed after the introduction of the heart-lung machine and then surgical skills allowed curing disease within the heart. Next, new tools became available to ease the surgical handling and surgery expanded toward smaller and thinner structures like the coronaries.

But all new technologies are worthless if the necessary skills are not acquired properly. A too steep learning curve might become an insurmountable hurdle to what could have been a very promising therapy (3,4). Therefore, strong emphasis has to be directed toward training as procedural success highly depends on mastering the new skills (5,6).

SIMULATOR-BASED TRAINING AND TRANSCATHETER SKILLS

The current surgical training practice is based on sheer volume exposure and caseload rather than being directed toward specific skill improvement. With the increase in health care costs and shorter residents' workweeks and higher operating room costs, efficiency training has become of uppermost concern. New training techniques focusing on breaking down complex procedures in easier step-by-step tasks are integrating the three-stage theory of motor skill acquisition (7,8). The trainee gains new skills by cognitive understanding followed by integration of understanding into mechanical tasks and finally repetitive performance reaching automation and refinement of precision. Each of the three phases is dependent on proper evaluation of performance as a mandatory feedback mechanism as the task most difficult to perform in the operating room.

Shifting training into simulation laboratories substantially increases performance scores of surgeons when comparing to non-simulator–trained surgeons (9). In a recent Food and Drug Administration panel, leading specialists recommend virtual reality simulators as an integral component of the training package for carotid artery stenting (10). Simulator-acquired skills translate into more rapid dissection, lesser errors, and higher economy of movement scores during laparoscopic procedures (11).

Training models can be classified as biological, including live animals and human cadavers, or nonbiological bench models. The latter have numerous advantages like safety, reproducibility and ready availability, greater mobility, and reusability. Nonbiological bench models allow data capture, are relatively cheap, and are free of ethical concerns. In this category fall two kinds of simulators: high fidelity and low fidelity. High fidelity being overall more expensive and dependent on software-generated electromechanical force feedback system, requiring enormous computing power for virtual reality simulation, for example, flight simulators. Surprisingly, except for some practical aspects, high-fidelity simulators are largely less realistic than low-fidelity simulators. But even videogames skills have been found to correlate with laparoscopic surgical skills. Training curricula that include video games might be of help to improve the screen-handling interface (12) with low fidelity only describing the software-based concept but not applying to anatomical accuracy. Transcatheter valve therapy (TCVT) low-fidelity simulators have been shown repeatedly to create extremely and superior realistic handling characteristics and by virtue of their nature forgive technical mistakes as little as the interventional or surgical reality. Altogether, fidelity might be less important at an earlier training level as shown in a randomized study (13).

ACCELERATED ACCEPTANCE OF NEW TECHNOLOGIES

Introduction

Designing a proper training model to most realistically simulate all technical aspects, including identical visualization aids as used in the clinical setting, is a vital aspect of peer acceptance but more importantly is a key measure to improve the patient's safety and the surgeon's confidence. Important segments of the learning curve are shifted to the simulator training and critical treatment decisions can repeatedly be simulated to trigger the optimal response pattern.

The author together with Elastrat (Geneva, Switzerland) has developed a see-through silicon transcatheter valve simulator to allow realistic training and device development. The bench model is composed of the left ventricular outflow tract, an exchangeable aortic valve, the aortic root with the left and right coronary orifices, the complete aortic arch with supraaortic vessels, and the descending aorta. All parts have been designed to reproduce most realistically clinical anatomical landmarks.

Method

Before designing the bench model, a specific request catalog is defined. The requested characteristics for simulator platforms are listed as follows:

1. Bidirectional transcatheter aortic valve bench test simulating as well remote retrograde transfemoral as well as the transapical procedure
2. Most realistic anatomical simulation
3. Most realistic imaging simulation
4. Allows periprocedural coronary flow measurement
5. Wet lab capable with most realistic hemodynamic reproduction
6. Simple device recovery after delivery
7. Permit device optimization and device as well as delivery system testing

8. See-through construction
9. Little maintenance needs and simple handling with fast setup and deconstruction
10. Reusable
11. Low cost
12. High mobility, low weight

Next, anatomical data are collected from two independent anatomical and pathoanatomical imaging studies of the author. The first is a transesophageal echographic comparison of the native and the calcified aortic roots and the second is a cardiac multislice computer tomography–based evaluation of the undiseased aortic root geometry (Chap. 7. Device-Related Insights into the Aortic Root Anatomy).

Illustrated Manufacturing Process of a TCVT Silicon Simulator

At first, a corrosion model is generated from an adult cadaver heart, including the ascending aorta, the aortic arch, and the thoracic aorta. This corrosion model is then duplicated into a wax model by using an intermediate cast copy. The latter wax model is then worked on by trimming and sculpturing to respect the data obtained from the described aortic root morphology studies (Fig. 1). Then the

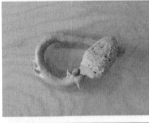
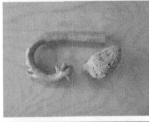
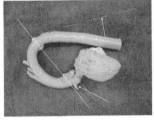
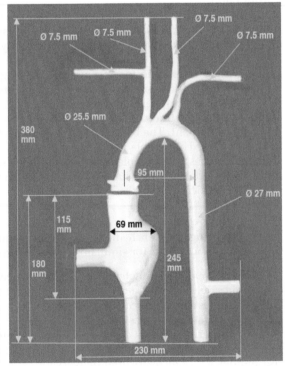

FIGURE 1 Anatomically corrected wax model of the left ventricle, aortic root and valve, and ascending and aortic arch in various development steps.

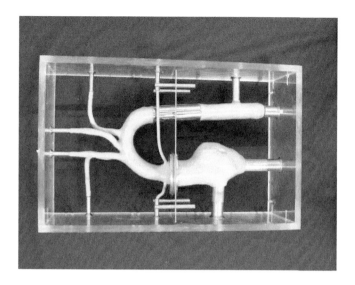

FIGURE 2 Wax model in silicon molding unit.

positive wax model is assembled into a two-block silicon molding unit (Fig. 2) to build the master silicon mold (Fig. 3). Once the mold is accomplished, the silicon models are created by silicon injection. All TCV silicon simulators then undergo a quality control process including, for example, dynamic leakage testing (Fig. 4). The aortic valve substituted is built from an identical setup as described earlier (Fig. 5). The two-block silicon and the exchangeable silicon valve then undergo x-ray imaging to allow silicon density adjustment to optimize fluoroscopic imaging. The final setup of the Elastrat TCV simulator (Fig. 6) was later validated in numerous international workshops (Fig. 7).

TCVT Silicon Simulator Characteristics
One of the distinctive features of the transcatheter valve simulation platform is the disposable aortic valve that can easily be exchanged after several implantations by a split-bloc construction. Further, the specific design makes recovery of the implanted device quick and simple. The system also provides the necessary connection to a continuous or pulsatile flow generator to create physiologic flow dynamics and wet lab functionality. Additionally, the unique design allows for a bidirectional approach including the antegrade transapical procedure as well as the retrograde percutaneous access. Finally, the see-through silicon concept not only supports and enhances interventional training but also provides an ideal platform for valved stent development and in vitro testing.

CREATING THE FAVORABLE ENVIRONMENT FOR TCVT
TCVT arises as a new treatment option for structural heart disease. Development is largely supported by cardiac surgeons and by interventional cardiologists. None of either specialty holds sufficient understanding, skills, and expertise to become an isolated player. Certainly some lonely cowboys have been identified since, but it is communally agreed that this novel, very powerful, and extremely promising therapy should be handled by a joint venture between both

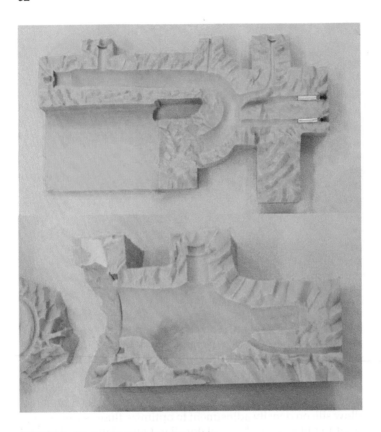

FIGURE 3 Reversed silicon master mold.

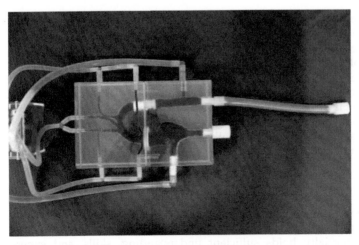

FIGURE 4 First silicon model of the TCVT TAP simulator filled with red dye for leakage testing and flow analysis.

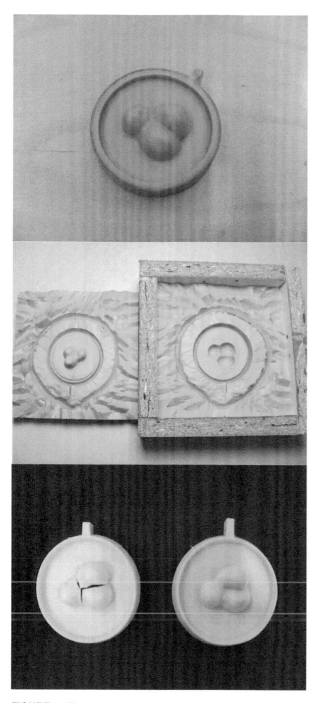

FIGURE 5 Three distinctive steps of aortic valve leaflet production, made from soft silicon with enhanced radio-opacity.

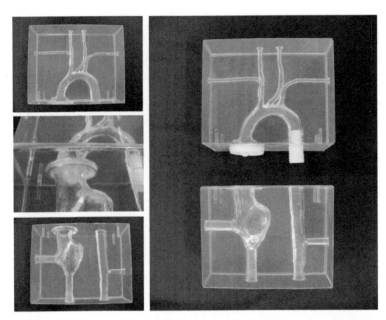

FIGURE 6 Final model build in the two-block principle to allow for rapid valve exchange and excellent sealing also under increase pulsatile workload. On the left, detailed views of the left ventricle, the aortic root and valve area, and the ascending aorta and arch.

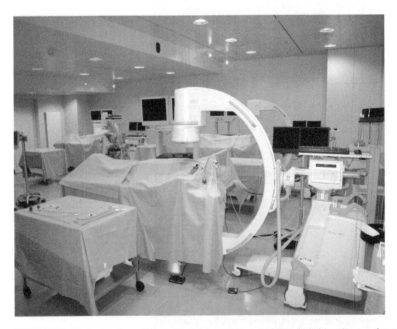

FIGURE 7 Typical setup of the simulator unit in a training hybrid suite as, for example, at the Medtronic facilities in Tolochenaz, Switzerland, on the occasion of the transcatheter EDGE course.

TABLE 1   Some Examples of Industry-Supported Training Programs

Title	Industrial sponsor	Specialty
Academia	Medtronic	Interventional cardiology
The Crossroad Institute	Abbott Vascular	Interventional cardiology
The Institute for Therapy Advancement	Boston Scientific	Interventional cardiology
The Cordis Cardiac and Vascular Institute	Cordis	Interventional cardiology
EDGE Course	Medtronic	Cardiac surgery

specialties in the patient's best interest (14). The key requisites can be separated into four large areas of interest:

1. Knowledge/understanding/skills
2. Materials and handling concepts
3. Access strategies
4. Environment and imaging

Industry-supported training programs have become more readily available (15) (Table 1). Training sessions are provided at an industrial level for device-specific training and at the respective society's level for basic or generic nondevice–related training. First, attempts of combined training seem identifiable at the horizon but remain rather seldom. Currently, the author is involved in organizing training opportunities and training curricula for the EuroPCR and for the European Association of Cardio-Thoracic Surgery—EACTS. Another new training concept called the EDGE course aims at teaching transcatheter skills by cross-trained cardiac surgeons and interventional cardiologists to interested peers. A specialist group, including the author, has designed a proposed curriculum within the Medtronic Academia EDGE course for TCVT skill training for cardiac surgeons. Emphasis is set on what were identified as the four key players:

1. Knowledge/understanding/simulated skill acquisition
2. Materials and handling concepts
3. Access strategies
4. New environment and imaging modalities

At present, this is the only nondevice-based transcatheter skill education program offered by the industry. The typical training curriculum is listed in Table 2. Table 3 lists an overview of basic and advanced procedures every interventionalist should be able to master.

Finally, the favorable environment as emphasized under point 4 requires modernization of catheter laboratories or operating theaters. The very dynamic developments might become a new opportunity to build the so-called hybrid suites. Some centers in the United States as well as in Europe have started to fuse interventional and surgical specialties to form cardiovascular centers as illustrated by the new Shapiro Center of the Brigham & Women's Hospital, Boston (Fig. 8), which became functional in the summer of 2008. Table 4 lists a nonexhaustive overview of international sites with functioning hybrid room facilities.

Within this new environment, imaging plays a key role in the success of percutaneous valve repair—starting with the need to appropriately identify eligible patients; precisely visualize and judge severity and anatomy of the lesion,

TABLE 2 EDGE Course Faculty Program Overview for 2008

Time	Topic	Training activity	Learning objectives
13:15–14:00	Arrival and welcome reception	None	Get known to each other
14:00–14:15	Quick welcome, introduce faculty, round table introduction	Everyone presents himself, his experience, and expectations	Get known to each other
14:15–14:30	Overview of transcatheter therapies for structural heart disease	Medtronic's vision of cardiovascular: Cardiac surgery presentation: vision & commitment to the cardiac surgeon. The future role in "structural heart disease"	1. Understand Medtronic's commitment to the cardiac surgeon's future and the investment Medtronic has made 2. Understand the future opportunity in structural heart disease (SHD) for the cardiac surgeon
14:30–14:14:40	Course introduction, objectives, expectations	Presentation of objectives and tools used to achieve them	Understand the course for the next 1.5 days, different learning objectives and how they will be achieved
14:40–14:50	Course pretest	Fill-in test	Self-assessment by participants: Where do I stand, what do I know about transcatheter techniques?
14:50–15:10	Vascular access and closure techniques and devices	Access-site, Seldinger technique and sheath introduction; alternatives and complications, sheaths	Understand different steps of Seldinger technique and where and how to create a port for access (using a sheath); name possible complications and how to avoid them; sheath construction and nomenclature
15:10–15:30	Hands-on vascular access training on tube simulator and vascular model	Train steps of access-creation on tube simulator, explain design and size	Train procedural steps, repeat tips and tricks
15:30–15:50	Break		
15:50–16:05	Guidewires	Introduction to guidewires, understand differences and construction, feel differences (hand down wires)	Understand construction, purpose and selection based on needs; understand lingo

(Continued)

TABLE 2 EDGE Course Faculty Program Overview for 2008 (*Continued*)

Time	Topic	Training activity	Learning objectives
16:05–16:20	Catheters	Function and features of catheters, construction, and curve selection	Understand what catheters are used for and why different tip shapes exist, compliance with sheaths
16:20–16:50	Hands-on tube simulator, catheter handling, overwire techniques rapid exchange	Create access and do one wire/catheter exchange	Handling of preparation and exchange
16:50–17:00	New environment—the hybrid room	Presentation about hybrid room considerations plus examples of already installed rooms in Europe. Followed by discussion	Understand rational for hybrid rooms, how they can be designed, what technologies is installed, and which procedures are done
17:00–17:25	New imaging modalities for transcatheter valve therapies	Techniques and technologies needed to do TCV/ endovascular procedures	Understand what is needed to perform an angiography, usage of contrast and projections used to visualize certain structures; other imaging tools used
17:25–17:40	The concept of hybrid procedures—is there a common denomination	Presentation about procedures that could be possible done and be considered hybrid procedures	Understand which hybrid procedures are currently performed
17:40–17:55	Break		
17:55–18:05	Basics of coronary imaging: angiography an overview	Presentation about manifold and injectors, contrast agents, angles and artifacts	Understand what is needed to perform an angiography, usage of contrast and projections used to visualize certain structures
18:05–18:10	Working with high-fidelity simulators the can/can't and the do's and don'ts	Intro of all components, explain limitations to real world and how simulation will be performed	Make them familiar with the workstation and different tasks they will have during the next simulation sessions; explain differences to real world; explain what they have to do in next part, divide in groups of three: operator, assistant, radiology technician

(*Continued*)

TABLE 2 EDGE Course Faculty Program Overview for 2008 (*Continued*)

Time	Topic	Training activity	Learning objectives
18:10–19:30	Simulated catheter working place: first angiography of left and right coronary system on high-fidelity simulator	Get basic camera angles: LAO, RAO; understand how imaging conduct first angiography; work with angles	Identify different components and how to use them, understand opportunities and limitations of simulation
08:30–08:40	Compliant and noncompliant angioplasty balloons	Presentation: coronary balloons	Understand construction, what they are used for, and what are the important features
08:40–08:50	Stents: an overview	Presentation: stents	Understand construction and which one to use for the different situations
08:50–09:00	Hands-on training—High-fidelity–simulated coronary angioplasty	Explain components and how to use	Understand the task and how to use all the components for a therapy
09:00–10:00	Hands-on training high-fidelity simulation aortic and pulmonary valve implantation and PCI simulated catheter working place: angiography and angioplasty; parallel: aortic and melody simulation?	Do multivessel procedure	Understand right usage of all components (guidewire, catheter, balloons, stents, projection angles); perform angioplasty on left and right coronary system
10:00–10:15	Break		
10:15–10:45	State of the art on aortic transcatheter valve therapies—current technologies and where do we stand and where is it going	Current technologies and trends and round table discussion	Understand which technologies are available/under development for TCV procedures. Understand indications and future options
10:45–11:15	Balloon aortic valvuloplasty—basic understanding	Perform BAV	When and how to perform BAV
11:15–13:30	Hands-on transapical and transfemoral aortic transcatheter valve implantation	Perform aortic and pulmonic TCV procedure	Understand tools needed and steps performed
13:30–14:15	Lunch		
14:15–14:35	State of the art on transcatheter mitral valve repair	Current available products	Understand technology used and procedural steps, precautions, and complications

(*Continued*)

TABLE 2 EDGE Course Faculty Program Overview for 2008 (*Continued*)

Time	Topic	Training activity	Learning objectives
14:35–14:55	Endovascular aortic aneurysm stenting: the EVAR approach	Presentation about TAA treatment with stents	Understand technology used and procedural steps, precautions, and complications
14:55–15:10	Hands-on EVAR basic techniques, crossover, aortic abdominal aneurysm stenting	Hands-on	Deploy a valiant stent in the bench model
15:10–15:20	Final test	Fill-in test	See what they have learned over the 2 d. Compare to test of first day
15:20–15:30	Last-minute case	Listen to case	Realize what they have learned over the 2 d
15:30–15:50	Discussion	Possible next steps	
15:50–16:00	Feedback and adjourn	Fill in feedback, receive certificates and other education material	

Source: With permission of Medtronic SARL, Tolochenaz, Switzerland.

of the entry point, and of the access path before the intervention; to estimate the needed device characteristics. Without direct visual guidance, navigation relies solely on imaging modalities (Chap. 6. Access to the Aortic Valves). Finally, quality control again is achieved by imaging assessment and clinical judgment, and the consecutive follow-up relies mostly on imaging as well.

For aortic TCVT, imaging is needed to identify and analyze valvular morphology and function, aortic valve quantification, aortic root configuration and coronary arteries setup, and to estimate the correct size of the future implant.

New Image Modalities

Transthoracic echocardiography detects and quantifies aortic stenosis, left ventricular hemodynamics, and concomitant lesions, for example, subaortic that might temper the procedural result significantly. Direct planimetric assessment can estimate the aortic valve area and the LVOT sizing can be achieved by Doppler calculation. The long axis view provides valuable information for TAP TCVT.

Of course, transesophageal echocardiography (TEE) offers a higher resolution, allows showing details and a better quantification, but also represents a more uncomfortable and more invasive procedure in the preoperative setup.

Multislice cardiac computer tomography (MSCT) that is due to high local resolution and very short scan time is the most promising imaging modality in regard to preprocedural planning. Of course the risk of x-ray exposure and the contrast medium have to balance with the benefit and the planning of a smooth TCVT. Measurement of the aortic valve area is most critical for successful device implantation. MSCT not only calculates the orifice size but also allows visualization of calcium distribution on the disease valve. An additional advantage of MSCT is visualization of the entire vascular path including degree of calcification, luminal narrowing, and tortuosity. Three-dimensional reconstructions further significantly enhance preprocedural planning. In regard to TAP, MSCT

TABLE 3   Armamentarium of Basic and Advanced Endoluminal Interventions and Techniques an Interventional Specialist Should Be Familiar with and Fully Able to Master

---

BASIC TECHNIQUES

Primary puncture
Basic tool handling and finger-play
Wire exchange soft/stiff/hydrophil
Crosstalk between wires and catheters and sheaths
Tortuous vessel crossing
Iliac crossover techniques

ACCESS

Transfemoral access
Transapical access
Bidirectional access
Transatrial access
Transseptal approach

Access Closure

Transapical
Vessel closure

PROCEDURES

Aortic

Aortic balloon valvuloplasty
DAVR via TAP
Remote-access retrograde valve replacement (femoral)

Pulmonary

DAVR via TAP
Remote-access antegrade replacement (transfemoral vein)

Mitral

Mitral balloon valvuloplasty
Percutaneous mitral valve repair

Transseptal

FOP closure
Transseptal left heart assistance placement

Endovascular

Descending aortic aneurysm repair
Abdominal aneurysm repair
Aortic arch aneurysm
Surgical antegrade with hybrid endoprosthetic supplementation
Dissection repair
Fenestration of a type B dissection

Coronary interventions

Handling of Judkins catheters/rapid exchange vs overwire
Navigation within coronaries/IVUS

Abbreviations: DAVR, direct access valve replacement; IVUS, intravascular ultrasound; TAP, transapical procedure.

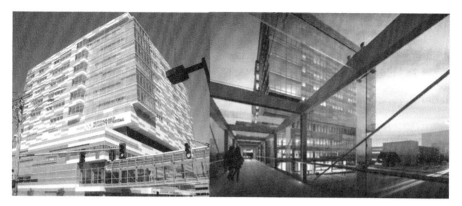

FIGURE 8 The Shapiro cardiovascular center extension of the Brigham & Women's Hospital, Boston, which opened in the summer of 2008.

offers access path information within the left ventricle and might be valuable in helping choose the ideal entry port.

With the recent progresses, magnetic resonance imaging (MRI) might become more and more attractive as supplementing imaging or as alternative to echocardiography and MSCT. MRI allows quantification of aortic valve area that is often overestimated. Software-supported angioSURF provides impressive new insights into the vascular three. MRI is very well tolerated and presents only minor auditive patient discomfort. The limiting factors are pacemakers, defibrillators, and claustrophobia. The currently improving picture quality still lacks local high resolution and is reduced significantly by calcifications.

The preprocedural planning ends with a detailed evaluation of peripheral vessels by angiography or angio-CT. Suitable vessels for the remote-access retrograde transfemoral approach require a diameter of at least 7 mm. The transapical procedure should be chosen if there is any doubt of the quality of the access path.

Periprocedural Imaging

X-ray and ultrasound imaging are the main imaging modalities used during the procedure. Fluoroscopy guidance with or without contrast is the first choice imaging for the operator. Therefore, only high-quality equipments should be used. Fluoroscopic imaging can be substantially enhanced by TEE assessment.

TEE enables analysis of the left ventricular function and end-diastolic changes. But, considering that most TCVTs nowadays are performed under local anesthesia and mild sedation, TEE remains a source of a patient's discomforts. Intracardiac echo provides high-resolution real-time images of the aortic valve

TABLE 4 List of Selected Sites with Hybrid Room Facilities

Children's Hospital, Boston
Vanderbilt University, Nashville
Sick Kids Hospital, Toronto, Canada
Beth Israel Hospital, Boston
University Hospital, Essen, Germany
Rhön Klinikum Heart Center, Leipzig, Germany
Saitama Medical University, Hidaka, Japan
German Heart Center, Munich, Germany

Source: Provided by Siemens AG, Medical Solutions.

and root and access can easily be gained by a femoral vein and, if at all, causes very little interference with the patient's comfort. The excellent image quality eliminates the need for contrast injections and the Doppler capability provides good postimplantation assessment of perivalvular leak and valve function as well as gradient. Intracardiac echo also can document and quantify postimplantation coronary flow (16).

Another future alternative visualization aid might rely totally on real-time MRI (17). But no clinical aortic MRI guidance experience exists for the time being. The future could bring MRI-guided TCVT but for the time being most catheters are not compatible with MRI use. A further development includes live overlay of a pre-procedurally gained 3D MRI reconstruction supplemented onto the fluoroscopic image during the intervention. A similar technique is currently being introduced with dyna-CT live overlay (periprocedural fluoroscopically gained 360 degree patient data, reconstructed into a digital 3D model). The reconstructed image of the aortic root is then superimposed and synchronized onto the fluoroscopic picture to follow the C-arm excursions. The screen live-overlay significantly eases the delivery process and reduces the amount of X-ray used throughout the procedure. MRI is brought a step further as proposed by Philipp Bonhoeffer using MRI-derived data to build implantation models by three-dimensional printing. A major limitation is the normalized geometry of the reconstructed model as images are acquired during multiples cycles and therefore measures are mean values between systolic and diastolic values and not actual systolic or diastolic measures. A further difficulty is that reconstruction is based only on the luminal data as provided from the MRI and the wall is added mathematically. Nevertheless, those developments represent a high level of interest and point toward stunning new results to be expected soon.

Postprocedural Imaging

Without doubt, for postprocedural follow-up, MSCT is technically the best imaging tool. This technique offers to visualize the aortic root as well as the LVOT but also gives remarkably good-quality pictures of the device. MSCT also allows calculating aortic valve orifice and can show the stent or strut's proximity to coronary ostia. As for EVAR procedure, MSCT is the technique of choice to follow device anchoring and integrity.

Transthoracic echo can supplement the data with estimates of LV function and aortic regurgitation from valvular incompetence or from paravalvular leaking as well as valve gradient over time and effective valve orifice.

Imaging plays an essential role for TCVT for all three phases: before, during, and after the procedure. Neither of the current imaging modalities is sufficient as stand-alone technique to cover all aspects and steps of the procedure setting. The optimum is a combination of the available and most appropriate imaging tools.

The Hybrid Suites—A New Environment

The hybrid suite is a synergistic combination of proven operating room concepts with catheter laboratory equipments. Its two most distinctive and important features are first and foremost the ideal hybrid suite requires more space ($\geq$85 m^2 or $\geq$900 ft^2) to fit in all the extra material in and second the hybrid suite integrates a very high-quality fluoroscopy sealing-, floor- or wall-mounted C-arm. All the additional equipment must be arranged around the improved OR table (Fig. 9).

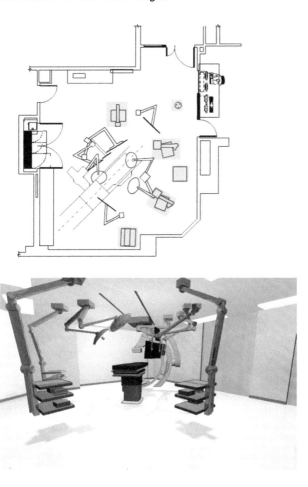

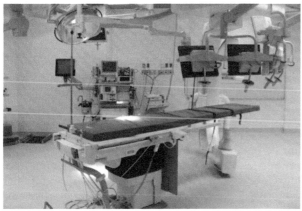

FIGURE 9 Planning, design, and final result of a hybrid operating room. (*Source*: Pictures provided by Dr. Fuchs, Siemens AG, Medical Solutions, Germany).

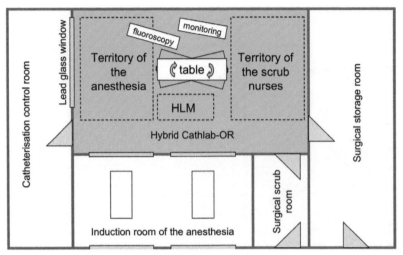

FIGURE 10 Room sectoring concept as proposed by Prof. Jacobs, West German Heart Center, Essen, Germany. (*Source*: Picture provided by Dr. Fuchs, Siemens AG, Medical Solutions, Germany).

The benefit of hybrid suites is to enable the combination of surgical therapy with state-of-the-art imaging–guided interventional procedures including periprocedural imaging in the OR. The following section provides an equipment-based analysis in regard to the hybrid suite setup.

Room sectoring concept (Fig. 10). The hybrid suite is partitioned into a centered working zone, including the patient's table, positioning the anesthesiology team at the patient's head and the interventional specialist team sideways beside the patient, and the scrub nurse close by toward the patient's feet. Around this center part are arranged the cardiotechnician area with the cardiopulmonary bypass, the parking slot for the preferentially ceiling-mounted fluoroscopy C-arm, the imaging technician control area, the anesthesia induction room, and the scrub sectors as well as the material storage spaces separating interventional and surgical equipment. The hybrid suite ceiling provides laminar flow not to be hindered by the additional ceiling-mounted equipment. Typical ceiling-mounted components might include the following:

- Laminar flow air conditioning with improved airflow and temperature regulation to compensate for the additional electrical material
- Slave monitors enabling multiples fields of view like life overlay of CT data and hemodynamic monitoring
- Surgical light
- Additionally movable surfaces for imaging and surgical equipment like echo, electric cautery and defibrillator, or the contrast injector
- Ceiling-mounted camera and audio equipment for scientific training and additional monitor systems might be optional

    Typical components of a cardiac OR include the following:

- Echo system (TEE, intracardiac echo, IVUS)
- Anesthesia setup and devices

- CPB machine
- Electrocautery
- Defibrillator
- Fiber-optic surgical headlight

Clinical information management. Additional monitors should be installed, where seamless information access is needed like access to the following:

- Preprocedural investigations (CT, MR, radiography, nuc, echo)
- Periprocedural images (road maps, angiography, echo, IVUS) allowing life overlay of various image modalities and real-time three-dimensional image reconstruction
- Continuous patient hemodynamic surveillance
- Additional space for portable units

The hybrid suite patient table's distinctive features should include the following:

- Collision protection
- Motorized tilting capabilities (15 degrees head up/down and 15 degrees lateral tilt)
- Floating table top
- Carbon fiber table top
- Preprogrammable positions

The ideal ceiling-mounted C-arm should present the following product characteristics:

- Close to 2 m free space between parking position and C-arm stand
- Imaging of all regions should be possible
- C-arm suspension should allow to be moved out of the surgery field without interfering with the anesthesiologist or other collaborating teams and equipments
- Collision protection cross-talking with the patient's table
- Preprogrammable positions

Ceiling-mounted equipment creates new challenges like limited possibilities to install surgical light above the OR field, requires customized (and expensive) solutions to install the laminar flow at the ceiling, and requires moving parts above the OR field what might temper with procedural sterility.

The image technician area should allow to work on imaging workstations and in room monitors for the following:

- Three-dimensional reconstruction
- Soft tissue imaging
- Image fusion

Optionally, create real-time three-dimensional models by three-dimensional printers for rapid prototyping and recreate real-time virtual three-dimensional access or vascular path of the patient. The hybrid suite should be in close proximity to the ICU and have access to full "tool-box" inventory for complicated endovascular repair and bailout procedures. Finally, one of the most essential features is personal and technician staff training within the new environment, the new team dynamics, and the additional materials.

ACCEPTANCE AND INTRODUCTION OF DISRUPTIVE NEW MEDICAL TECHNOLOGY

A typical example of smooth transition of a new technology is to permit extensive device handling. A step further to familiarize the user is achieved by implementing them into the device construction process. A recently published paper by the author describes a possible way to familiarize with TCVT (18).

The following study is in part reproduced from Huber CH, et al. Acceptance and introduction of disruptive technologies—Simple steps to build a fully functional pulmonary valved stent. Interact Cardiovasc Thorac Surg 2007; 6(4):430–432.

Introduction

Transcatheter therapy of structural heart disease is an emerging alternative for the treatment of heart valve disease. Pioneering interventional cardiologists and cardiac surgeons are the driving forces constructing the fundamentals of what might become the next choice for the treatment of cardiac valvulopathies (19–21). For most cardiac surgeons, endoluminal therapies still present untouched new land even though the direct access valve replacement via the transapical procedure—a surgery-based technique—has first been proposed by a cardiac surgeon (22) and gained wide popularity after validation by peer-reviewed position statement (23,24). To further sensitize and to ease introduction of those promising new technologies, Med-Tech meetings have set out to expose surgeons with the new devices. One way to familiarize with valved stents is presented in this paper by disclosing some simple steps to build a patient-specific pulmonary valved stent. The design concept has first been tested in an acute animal study (data previously presented) (25) and then by random participants at two consecutive Swiss Med-Tech meetings, the HeartLAB 2005 and 2006 in Zurich, Switzerland. Participants were asked to build and implant a self-made valved stent in a porcine model via a transinfundibular approach.

Methods and Techniques

The pulmonary valved stent is constructed from two components: an endoprosthetic graft and a valved jugular vein conduit. Both parts are chosen to approximate their respective diameter and trimmed to equal length. Then the adapted valved conduit cylinder is inserted into the carrier stent cylinder. Following, two sutures lines are created, one at the distal and one at the proximal device end. Next, the valve is inspected visually and tested by filling with saline solution. Next, the valved stent is crimped and loaded manually into the delivery device constructed from a 5-mm syringe (Chap. 9, Experimental Data).

To validate the concept, a total of 72 participants of two consecutive Med-Tech meetings in Switzerland in the years 2005 and 2006 (HeartLab, Zurich) were asked to build and implant the self-made device in the pulmonary position of a porcine heart. After a 30-minute introduction on the topic and a live demonstration on how to build the device in each meeting, every six participants were joined into six groups and invited to join the workbenches for the hands-on session. The allocated time for construction and insertion was set to 45 minutes. All implants were tested for adequacy of delivery and anchoring capacity within their delivery location by simple pull-test as well as correctness of construction and valve function by static leakage testing after explantation. Finally, the overstented native pulmonary valve was macroscopically assessed for traumatic lesions.

Results

This pulmonary valved stent concept was first validated in vitro and in vivo within an experimental animal setting (data previously presented) (26). Subsequently, the simplicity of the design concept was further challenged by integration into a hands-on session of two Med-Tech events. Within an allocated time window of 45 minutes, 11 of 12 groups of participants successfully built their own pulmonary valved stent. A total of 10 groups implanted the device into the targeted pulmonary position by using the self-made delivery tool. Only one group delivered the valved stent too distally, above the native valve. Anchoring capacity of all 10 implanted valved stents was excellent; none could be dislodged back into the right ventricle. On gross inspection, 11 valved stents were correctly constructed and showed no obvious signs of malfunction. At static leakage testing, 2 of the 11 valved stents were identified to have a minor valve insufficiency because of size mismatch between the graft and the valved conduit. None of the native pulmonary valves showed macroscopic signs of trauma.

Methodical Considerations

The device-specific design limits its use strictly to the right side of the heart as the covered stent might occlude the coronaries. The described valved stent/delivery device setup is to be used only in an experimental setting, as there are no long-term or clinical data available. The mild valvular insufficiency of 2 of the 11 devices at the post-implantation static leakage test might have resulted from size-mismatch of the used components while assembling the device or from traumatic handling of the device during retrieval.

All surgical therapy is a "hand-made" activity and as such fully recognized as a rather major advantage by allowing precise and individualized patient-adapted therapy. Custom-built prosthesis is a further advantage to allow quick and effective production of a patient-adapted prosthesis and furthermore avoids the off-the-shelf bottleneck. The authors very strongly believe device construction to be simple and safe enough to be introduced into clinical practice when handled by an experienced surgeon. Regarding biotolerance, functionality, and approval of all components, no issues are expected to arise as the endograft and the bovine jugular vein conduit have widely been implanted clinically—the former for endoluminal aortic aneurysm grafting and the latter for right ventricular outflow tract reconstruction in congenital cardiac surgery. The valve has also shown its validity in percutaneous procedures in more than 100 patients within a commercially available device. The primary indication for this device is to be found in congenital cardiac surgery.

One of the most frequent procedures, the repair of tetralogy of Fallot, might have an important benefit from the device. An insufficient pulmonary valve after right ventricular outflow tract enlargement could temporarily be replaced by this pulmonary valved stent until reoperation for graft outgrowth becomes necessary. Slight oversizing of the device with successive later balloon dilation or even percutaneous reinsertion of a second valved stent could further delay the point of outgrowth and successive surgery. Two groups have reported their clinical results of a similar device manufactured by Shelhigh recently (27,28). The device is based on a valved stent first published in 2003 by our group, constructed from a valved conduit scaffold by two rows of self-expanding stents (29).

The clinical results confirm the clinical feasibility of intraoperative implantation for pulmonary regurgitation. Six patients (9–27 years) received an injectable porcine pulmonary valved stent after total correction of tetralogy of Fallot at 4.2 ± 4.0 years. All implantations were uneventful and except for one patient with a major paravalvular leak requiring surgical reintervention, the 6 to 12 months follow-up was very promising. Unfortunately, the valved stent insertion requires surgical access to the right ventricular outflow tract for device insertion. The valved stent reported in this publication is designed to be inserted via a guidewire to allow for a minimally invasive insertion via the previously reported direct access transapical procedure by puncturing the right ventricle via a small thoracotomy. Visualization for delivery monitoring is achieved either by intracardiac or transesophageal echo with or without contrast-enhanced fluoroscopy.

Summary

Valved stents are slowly moving into clinical practice. Availability and familiarity are limiting factors for their acceptance. This study shows the feasibility to hand-build a valved stent and the simplicity of implantation. Furthermore, the off-the-shelf bottleneck is avoided by the self-constructed and custom-made design of the device. The above-mentioned key element must be applied in the widest extent possible for the supportive staff, for example, nursing and technical staff including hands-on session for everyone involved in such a novel technology. Finally, on-site technical support throughout the procedure is an indispensable strategy for successful procedural outcome.

REFERENCES

1. Lillehei CW. New ideas and their acceptance—As it has related to preservation of chordae tendinea and certain other discoveries. J Heart Valve Dis 1995; 4(suppl II):S106–S114.
2. Bower JL, Christensen CM. Disruptive technologies: Catching the wave. Harv Bus Rev 1995; 43–53.
3. Dobrow S, Pisano G, Heartport Inc. Harvard Business Review. 2000; 9-600-020;1–19.
4. Edmondson AC. Framing for learning: Lessons in successful technology implementation. Calif Manageme Rev 2003; 45(2):34–54.
5. Stuge O, Liddicoat J. Emerging opportunities for cardiac surgeons within structural heart disease. J Thorac Cardiovasc Surg 2006; 132:1258–1261.
6. Wheatley GH III, McNutt R, Diethrich EB. Introduction to thoracic endografting: imaging, guidewires, guiding catheters, and delivery sheaths. Ann Thorac Surg 2007; 83:272–278.
7. Reznick RK, MacRae H. Teaching surgical skills—Changes in the wind. N Engl J Med 2006; 355:2664–2669.
8. Fitts PM, Posner MI. Human Performance. Belmont, CA: Brooks/Cole, 1967.
9. Scott DJ, Bergen PC, Rege RV, et al. Laparoscopic training on bench models: Better and more cost effective than operating room experience? J Am Coll Surg 2000; 191(3):272–283.
10. Gallagher AG, Cates CU. Approval of virtual reality training for carotid artery stenting: What this means for procedural-based medicine. JAMA 2004; 292:3024–3026.

11.

12. Rosser JC Jr, Lynch PJ, Cuddihy L, et al. The impact of video games on training surgeons in the 21st century. Arch Surg 2007; 142(2):181–186; discussion 186.

13. Matsumoto ED, Hamstra SJ, Radomski SB, et al. The effect of bench model fidelity on denourological skills: A randomized controlled study. J Urol 2002; 167:1243–1247.

14. Vahanian A, Alfieri OR, Al-Attar N, et al, in collaboration with the European Association of Percutaneous Cardiovascular Interventions (EAPCI). Transcatheter valve implantation for patients with aortic stenosis: A position statement from the European Association of Cardio-Thoracic Surgery (EACTS) and the European Society of Cardiology (ESC) [published online ahead of print May 12, 2008]. Eur Heart J 2008; 29(11):1463–1470.

15. Wijns W. EAPCI: Education and training programmes in interventional cardiology today. EuroInterv 2007; 3:301–303.

16. Huber CH, Tozzi P, Corno AF, et al. Do valved stents compromise coronary flow? Eur J Cardiothorac Surg 2004; 25(5):754–759.

17. McVeigh E, Guttman MA, Lederman RJ, et al. Real-time interactive MRI-guided cardiac surgery: Aortic valve replacement using a direct apical approach. Magn Reson Med 2006; 56:958–964.

18. Huber CH, Marty B, von Segesser LK. Acceptance and introduction of disruptive technologies—Simple steps to build a fully functional pulmonary valved stent. Interact Cardiovasc Thorac Surg 2007; 6(4):430–432.

19. Bonhoeffer P, Boudjemline Y, Saliba Z, et al. Percutaneous replacement of pulmonary valve in a right-ventricle to pulmonary-artery prosthetic conduit with valve dysfunction. Lancet 2000; 356(9239):1403–1405.

20. Cribier A, Eltchaninoff H, Bash A, et al. Percutaneous transcatheter implantation of an aortic valve prosthesis for calcific aortic stenosis: First human case description. Circulation 2002; 106:3006–3008.

21.

22. Huber CH, Nasratulla M, Augstburger M, et al. Ultrasound navigation through the heart for off-pump aortic valved stent implantation: New tools for new goals. J Endovasc Ther 2004; 11:503–510.

23. Vassiliades TA, Block PC, Cohn LH, et al. The clinical development of percutaneous heart valve technology. A position statement of the Society of Thoracic Surgeons (STS), the American Association for Thoracic Surgery (AATS), and the Society for Cardiovascular Angiography and Interventions (SCAI). J Am Coll Cardiol 2005; 45:1554–1560.

24. Huber CH, Cohn LH, von Segesser LK. Direct-access valve replacement a novel approach for off-pump valve implantation using valved stents. J Am Coll Cardiol 2005; 46(2):366–370.

25. Huber CH, Zhou J, von Segesser LK. Transapical implantation of valved stents—Or how to prevent reoperation for postoperative pulmonary regurgitation. Cardiology in the young, Abstract book. 2006 May O-18:7 Data presented at the 41st Annual Meeting of the Association for European Pediatric Cardiology in Basel, Switzerland, 2006.

26. Oechslin EN, Harrison DA, Harris L, et al. Reoperation in adults with repair of tetralogy of Fallot: Indications and outcomes. J Thorac Cardiovasc Surg 1999; 118:245–251.

27. Berdat PA, Schönhoff F, Pavlovic M, et al. Cardiology in the Young. Abstract book. 2006:O-39:15.

28. Schreiber C, Hörer J, Vogt M, et al. A new treatment option for pulmonary valve insufficiency: First experiences with implantation of a self-expanding stented valve without use of cardiopulmonary bypass. Eur J Cardiothorac Surg 2007; 31:26–30.

29. Zhou JQ, Corno AF, Huber CH, et al. Self-expanding valved stent of large size: Off-bypass implantation in pulmonary position. Eur J Cardiothorac Surg 2003; 24:212–216.

6   Access to the Aortic Valves

There is no single ideal approach to the aortic valve. Several techniques allow gaining access to the aortic valve and each has its own pros and cons. Figure 1 presents a decision tree to access the aortic valve. Listed below is a prioritized overview of the ten most important characteristics for the optimal access route weighted by the author.

1. Allow safe access to the target location
2. Permit highest quality valve replacement or repair with best possible procedural and long-term outcome
3. Lead to high degree of patient satisfaction
4. Requires minimal invasiveness
5. Smallest impact on financial resources
6. Applicable to a widest patient's population
7. Permit early hospital discharge and rapid gain of patient mobility
8. Multipurpose access and accepts repeat procedures
9. Short learning curve and allows for off-patient simulator training
10. High degree of operator satisfaction

THE SURGICAL APPROACH—A RETROGRADE DIRECT OR LOCAL ACCESS

The only widespread technique is the surgical valve replacement most commonly performed via a midline sternotomy, under cardiopulmonary support and with cardioplegia induced cardiac arrest. Less invasive variants have been described including smaller skin incisions hemisternotomies, thoracotomies, port access, and robotic-assisted surgery. Furthermore, various cannulation techniques might further decrease invasiveness of surgery, for example, percutaneous cannulation for cardiopulmonary bypass or beating heart valve replacement.

Regarding the above-mentioned list of requirements for the ideal replacement, it seems that surgical replacement positions itself in the midrange of optimal therapy requirements. Surgical replacement remains highly invasive but allows safe access to the aortic valve in the hands of an experienced surgeon. The surgical technique might be considered easy after several years of training in the OR but the learning curve is steep and long. The results are without doubt very good and the surgical approach is the only one to effectively provide long-term data. Obviously, the cost of surgical aortic valve replacement is high because of the required highly specialized personnel and the cost-intensive OR environment. Further substantial contributing cost factors are the postoperative care requiring intensive care facilities as well as the overall length of stay in the hospital. Finally, patient recovery eventually will be complete by two to three months after surgery, the amount of time needed for the sternum to heal, what also implies a prolonged absence from work. A major advantage of surgery is

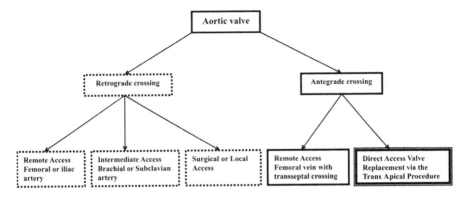

FIGURE 1 Access classification in regard to distance from target site and delivery direction.

the wide patient applicability in respect to what is called the operable patient, missing out on close to double the number of patients with aortic valve disease classified as to be not eligible for surgery.

Quality of life after surgical aortic valve replacement is without doubt excellent even in the elderly patients (1) but the interventions remains a traumatic life event. Surgical replacement is the best treatment currently available but is far from what could be called an ideal therapy.

⊕ *The Pros*
Longest clinical experience
Very good postoperative results
Excellent exposure
Direct visual control during implantation
Applicable to most patients
Allows combined procedures
Widest choice of devices

⊗ *The Cons*
Surgical approach requiring a full or partial sternotomy or thoracotomy
Need for cardiopulmonary bypass
Cardiac arrest and aortic cross-clamping mandatory
Increased level of postoperative pain
Overall longer ICU and in-hospital length of stay
Delay in getting back to work and to daily self-care
Increased risks in the reoperative setting

NEW APPROACHES

Alternative delivery routes can be categorized by various parameters, two have been shown to be most useful and are clinically well established. The first classification is the direction of implantation in regard to the blood flow—antegrade or retrograde. The second classification is relating to the distance of the insertion site from the delivery site and is named direct access and remote access. All of these approaches have specific strengths and weaknesses.

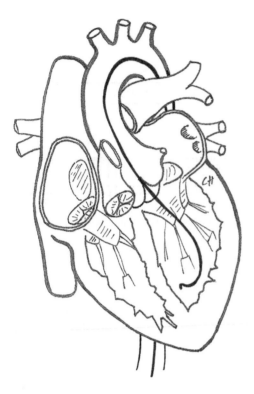

FIGURE 2 Remote retrograde transfemoral artery access. Note the short
guidewire part within the dead-ended left
ventricle swinging freely without further
possible stabilization options.

The Remote Retrograde Approach

The remote retrograde approach (Fig. 2) was the first route used for experimental transcatheter aortic valve replacement (2) and remains the approach with
the widest clinical experience. Obviously, this approach represents a proprietary
familiarity for every interventional specialist. Nevertheless, this remote access
harbors many pitfalls and suffers from several nonsolved difficulties. Safe access
to the target location widely depends on the quality of the access vessel, in most
cases, a calcified common femoral artery with a restricted inner diameter of only
a few millimeters. To insert the device, the valved stent has to be crimped down
tightly to a diameter as small as 24 to 26F, and more recently 18F is what represents high compression forces from the stent struts onto the future valve leaflets.
After mastering the insertion follows an often torturous and calcified long vascular path up into the thoracic aorta. Next, the delivery device is advanced further curving around the aortic arch and finally pushed into the ascending aorta.
The last challenge is still to come—the retrograde crossing of the stenotic aortic
valve. Manipulation within the ascending aorta and the crossing of the highly
calcified aortic valve bears the risk of embolization and consecutive stroke. A
prospective German study published in *Lancet* in 2003 analyzed the risk of silent
and apparent cerebral event after retrograde catheterization of the aortic valve in
valvular stenosis, presenting a surprising 22% radiologically confirmed cerebral
event, even though only 3% of patients presented with clinically apparent neurological symptoms (3). The stroke risk associated with retrograde aortic valve
crossing becomes apparent in the recent retrograde remote access aortic TCV

studies reporting from 5% (4) to 10% (5) versus 0% stroke rates in the transapical access (6).

Another consideration is of mechanical nature. In construction, flexibility is typically opposing to stability. But to allow remote insertion, the device not only needs to be small and tightly compressed but also highly flexible and short enough to travel all the way to its destination. The highest quality valve replacement is compromised by the necessary design modifications. Fish recently published a nonexhaustive overview of these limitations (7). First and foremost, the complication profile is high for the insertion of large introducer systems, such as would be needed to navigate through and work on diseased valves. Two complication profiles were identified; local complications included vessel rupture, dissection, pseudoaneurysm formation, bleeding, vessel stenosis, and thrombus formation. Transcatheter aortic valve replacement also creates new complications associated with traversing implements and devices through a long vascular path to reach the desired target in the heart. These complications include increased risk of kinking, higher shear stress on the vessel wall, and a demanding and cumbersome delivery process that hinders the precise delivery of the implantation device. Small vessel diameter also limits the size of the delivery device making removal of diseased valves nearly impossible.

⊕ *The Pros*
Preferred access method for percutaneous coronary interventions with long-standing clinical experience
Full percutaneous technique
Easy-to-handle local complications
Very well tolerated by the patients
Well suited for inoperable patients
Might be performed in local anesthesia
Virtual absence of postinterventional pain

⊗ *The Cons*
Allows only very low-profile devices and delivery systems
Retrograde eccentric crossing of the diseased valve
Requires preinterventional diagnostic assessment of the vascular path
High local complication profile
Increased risk for mobilization of calcified plaques of the ascending aorta and aortic arch
Remote locations make handling of long catheter and delivery systems mandatory and decrease precision of device deployment
Free-floating wire end within the left ventricle, no true wire stabilization

The Remote Antegrade Approach
The remote antegrade approach (Fig. 3) first clinically introduced by Alain Cribier seemed to become a very promising approach at first overcoming several of the before mentioned shortcomings. The fast-spreading enthusiasm led to the first clinical study for transcatheter aortic valve replacement. Shortly after, the same study was discontinued by Edwards Lifescience in accordance with the FDA. The major advantage of the antegrade aortic valve crossing and delivery direction was overshadowed by the poorly tolerated interference of the

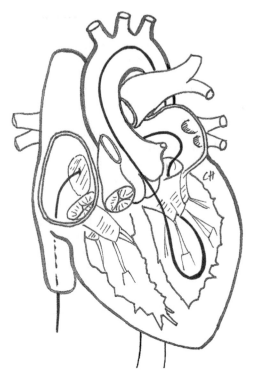

FIGURE 3 Remote antegrade transfemoral vein access. Good wire stability
but interference with the anterior mitral
valve. This approach requires a transseptal crossing.

guidewire with the anterior mitral valve leaflet. Technically, the guidewire is
inserted into the femoral vein and then advanced into the right atrium. By
transseptal crossing and after septal dilatation, the wire accesses the left atrium
and is then advanced by helping a floatation balloon over the mitral valve to loop
up from the left ventricle through the aortic valve into the ascending aorta in an
antegrade fashion. Finally, the wire is snared from the opposite femoral artery
and externalized to create a venous arterial loop.

Some of the potential problems of the antegrade remote access for aortic
valve disease were identified by Cribier in 2004 (8). He reported significant complications in end-stage inoperable patients with calcified aortic stenosis, using
the transseptal approach. One-third of patients developed severe mitral incompetence from injury caused by passing the guidewire through the mitral valve,
and in a substantial number of patients the valved stent showed severe paravalvular leakage. Progressive length of the delivery system increases the risk
of kinking, puts higher shear stress onto the vessel wall, and makes precise
device delivery more demanding and handling more cumbersome. The transept
puncture and dilatation carries the risk of pericardial tamponade. Further atrial
and ventricular arrhythmias are frequently generated by the interfering wire
and delivery system. Overall, the technical complexity of the procedure severely
restricts its use.

⊕ *The Pros*

Venous pathway with very compliant vessel walls, bigger-sized vessels, and
virtually no calcifications

Antegrade valve crossing
Allows intermediate-sized delivery systems and devices
Full percutaneous technique
Little risk of local complications
Might be performed in local anesthesia
Virtual absence of postinterventional pain
Potential for bidirectional wire use

⊗ *The Cons*

Demanding transseptal puncture which creates the need for periprocedural ASD closure

Intermittently poorly tolerated periprocedural mitral valve insufficiency

Of all three access methods, longest wires and delivery systems with increases wire slag and loops precludes axial and rotational handling precision

Requires devices and delivery systems with higher flexibility for better compliance with tighter wire curves

The Direct Access Antegrade Approach—The Transapical Procedure

New technology creates the need for new applications and vice versa. Direct access valve replacement (DAVR) via the transapical procedure (TAP) has been first introduced by the author in 2004 (9–11). The major advantage of this approach (Fig. 4) is to circumvent the majority of the limitations and drawbacks of the before described techniques while preserving and improving upon the low

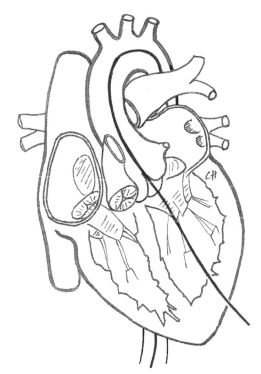

FIGURE 4 Direct antegrade access by the direct access valve replacement technique via the transapical procedure combines the advantages of both remote access approaches within a straightforward procedure.

patient morbidity and mortality rates associated with cardiac surgery. The capability of using embolic filters, temporary valve-tipped catheters, or short-term axial ventricular-assist devices could in future leverage DAVR via TAP to become the new therapy of choice for patients with structural heart disease. This technique represents a true convergence of the interventional and standard surgical approaches and has the potential to be applied to the widest patient population, including very severe forms of aortic valve disease, high-risk patients, but also early disease stages within younger patients. DAVR via TAP involves the percutaneous transmyocardial entry of any cardiac cavity through the respective ventricular apex. Alternatively, DAVR might be useful for access to the mitral valve via direct puncture of the left atrium (12). Further, major advantages of DAVR via TAP include the straight-line access to the target site (Fig. 4), which improves handling and permits insertion of long-handled delivery or decalcification tools, increased caliber delivery systems, and simultaneous use of other interventional tools, for example, embolic projection devices, temporary valve-tipped catheters, or short-term-use ventricular support pumps.

⊕ *The Pros*
Short and straight access to the target location
Antegrade crossing of the diseased valve
Little risk of local complication
Increases access diameter, enables bigger-sized delivery devices
Potentially further developed to a full percutaneous procedure
Ideal for bidirectional wire use with distal stabilization
Permits simultaneous insertion of multiple procedure-associated devices
Sole technique to harbor potential to become a real alternative to surgical valve replacement
Wide applicability to expanded therapies of structural heart disease

⊗ *The Cons*
Currently, DAVR requires a keyhole thoracotomy with purse-string sutures placement onto the myocardium
Local complication more difficult to manage
Limited clinical experience as access route in the nonsurgical specialties

DIRECT ACCESS PERCUTANEOUS VALVE REPLACEMENT VIA TAP

Introduction
Surgical valve repair or replacement has become the only and most adequate treatment option for stenotic or insufficient valvular disease over time. However, undergoing valve surgery remains a major trauma for the patients associated with a large number of limitations and risks.

Recent progress in interventional cardiology and cardiac surgery has placed transcatheter valve therapies (TCVT) into a new focus of interest of emerging cardiovascular therapies (13–16). More than 10 years after Henning Anderson (2) and the same year Dusan Pavcnik (17,18) published the concept of integrating a valve into a stent to build a valved stent device (Fig. 5), the overall interest has sharply risen since. The first successful human percutaneous

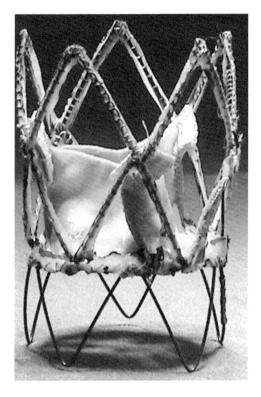

FIGURE 5 Aortic valved stent made from three linked nitinol Z-stents and a pericardial tissue valve—ready to use.

implantation of a valved stent into a pulmonary artery conduit by Bonhoeffer et al. in 2000 (19) was followed two years later by Cribier's first clinical percutaneous implantation of a valved stent into a severely diseased aortic valve (20).

Various access techniques have been advocated, in particular the percutaneous remote access, but recent drawbacks have tempered the optimism toward these techniques (7). Remote retrograde access has proven its validity since the very beginning of interventional cardiology, however yields a high complication profile for insertion of large introducer systems including local complications like vessel rupture, dissection, pseudoaneurysm formation, bleeding or vessel stenosis, and thrombus formation, but furthermore creates new types of complications while traveling through a long vascular path to reach the desired target location in the heart. As experienced by Cribier (8), using a transseptal approach and placing the guidewire through the mitral valve caused severe mitral incompetence in up to one-third of the reported patients.

Progressive length of the delivery system increases the risk of kinking, puts higher shear stress onto the vessel wall, makes precise device delivery more demanding, and handling more cumbersome. Not to mention that access vessel diameter highly limits the size of any delivery device and makes removal of the diseased valve close to impossible. Finally, looking at further development options, remote access techniques do not qualify for off-pump surgical aortic valve replacement with prior removal of the diseased valve.

The following study is in part reproduced from Huber CH, Cohn LH, von Segesser LK. Direct-access valve replacement a novel approach for off-pump valve implantation using valved stents. J Am Coll Cardiol 2005; 46(2):366–370.

The Concept of a Novel Approach—DAVR

DAVR is based on percutaneous transmyocardial entry into any cardiac cavity, preferably through either ventricular apex for aortic or pulmonary valve procedures or through the atrial wall for mitral or tricuspid interventions. Access through the left ventricular (LV) apex combined with the routine use of intravascular ultrasound (IVUS) and intracardiac echocardiography (ICE) providing real time out of the lumen dimensions and identification of the coronary configuration are promising new elements to overcome the shortcomings of a percutaneous approach. Those new tools allow for periprocedural valved stent delivery monitoring and quantitative assessment of postimplantation coronary flow despite the highly echodense structure of the implanted stent. Obvious advantages over remote access percutaneous techniques are straight-line access to the target location alleviating handling, allowing for insertion of long-handled decalcification tools, and delivery system with increased caliber as well as simultaneous positioning of multiple interventional devices, for example, embolic protection devices or temporary ventricular support pumps. DAVR eliminates virtually all the mentioned complications of remote access TCVT and yet still yields the advantages of a percutaneous technique with typical low patient mortality and morbidity in comparison to cardiac surgery. The use of embolic filters and of temporary valve-tipped catheters or brief-use axial ventricular-assist devices makes DAVR become a low-risk operation and possibly compete with surgical valve replacement soon. It might benefit not only highly selected patients population but be applicable to most of the valvular cardiomyopathy patients.

From Remote Access to DAVR

The author first introduced DAVR via TAP in 2004. The author's research program started in 2001 and evolved continuously throughout. Based on the good results of remote pulmonary TCVT (Figs. 6 and 7) and the high failure rate of remote access TCVT aortic valve replacement, the author set out to develop a new approach combining the obvious advantages of a percutaneous technique with the extended therapeutic options of the surgical procedure. Initially, the concept of DAVR was validated for right heart valve interventions, namely, for pulmonary valve replacement (21).

Considering the highly complex anatomy of the aortic root, more ingenious methods are required for relief of aortic valve disease. The most common aortic valve pathology is the highly calcified and stenotic valve. To implant a new valve with the least patient prosthesis mismatch, the disease valve needs to be predilated (7,20), decalcified, or removed (9,22,23). Furthermore, the close relationship of the aortic valve to the mitral valve apparatus and the coronary ostia severely restricts the valved stent design (22) and limits the possibilities for the safe anchoring of the device in the subannular region. It is essential to avoid any interference with the coronary blood flow by direct obstruction or indirect flow modifications while or after implantation (17,19,22,24).

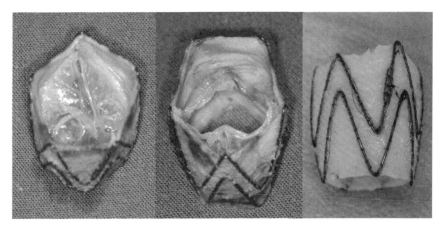

FIGURE 6 First valved stent used for pulmonary valve implantation using the DAVR technique. A 22-mm valved bovine jugular xenograft was mounted into two self-expanding nitinol Z-stents.

Considering the given facts, it seems evident that safe and successful aortic valve replacement requires more than what can be done by current remote access transcatheter-based techniques.

Intracardiac Echo for Adequate Visualization

The outcome of TCVT relies on adequate visualization (Fig. 8) of the target area and precise monitoring of the valved stent delivery. To avoid dye load together with the previous excellent results using IVUS for endovascular aneurysm repair (25) prompted into extending the use of IVUS to endoluminal cardiac valve

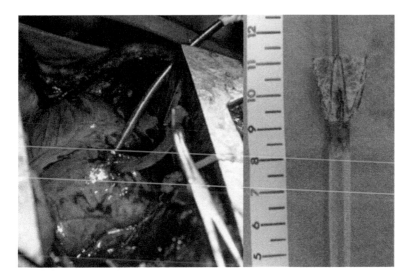

FIGURE 7 Through a small right-sided thoracotomy, a purse-string suture is placed onto the right ventricular apex to allow for safe introduction of the valved stent delivery system. Valved stent halfway loaded into the delivery device.

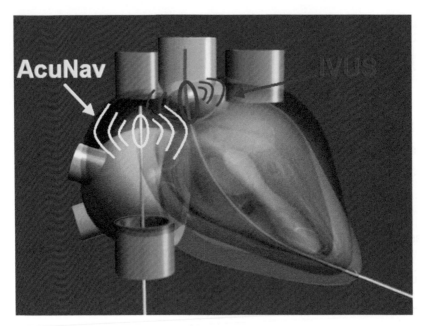

FIGURE 8 Ultrasound-guided intracardiac navigation. ICE probe placed in the right atrium and the IVUS probe is placed through the left apex into the aortic valve annulus. *Abbreviations*: ICE, intracardiac echo; IVUS, intravascular ultrasound.

procedures. Adding intracardiac echo did allow to enhance visualization despite the echodense stent structure and to monitor postimplantation coronary flow. Furthermore, it supports three-dimensional assessment and helps adequately monitor delivery of the valved stent into the target location (9).

   Direct left ventricular apex access (Fig. 9) in combination with either fluoro-scopic and transesophageal echo or intravascular (IVUS) and intracardiac (ICE) ultrasound can overcome the shortcomings of the remote access percutaneous approaches.

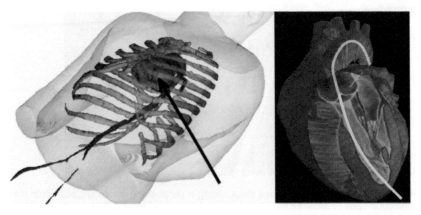

FIGURE 9 Three-dimensional model showing relationship between thoracic cage and left/right ventricular apex (*left*). Illustrating the left ventricular path via a transapical access (*right*).

How-To-Do—Technical Aspects of DAVR
The method is outlined as follows.

Surgical Access
After full equipment of the animals, including Swan-Ganz catheters for continuous cardiac output measurement, access for the ICE is prepared by exposure of the proximal right femoral vein and placement of an 11F introducer. Then a 10- to 15-cm incision is made for a left-sided thoracotomy (Fig. 9) and a Xylocaine drip (1.5 mg/kg) started to minimize arrhythmias. Next, two purse-string sutures are placed on the LV apex and heparin (300 IU/kg) given. Then the ICE probe is inserted and advanced into the right atrium (Fig. 8) to visualize and measure the native aortic valve as well as the aortic root including annular diameter, valvular surface and length of the leaflets, the size of the sinuses of Valsalva and the coronary orifice diameter, the diameter and height of the sinotubular junction, diameter and height of the ascending aorta, as well as the distance from the valvular plane to the brachiocephalic trunk. Special attention should be given to the coronary orifice region to identify and quantify the residual sinuses (sinuses of Valsalva) in front of the proper coronary arteries.

Off-Pump Aortic Valved Stent Implantation
Next, the valved stent is prepared and hand-crimped onto the delivery system. An over-the-needle catheter is inserted into the left ventricle via the apex and the correct position confirmed by fluoroscopy. An 8F introducer is then advanced and a soft-tip guidewire advanced beyond the aortic valve aortic valve. Next, the guidewire is exchanged for an ultrastiff guidewire. The monorail wire-guided disposable IVUS 6F catheter transducer providing a cross-sectional view with 80-mm diameter is inserted next and the aortic target site identified. The IVUS probe location is simultaneously tracked with the ICE and fluoroscopy. Four radioopaque markers are placed to temporarily define the target zone at the level of the aortic annulus, the end of the native leaflet in systole, the sinotubular junction, and the beginning of the brachiocephalic trunk. The fluoroscopic C-arm and operating table are locked into position to avoid parallaxes.

Simultaneous Periprocedural Valved Stent Position Assessment with ICE and Fluoroscopy
After removal of the IVUS and the 8F introducer, the valved stent delivery system is advanced over the guidewire under fluoroscopy and simultaneous ICE guidance. When fluoroscopic and sonographic target sites are congruent, the valved stent is deployed over the native valves in a two-step procedure. First the distal, and if the location stayed unchanged, the proximal end was released. To be able of minor position corrections, the valved stent initial landing site was chosen slightly above the prior identified target site. Therefore, after opening the first row of Z-stent, the hall device could be pulled back until fluoroscopic and sonographic landings and target site match.

Animal Study and Device Implantation

Valved Stent Design and In Vitro Testing
The valved stent custom-designed for this study (Fig. 5) is based on a previously described prototype (21).

Animal Studies

Direct access valved stent implantation was performed in 12 pigs (68.5 ± 7.3 kg). All animals received humane care in compliance with the principles of the Guide for the Care and Use of Laboratory Animals (26). All data are expressed as mean ± standard deviation.

Direct Access Implantation Technique

The detailed implantation techniques described earlier following some specific steps are briefly outlined. The jugular veins and carotid arteries are mobilized and animals fully equipped for complete invasive monitoring. Next, the 11F introducer is inserted into the right femoral vein to provide ICE access. The mini left-sided thoracotomy incisions are made and the sixth intercostal space is entered. Two Teflon-reinforced purse-string sutures are placed on the LV apex. After full heparinization (300 IU/kg), the 10F ICE probe is inserted into the right atrium (Fig. 8).

Measures

Predeployment measurements of the aortic valve, root, and coronary ostia configuration are made by ICE to allow for postdeployment comparison without interference caused by the echodense stent struts, a disadvantage of transesophageal echocardiography.

LV Valved Stent Implantation

The implant is hand-crimped to the delivery device (Fig. 10). The LV apex is punctured and an introducer and guidewire are inserted into the descending aorta. Catheter location is confirmed by ICE and fluoroscopy. The monorail wire-guided disposable IVUS is advanced for aortic road mapping. The advancement and positioning of the IVUS probe is monitored by ICE and fluoroscopy for target site identification. Three to four radioopaque markers are placed to reference

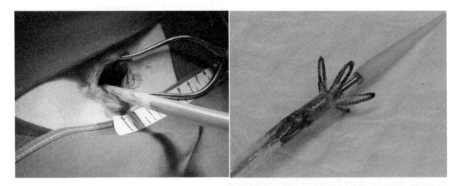

FIGURE 10   Valved stent and delivery system. The off-pump valved stent is manually crimped and loaded into a standard endoprosthetic delivery device with a max diameter of 9.2 mm. Insertion of a 2-cm minithoracotomy for TAP access to the left heart.

the level of the aortic annulus, end of the native leaflet in systole, sinotubular junction, and beginning of the brachiocephalic trunk.

ICE and Fluoroscopy for Real-Time Valved Stent Deployment Monitoring

After removing the IVUS and 8F introducer, the valved stent delivery system is advanced over the guidewire under fluoroscopic and ICE guidance (Fig. 10). When fluoroscopic and sonographic target sites reach congruency, the valved stent is deployed orthotopically over the native valve leaflets releasing the distal end first. If the location remains unchanged, the proximal end is released. The valved stent is targeted to land slightly above the optimal site to ensure that the entire device can be pulled back if needed after opening the first line of the Z-stent. The self-expanding nitinol stent has a low metal-to-stent ratio with minimal contact area between the interface of the stent and aortic wall. These features increase the expansion force at the interface, creating a firm attachment to the aortic root, without injuring the aortic wall. This stent design is being used clinically for aortic endovascular procedures.

The Residual Coronary Sinus Stent Index

This study used the residual coronary sinus stent index (RCSSI) to evaluate CBF impairment (Chap. 8. Physiologic Response to Aortic Valved Stent with Emphasis on Coronary Flow). This index compares the flow ratio between the native coronary flow with the blood flow required to pass through the valved stent after implantation. More specifically, RCSSI is a comparison between the coronary cross-sectional surface area and the plane defined by the valved stent and the native aortic wall (Fig. 11). Coronary diameter was measured at the termination of the sinus portion. The residual stent aortic wall plane was measured at the level of the coronary orifice. All measurements were made using intracardiac ultrasound. To calculate the index value, the distance of the stent from the aortic wall (residual gap at the level of the aortic sinus portion) is divided by the coronary diameter. CBF impairment was not observed for index values >1.

Acute Outcome Assessment

In vivo assessment included leaflet motion, planimetric valve orifice, RCSSI, CBF, characteristics of the left coronary artery, transvalvular gradient, regurgitation, and paravalvular leaking. After the experiments, animals were sacrificed and a macroscopic analysis was performed at necropsy (Fig. 12).

Results

In Vitro Study

All valved stents demonstrated good function with a pressure gradient of 5.2 ± 2.6 and mean flow rate of 4.7 ± 1.5 L/min. IVUS imaging exhibited full opening and closing of the pericardial leaflets in all valves. Mild paravalvular leakage was observed in 2/12 valved stents. No valved stent migration occurred inside the silicon valved stent chamber.

In Vivo Study

ICE measurements revealed aortic diameter 23.0 ± 2.2 mm, valve area 3.76 ± 1.3 cm^2, height of the native leaflets 11.4 ± 2.4 mm, depth of the coronary sinuses

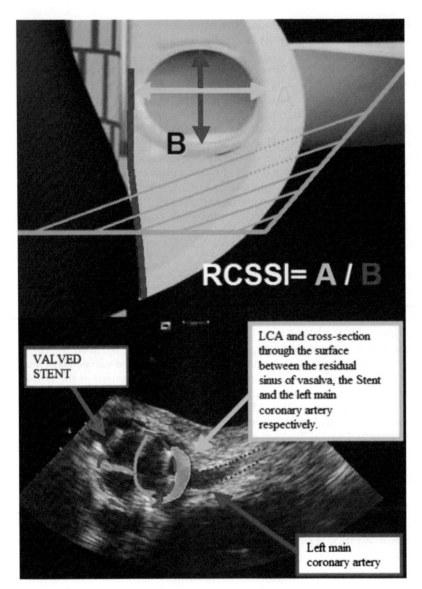

FIGURE 11 Aortic root reconstruction illustration. The RCSSI and aortic DAVR valved stent implantation as seen by two-dimensional ICE. *Abbreviation*: RCSSI, Residual Coronary Sinus Stent Index.

of Valsalva 4.2 ± 1.3 mm, height of the sinus portion 14.6 ± 1.7 mm, and diameter at the sinotubular junction 25.2 ± 2.8 mm. Eight of twelve implanted valved stents were delivered accurately. Two were deployed in supraannular position and occluded the RCA. Another two dislodged into the LV, one because of size mismatch and the other because of failure to fully deploy.

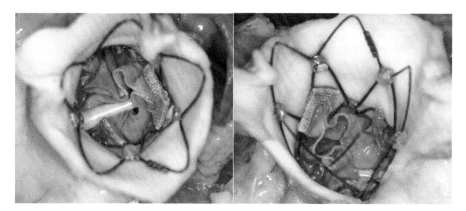

FIGURE 12   Postmortem implantation shows fully deployed and precisely placed valved stent. The catheters show the coronary orifice, free of any obstruction.

ICE demonstrated good leaflet motion, with full valvular opening and closing in all correctly delivered, deployed, and sized valved stents. The overall planimetric valve orifice area was 2.6 ± 0.8 cm^2. Of the eight correctly deployed valved stents, one had mild-to-moderate paravalvular leakage because of size mismatch and one exhibited mild regurgitation. All eight valved stents had a low transvalvular gradient of 5.3 ± 3.9 mm Hg (mean, peak-to-peak) on invasive measurement and 5.6 ± 4.7 mm Hg on noninvasive measurement. Continuous cardiac output remained stable (5.2 ± 0.6 L/min valved stent 4.7 ± 0.4 L/min) for the eight correctly delivered valved stents. Intracardiac color Doppler imaging revealed laminar blood flow.

Procedure time was typically 120 minutes (range, 90–180 minutes) and duration of delivery and deployment was 4 to 6 minutes. The postimplantation CBF pattern using ICE color Doppler and M-mode (Fig. 13) indicated no signs of CBF impairment in the valved stents deployed exactly on target. RCSSI was obtained to evaluate potential flow impairment in the left coronary artery (Fig. 11). The mean distance between the coronary orifice and aortic wall was 8.1 ± 2.4 mm and the mean diameter of the left coronary artery was 5.7 ± 1.2 mm, yielding an RCSSI value of 1.6 ± 0.5. The postimplantation observation period was 4.5 ± 1.8 hours. Postmortem examination (Fig. 12) confirmed that $8/12$ valved stents were correctly positioned and firmly anchored to the aortic wall. No implants showed signs of coronary obstruction. Necropsy confirmed that the two supraannular deployments occluded the RCA. The two dislodged valved stents were found in the LV. Macroscopic analysis provided no evidence of damage to the aortic wall, signs of dissection, or hematoma. Eight valved stents were structurally sound. All were thrombus-free.

Promising Results of Aortic DAVR

The acute animal study confirms that antegrade direct access orthotopic aortic valve implantation via the LV apex is feasible. Recent reports show promising results with remote access percutaneous antegrade and retrograde valved stent implantation in the pulmonary or aortic position in selected patients (4,6,14) However, the remote access technique is not a viable alternative to surgical AVR,

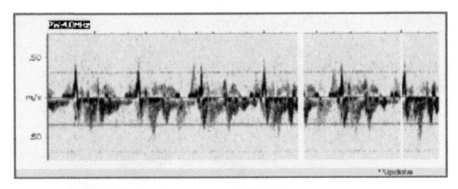

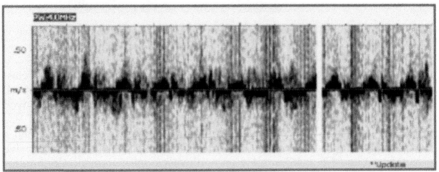

FIGURE 13 Postimplantation coronary blood flow pattern as assessed with ICE color Doppler and M-mode.

for example, it will not allow prior diseased valve removal as might be feasible by the TAP. Innovative surgical techniques are becoming increasingly less invasive (27). These innovations are likely to improve measurable parameters such as patient outcome, length of hospital stay, and perioperative mortality and morbidity, but more data are needed to establish their true benefits.

Development of an off-pump surgical AVR technique began at the laboratory of the Centre Hospitalier Universitaire Vaudois, Lausanne, in 1999. The author's early experience with direct RV access for antegrade pulmonary valved stent implantation reinforced his research project to develop an analog procedure for the left heart. The advantages of direct access via the LV apex DAVR-TAP include avoidance of the cardiopulmonary circulation, antegrade less traumatic aortic valve crossing, decreased distance to the target site, and ability to deliver larger devices for valve removal as well as bidirectional guidewire stabilization and access. Design features for optimal implantation or replacement of the aortic valve include the following:

- Antegrade access through the LV apex
- A delivery system with directional guidance to eliminate the risk of coronary orifice obstruction
- A mechanism for reloading malpositioned valved stents

Intracardiac echo in combination with fluoroscopy can locate the level of deployment with precision, but is not sufficient to monitor rotation of the device within the aorta before deployment. Currently, we are developing a radioopaque marker for the delivery envelope that contains the collapsed valved stent.

Four of twelve valved stents were incorrectly placed at necropsy. Two dislodged, one because of failure to fully expand attributed to difficulties in collapsing and loading the device into the delivery system and the other because an undersized valved stent was used in a larger than anticipated aortic root. Both animals remained stable during the operation, but all attempts to recover or reposition the device without going on pump failed. Only one valved stent dislodged after it was initially correctly placed. Similar difficulties have been described (23,28). Two valved stents were deployed in a supraannular position and occluded the RCA.

No interference with CBF was found in correctly placed and deployed devices. Previous studies lack data on postimplantation CBF secondary to interference from echodense stent struts. ICE eliminated much of this interference in the present study, permitting reliable postimplantation CBF analysis. The RCSSI was a useful indicator for absence of CBF flow interference for all index values >1. In the eight valved stents, the mean RCSSI values was 1.6 ± 0.5. Moreover, leaving the native leaflets in place did not cause coronary ostia obstruction. These findings conflict with other published data (20) that demonstrate a high failure rate with valved stent implants in the annular aortic position (orthotopic) consequent to flow restriction caused by the native leaflets.

Further measures to ensure the safety of valved stent aortic valve implantation and replacement include the development of embolic devices to protect the coronary orifices and aortic arch, similar to the devices used for percutaneous carotid endarterectomy or the aortic filter cannulae used in cardiac surgery. Specialized tools for remote decalcification and tissue removal are also needed. Several have been proposed, such as, laser ablation, ablation chambers, or cutting catheters, but experimental data are lacking to support their feasibility. A temporary valve to support LV function during the removal/replacement interval and to overcome increased afterload caused by embolic filters and intraaortic tools used for decalcification will also be required. Previous publications have proposed valve-tipped catheters as a temporary solution. LV-assist devices placed in the LV outflow tract, such as the Impella VAD catheter, might also work.

The necessity of placing valved stents in patients with heavily calcified aortic valves calls for new strategies and techniques such as the proposed by the direct access approach via TAP. These experimental data demonstrate that direct access antegrade off-pump aortic valved stent implantation through the LV apex is feasible in animals with normal, noncalcified leaflets. The absence of CBF impairment or mitral valve hindrance in properly placed and sized devices makes the direct access valved stent a promising new technology.

Entering the Era of Percutaneous Valve Therapies and Future Clinical Applications

The recent achievements in interventional cardiology and ingenious new devices are opening the gate to an exciting new field of percutaneous valve therapies including the aortic, pulmonary, and the mitral valves. At the same time, enormous progress has been made in cardiac surgery. Innovative surgical techniques are less and less invasive, as they are being carried out through smaller incisions (26,29–32) endoscopically (33) or being assisted by robotics (34,35). This is likely to further increase patient outcome, shorten hospital stay, and decrease peri- as well as postoperative mortality and morbidity, but only more data will show true patients benefits. Despite all mentioned breakthroughs, undergoing surgical aortic valve replacement remains a major trauma for the patients associated with a large number of risks.

Percutaneous aortic valve procedures have been burdened with considerable difficulties. The complex aortic root configuration generates the need for more sophisticated technologies with self-orienting valved stents and safe anchoring yet atraumatic implantation into the aortic annulus. Removal of the often highly calcified and stenotic aortic valve needs ingenious combined use of support and embolic protection devices to increase patient safety. Joining transcatheter-based principles (36,37) of interventional cardiology with the advantages of surgical keyhole access (Fig. 5) might be the right approach to the aortic and the mitral valves.

DAVR decreases the working distance from remote access to "surgical dimensions" and allows working in close proximity to the aortic target location. Furthermore, DAVR offers enormous advantages to permit simultaneous insertion of decalcification or valve removal tools, embolic protection, and ventricular-assist devices as well as bigger-sized delivery systems and joins all the advantages of a transcatheter-based percutaneous approach.

A Bright Future for DAVR

Many obstacles in percutaneous valve replacement still remain asking for new answers. Only new ingenious approaches merging surgical and interventional advantages and novel technologies will overcome the current shortcomings (10). Experimental and clinical studies have shown that percutaneous aortic valve implantation is feasible and well tolerated by the patients. These early results are very encouraging to further pursue and develop valved stent–based techniques.

DAVR for the treatment of aortic valve disease unites major advantages of a transcatheter and of a surgical approach and might offer the potential to increased patient's safety and compete with the current gold standard—the surgical aortic valve replacement. In the future, aortic DAVR via TAP might become the therapy of choice for aortic valve replacement.

REFERENCES

1. Huber CH, Goeber V, Berdat P, et al. Benefits of cardiac surgery in octogenarians—A postoperative quality of life assessment [published online ahead of print March 19, 2007]. Eur J Cardiothorac Surg 2007; 31(6):1099–1105.
2. Andersen HR, Knudsen LL, Hasenkam JM. Transluminal implantation of artificial heart valves. Description of a new expandable aortic valve and initial results with implantation by catheter technique in closed chest pigs. Eur Heart J 1992; 13(5):704–708.
3. Omran H, Schmidt H, Hackenbroch M, et al. Silent and apparent cerebral embolism after retrograde catheterisation of the aortic valve in valvular stenosis: A prospective, randomised study. Lancet 2003; 361(9365):1241–1246.

4. Cribier A, Eltchaninoff H, Tron C, et al. Treatment of calcific aortic stenosis with the percutaneous heart valve: Mid-term follow-up from the initial feasibility studies: The French experience. J Am Coll Cardiol 2006; 47(6):1214–1223.
5. Grube E, Schuler G, Buellesfeld L, et al. Percutaneous aortic valve replacement for severe aortic stenosis in high-risk patients using the second- and current third-generation self-expanding CoreValve prosthesis: Device success and 30-day clinical outcome. J Am Coll Cardiol 2007; 50(1):69–76.
6. Walther T, Falk V, Borger MA, et al. Minimally invasive transapical beating heart aortic valve implantation—Proof of concept. Eur J Cardiothorac Surg 2007; 31:9–15.
7. Fish R. Percutaneous heart valve replacement: Enthusiasm tempered. Circulation 2004; 110:1876–1878.
8. Cribier A, Eltchaninoff H, Tron C, et al. Early experience with percutaneous transcatheter implantation of heart valve prosthesis for the treatment of end-stage inoperable patients with calcific aortic stenosis. J Am Coll Cardiol 2004; 43: 698–703.
9. Huber CH, Nasratulla M, Augstburger M, et al. New tools for new goals: Ultrasound navigation through the heart for off pump aortic valved stent implantation. J Endovasc Ther 2004; 11(4):503–510.
10. Huber CH, Cohn LH, von Segesser LK. Direct-access valve replacement a novel approach for off-pump implantation using valved stents. J Am Coll Cardiol 2005; 46:366–370.
11. Huber CH, von Segesser LK. Direct access valve replacement. Intervent Cardiol Mon 2005; 12(2):29–34.
12. Ma L, Huber CH, Taub S, et al. Double-crowned valved stents for off-pump mitral valve replacement. Eur J Cardiothorac Surg 2005; 28:194–199.
13. Palacios IF. Percutaneous valve replacement and repair: Fiction or reality? J Am Coll Cardiol 2004; 44(8):1662–1663.
14. Hijazi ZM. Transcatheter valve replacement: A new era of percutaneous cardiac intervention begins. J Am Coll Cardiol 2004; 43(6):1088–1089.
15. von Segesser LK. Direct percutaneous valve replacement: The next step? Eur J Cardiothorac Surg 2004; 26(5):873–874.
16. van Herwerden LA, Serruys PW. Percutaneous valve implantation: Back to the future? Eur Heart J 2002; 23(18):1415–1416.
17. Pavcnik D, Wright KC, Wallace S. Development and initial experimental evaluation of a prosthetic aortic valve for transcatheter placement: Work in progress. Radiology 1992; 183:151–154.
18. Sochman J, Peregrin JH, Pavcnik D, et al. Percutaneous transcatheter aortic disc valve prosthesis implantation: A feasibility study. Cardiovasc Intervent Radiol 2000; 23(5):384–388.
19. Bonhoeffer P, Boudjemline Y, Saliba Z, et al. Percutaneous replacement of pulmonary valve in a right-ventricle to pulmonary-artery prosthetic conduit with valve dysfunction. Lancet 2000; 356(9239):1403–1405.
20. Cribier A, Eltchaninoff H, Bash A, et al. Percutaneous transcatheter implantation of an aortic valve prosthesis for calcific aortic stenosis: First human case description. Circulation 2002; 106(24):3006–3008.
21. Zhou JQ, Corno AF, Huber CH, et al. Self-expandable valved stent of large size: Off-bypass implantation in pulmonary position. Eur J Cardiothorac Surg 2003; 24(2):212–216.
22. Huber CH, Tozzi P, Corno AF, et al. Do valved stents compromise coronary flow? Eur J Cardiothorac Surg 2004; 25(5):754–759.
23. Lutter G, Kuklinski D, Berg G, et al. Percutaneous aortic valve replacement: An experimental study. I. Studies on implantation. J Thorac Cardiovasc Surg 2002; 123(4):768–776.
24. Quaden R, Attmann T, Schünke M, et al. Percutaneous aortic valve replacement: Endovascular resection of human aortic valves in situ. J Thorac Cardiovasc Surg 2008; 135(5):1081–1086.

25. von Segesser LK, Marty B, Ruchat P, et al. Routine use of intravascular ultrasound for endovascular aneurysm repair: Angiography is not necessary. Eur J Vasc Endovasc Surg 2002; 23:537–542.
26. Guide for the Care and Use of Laboratory Animals. Institute of Laboratory Animal Research, Commission on Life Sciences, National Research Council. 140p. 1996.
27. Yacoub MH, Cohn LH. Novel approaches to cardiac valve repair: From structure to function: Part II. Circulation 2004; 109:1064–1072.
28. Boudjemline Y, Bonhoeffer P. Steps toward percutaneous aortic valve replacement. Circulation 2002; 105:775–778.
29. Cohn LH, Adams DH, Couper GS, et al. Minimally invasive cardiac valve surgery improves patient satisfaction while reducing costs of cardiac valve replacement and repair. Ann Surg 1997; 226(4):421–426, discussion 427–428.
30. Byrne JG, Karavas AN, Cohn LH, et al. Minimal access aortic root, valve, and complex ascending aortic surgery. Curr Cardiol Rep 2000; 2(6):549–557.
31. Sharony R, Grossi EA, Saunders PC, et al. Minimally invasive aortic valve surgery in the elderly: A case-control study. Circulation 2003; 108(suppl):II43–II47.
32. Gillinov AM, Cosgrove DM. Minimally invasive mitral valve surgery: Mini-sternotomy with extended transseptal approach. Semin Thorac Cardiovasc Surg 1999; 11(3):206–211.
33. Casselman FP, Van Slycke S, Dom H, et al. Endoscopic mitral valve repair: Feasible, reproducible, and durable. J Thorac Cardiovasc Surg 2003; 125(2):273–282.
34. Kypson AP, Nifong LW, Chitwood WR Jr. Robotic mitral valve surgery. Semin Thorac Cardiovasc Surg 2003; 15(2):121–129.
35. Mohr FW, Falk V, Diegeler A, et al. Computer-enhanced "robotic" cardiac surgery: Experience in 148 patients. J Thorac Cardiovasc Surg 2001; 121(5):842–853.
36. Liddicoat JR, Mac Neill BD, Gillinov AM, et al. Percutaneous mitral valve repair: A feasibility study in an ovine model of acute ischemic mitral regurgitation. Catheter Cardiovasc Interv 2003; 60:410–416.
37. St. Goar FG, Fann JI, Komtebedde J, et al. Endovascular edge-to-edge mitral valve. repair: Short-term results in a porcine model. Circulation 2003; 108:1990–1993.

7 Device-Related Insights into the Aortic Root Anatomy

The author has initiated two studies analyzing the native and diseased aortic root in regard to valved stents or aortic root devices. The first is a transesophageal study comparing disease-induced changes in aortic root geometry in 48 cardiac surgery patients and the latter is a multislice computer tomography (CT) pilot study coauthored by the author.

ECHOGRAPHIC INSIGHTS FROM THE AORTIC ROOT IN REGARD OF TRANSCATHETER VALVE THERAPIES

Introduction
Several aortic valved stent designs have been proposed; the majority is still under experimental investigation for suitability and only two early valved stent designs have reached the state of controlled clinical application. Nevertheless, none of the valved stents have been designed to explicitly fit the complex aortic root anatomy.

Hardly any device-specific data on the aortic root are available, but knowledge and functional understanding of the aortic root anatomy are essential for the design of an aortic valve device. This study analyzes the aortic valve and root geometry in regard of an optimized valved stent design to improve function, sealing, and anchoring of the device.

Technical Considerations
In a prospective study of a total of 48 patients undergoing either coronary artery bypass graft surgery (CABG) with a normal aortic valve or undergoing aortic valve replacement (AVR) for aortic stenosis, extensive transoesophageal echographic measures were taken. The aim of the study was to assess normal aortic root dimensions and compare the data with the geometry of aortic root exposed to stenotic aortic valves. These data were then integrated into aortic valve device design considerations to improve and refine the current device concepts.

The measures included aortic–annular diameter, the maximum depth of each sinus pouch, the diameter of the coronary orifices, the diameter at the sinotubular junction (STJ), the intercommissural distances (ICDs), the aortic diameter at the crossing with the pulmonary artery, the length of aortic leaflets, the heights of the right coronary (RC) orifices, and the height of STJ and the length of the ascending aorta (depending on the echographic window). The body mass index (BMI) was calculated from the collected length and weight data. The body surface area (BSA) was calculated based on the Mosteller formula.

Statistical Analysis
Data were analyzed with GraphPad Prism (version 3.02). Data are presented as absolute numbers, mean ± standard deviation or percentages where appropriate. Where adequate, dimensional data are expressed as mean ±1 SD for the CABG patients followed by the AVR patients and separated by the backslash sign. If significance is reached ($p < 0.05$), the data are followed by the p value in brackets. Nonparametric analysis of variance was performed using the Mann-Whitney test.

Results
In 48 consecutive patients aged 65.0 ± 13.6 years undergoing either CABG or AVR for isolated coronary artery disease or isolated stenotic aortic valve disease respectively, extensive echographic measures were taken. The patient population split into 24 CABG patients with native aortic roots and 24 AVR patients with diseased aortic valves, and included 26 male patients and 16 female patients. The average age, weight and length, as well as BMI and BSA of the male patients was 62.4 ± 14.0 years, 77.7 ± 15.7 kg for 173.3 ± 7.7 cm, 26.0 ± 5.6 kg/m^2, and 1.93 ± 0.21 m^2. For the female patients, age was 72.3 ± 9.5 years, weight 71.3 ± 20.3 kg for 163.1 ± 6.9 cm, and BMI was 26.8 ± 7.9 kg/m^2 with a BSA of 1.78 ± 0.21 m^2. For further preoperative variables, see Table 1.

Transverse Dimensions
The diameter of the aortic root at the level of the aortic annulus measured 22.6 ± 2.0 mm/23.5 ± 3.3 mm. At the sinotubular level, the transverse diameter increases by close to 12% to 26.0 ± 2.7 mm/28.2 ± 0.7 mm. At the level of the pulmonary artery, crossing the aorta measures 31.4 ± 4.6 mm/33.8 ± 7.8 mm (Fig. 1).

The Sinus Portion
Systolic measures in both groups revealed very little variation of the ICD. The RC ICD measures 23.4 ± 2.5 mm/24.2 ± 1.4 mm compared to the noncoronary

TABLE 1 Preoperative Patient Characteristics

	No. of patients (%)		
Variables	All ($n = 48$)	CABG ($n = 24$)	AVR ($n = 24$)
Males	26 (61)	14 (58)	12 (50)
Age	65.0 ± 13.6	65.3 ± 11.3	64.8 ± 16.3
NYHA or CCS ≥ III	12 (27)	5 (21)	7 (29)
Hypertension	32 (76)	17 (71)	15 (63)
Creatinine ≥ 120 μmol/L	7 (17)	5 (20)	2 (8)
Tobacco abuse	22 (52)	12 (50)	10 (42)
Weight (kg)	75.6 ± 17.3	73.2 ± 14.7	78.3 ± 19.8
Length (cm)	169.9 ± 8.8	168.8 ± 6.2	171.3 ± 11.2
BMI (kg/m^2)	26.3 ± 6.4	25.8 ± 5.6	26.8 ± 7.3
BSA (m^2)	1.9 ± 0.2	1.8 ± 0.2	1.9 ± 0.3

Abbreviations: NYHA, New York Hear Association; CCS, Canadian Cardiovascular Society; BMI, body mass index; BSA, body surface area.

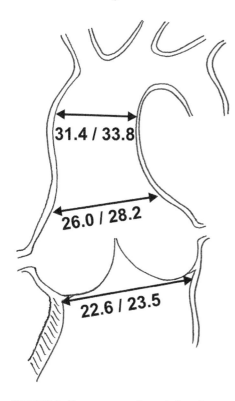

FIGURE 1 Transverse aortic root diameters.

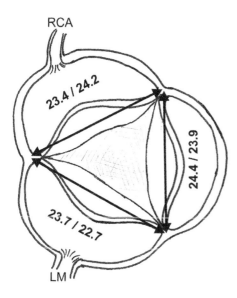

FIGURE 2 Intercommissural distance in systole.

(NC) ICD with 24.4 ± 2.5 mm/23.9 ± 3.9 mm and to the left coronary (LC) ICD of 23.7 ± 1.7 mm/22.7 ± 3.2 mm dimension (Fig. 2). In contrast, the ICD varies more in diastolic measures of the patients undergoing AVR (Fig. 3). The RC ICD dimensions are 24.5 ± 2.6/27.0 ± 4.6 compared to the NC ICD 23.6 ± 2.1/26.3 ± 4.6 and to the LC ICD 23.2 ± 2.8/24.7 ± 3.3.

A similar pattern can be identifiable regarding the depths of the sinus pouches. While hardly variable during systole and diastole in the CABG group, measurements showed a more pronounced variation from each sinus pouch relative to the heart cycle in the AVR group. In systole, the sinus depth from a constructed line of the ICD (Fig. 4) measured as follows: RC sinus 10.9 ± 2.4 mm/9.3 ± 1.5 mm, NC sinus 10.4 ± 1.0 mm/ 10.6 ± 3.3 mm, and LC sinus 10.8 ± 1.1 mm/8.3 ± 1.0 mm. In early diastole, all sinus pouches increased with a maximum depth for the RC sinus of 11.1 ± 2.2 mm/10.2 ± 0.6, an NC sinus depth of 11.7 ± 2.0 mm/12.5 ± 2.4 mm, and LC sinus of 11.0 ± 2.2 mm/9.1 ± 1.4 mm (Fig. 5).

Coronary artery bypass patients showed a more important decrease of the intercommissural sinus area (ICSA) compared to AVR patients during the heart cycle. In systole, the RC-ICSA measured 14.9 ± 6.0 mm^2/16.2 ± 3.9 mm^2, the NC-ICSA measured 14.7 ± 4.7 mm^2/19.0 ± 4.9 mm^2 and the LM-ICSA measured 16.3 ± 5.4 mm^2/18.1 ± 4.7 mm^2. In contrast, during diastole, the RC-ICSA was calculated at 19.3 ± 4.6 mm^2/18.3 ± 4.1 mm^2, the NC-ICSA at 18.9 ± 4.6 mm^2/19.4 ± 6.0 mm^2 and the LC-ICSA at 20.0 ± 3.3 mm^2/18.3 ± 3.5 mm^2 (Fig. 6). No such pattern could be found for the sinus surface circumference (SSC). But in the AVR group, all SSC decreased from systole to diastole, while in the CABG group only the RC-SSC decreased from systole to diastole in both groups from 58.5 ± 8.4 mm/57.7 ± 4.0 mm to 57.2 ± 8.7 mm/51.6 ± 46.7 mm (Fig. 7).

Coronary Measures

The left main artery ostium is significantly larger ($p < 0.001$) than the RC offspring measuring 4.1 ± 0.9 mm /4.3 ± 1.3 versus 3.0 ± 0.9 mm/2.8 ± 0.7 mm respectively.

Axial Measures

The STJ is defined by the highest point of the three commissures. For technical reasons, the RC and the NC only were assessed. There is a more pronounced difference in the height of the RCA sinus compared to the noncoronary sinus in the nondiseased aortic root. The STJ of the RC sinus levels at 21.5 ± 3.9 mm/22.3 ± 6.2 mm from the aortic valve. The NC sinus height is slightly lower, elevating 20.4 ± 3.9 mm/22.0 ± 4.6 mm above the valvular plane.

The RCA orifice originates 16.2 ± 3.1 mm/16.6 ± 4.8 mm above the annulus. The LC height could not be measured because of technical limitations. During systole, the aortic valve leaflets stretched over 68% in CABG patients, but reached higher in the AVR groups to overlap 71% to 74% for the right and the noncoronary sinuses respectively and therefore remaining 2 mm underneath the RCA ostium. The RC leaflet height reached 14.7 ± 2.6 mm/14.9 ± 3.7 mm compared to the noncoronary leaflet reaching 13.9 ± 2.8 mm/15.6 ± 5.3 mm. Finally, the length of the ascending aorta at the level with the pulmonary artery crossing is 48.7 ± 6.4 mm/ 53.8 ± 14.6 mm (Fig. 8).

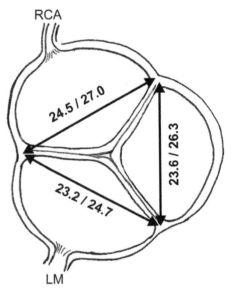

FIGURE 3 Intercommissural distance in diastole.

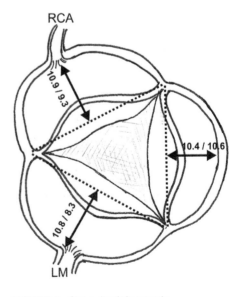

FIGURE 4 Sinus depth in systole.

Discussion

Innovative transcatheter valve therapies are challenging the current concept of surgical valve repair or replacement. A growing number of patients undergo investigation for suitability of transcatheter valve treatment. Nevertheless, indications are still few and limited to specific anatomical considerations.

In contrast to the open surgical approach, endoluminal techniques very much rely on the device on one hand and the anatomopathological setting on the other. Restricted by the narrow entry site and limited by a defined endovascular pathway, interventions within the cardiovascular system represent a trade-off, negotiating the benefits of the least invasive technique with the limitations of the device to target site interaction. The better adapted the device is to the landing zone, the better it will perform its function. The first step toward improved outcomes might be a detailed description of the aortic root anatomy in regard to transcatheter-aided AVR.

As a matter of fact, the early enthusiasm of endoluminal aortic aneurismal techniques (1) quickly tempered because of the growing evidence that this promising new treatment modality was limited to benefit fewer patients than expected. Anatomical characteristics like a short aneurismal neck or various aortic configurations including strongly kinked pre-/postaneurismal landing zones or tortuous and highly calcified access vessels restricted its use and downscaled the wide applicability (2).

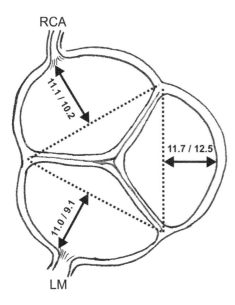

FIGURE 5   Sinus depth in diastole.

The striking familiarity of aortic valve transcatheter therapies and endovascular aortic repair suggests that similar limitation might appear on the horizon. Therefore, careful consideration should be given to the aortic valve and root configuration to determine device specifications and predict horizontal penetration.

The complex aortic root is composed by the fibrous structure of the aortic annulus, the aortic cusps, the aortic sinuses, and the coronaries orifices. The aortic root lies between the left ventricle in continuity with the anterior mitral leaflet proximally and the ascending aorta linked by the STJ distally. Above the STJ extents the ascending aorta and becomes the aortic arch after branching off the brachiocephalic artery. The aortic valve is wedged between the pulmonary, the mitral, and the tricuspid valves and forms "the centrepiece of the heart" (3). All chambers of the heart relate to the aortic valve. In contrast to the pulmonary leaflets, supported by the subpulmonary infundibular portion of the right ventricle, the aortic leaflets are only partially sustained by the muscular part of the left ventricle. The aortic leaflets are attached in a trisegment semilunar or coronet fashion within the barrel-shaped aortic root. Each of the commissures is forming the lateral boarders of the three sinus pouches. One of the pouches contains the LC and one the RC orifice—altogether an anatomically and functionally complex structure that has recently become the main target for transcatheter therapies.

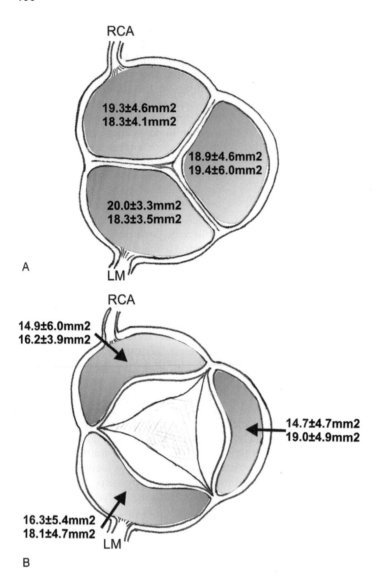

FIGURE 6 Sinus surface in systole and diastole.

Surprisingly, few in vivo studies have aimed at establishing a normative aortic root database and none has specifically looked at device-related character-istics in relation to calcified aortic stenosis.

Imaging modalities included x-ray–based angiographic assessment (4,5) requiring an invasive approach and are largely limited by summation images dependent of the chosen projection leading to overlapping and possibly geomet-rical distortion (6). A further x-ray–based technique is CT. Previous studies by

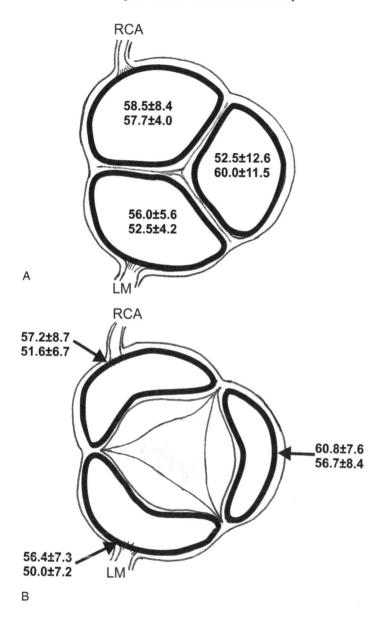

FIGURE 7 Sinus circumference in systole and diastole.

nongated CT in adults provided some normative insights (7,8) but precise measurements are hampered by frequent motion artifacts.

High-resolution ECG-gated tomography offering better temporal resolution compared to nongated CT has become widely available and some device-related studies are currently on their way.

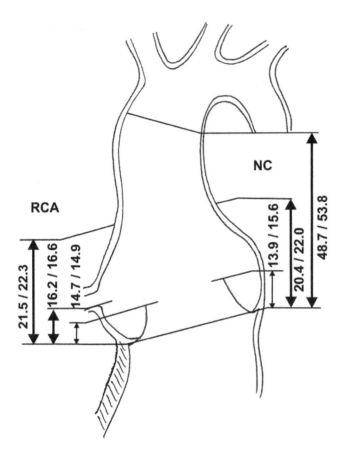

FIGURE 8 Axial aortic root measures.

Cardiac magnetic resonance angiography requires fast acquisition protocols like echoplanar imaging offering sufficient imaging quality versus acquisition times. But ghosting and geometrical distortion artefacts might result (9) and require multistep postprocessing reconstructions. Stronger magnetical fields partially overcome those technical limitations but create new ones based on the magnetohydrodynamic effect that is deflecting the polarized blood particles and creates parasiting potentials interfering with the ECG triggering (10). Only few magnetic resonance imaging aortic dimensional data exist (11).

Echo-based imaging modalities have studied the aortic root in regard to either surgical techniques focusing on aortic valve sparing techniques (12) or disease progression (13). Some data were also obtained from transthoracic echographic measures in children and the young adults (14) but lack image quality in adult patients and more so in calcified root by interfering with the echo pattern. Transesophageal echocardiography results in a much improved image quality allowing millimetric measurements. Although readily available, echographic studies are certainly not exempt of limitations. Image acquisition and interpretation is highly operator-dependent (15) and echodense calcifications might interfere with precise visualization. Further structural artifacts can appear from atrio–aortic interface and can cause false-positive findings as seen in diagnosing aortic dissection (16).

To the authors best knowledge, no previous study aimed at obtaining device-related aortic root and valve dimensional data comparing calcified and native aortic root anatomy.

Only limited data allow direct comparison as variables were assessed differently aiming at other questions. For example, one ex vivo study (17) showed overall smaller-dimensional data. The reasons for this difference might be threefold. First, the absence of hydrodynamic parameters in the cadaver studies, second, the postmortem diminution of tissue elasticity and decreased water content leading to a possible shrinking of the anatomic structures, and finally, the impact of tissue fixation processes on tissue characteristics.

In the linear regression analysis, the age became the most impacting factor on the aortic root geometry in AVR patients. A significant correlation was found between age and the annular diameter ($p = 0.005$), the diameter at the STJ ($p < 0.0001$), the ICD ($p = 0.002$–0.004), as well as the depth of the non- and RC sinus. In the same patient population, further significance was reached for height correlating with the aortic annulus ($p < 0.001$), the non- ($p = 0.005$) and RC sinus height ($p = 0.01$) as well as the height of the RCA ($p = 0.001$). A weak correlation was also identified between height and the systolic residual sinus depth for the NC ($p = 0.01$), LC ($p < 0.05$), and RC sinus ($p = 0.003$).

In the CABG population, these study results are very much in concordance with previous echographic studies where the measured parameters were independent of body weight, BMI, BSA, gender, and age. In particular, there is no dependence on body height in this older patient population in contrast to that in children and younger adults (12,18).

Implications for Transcatheter Aortic Valve Therapies

The central question is how many of the patients present a suitable aortic root configuration to allow for a transcatheter AVR and how large is the interindividual anatomic variability. Normative measures as well as measures of calcified aortic root configurations will provide the answer if rather the "one size fits all" rule applies or individual device construction becomes necessary. Regarding the valved stent design specifications, the critical aortic root in vivo dimensions are the diameter at the lowest portion of the semilunar hinges (equivalent to aortic annulus), the depth of the three sinus pouches, the diameter of the coronary orifices (19), the ICD, the diameter of the STJ, and the aortic diameter proximal to the brachiocephalic artery. In longitudinal arrangement, the key measures in relation to the aortic annulus are the heights of each of the coronary orifices, the length of aortic leaflets and the minimal heights of the sinus pouches as described by the height of the STJ, and finally the length of the ascending aorta.

The ideal valved stent anchors firmly to the supporting aortic root and creates an effective circumferential seal with stable valve suspension avoiding any coronary or hemodynamic interference. Anchoring and sealing go hand in hand as both functions are dependent upon contact with the native aortic wall. The lower the stent profile, the lower the risk for coronary interference but the higher the risk of axial misalignment and of perivalvular leek because of limited overlap of the device sealing zone and the irregular and calcified landing zone.

Designing a second anchor portion lying at or above the STJ portion presents two advantages: first, the axial stability is increased and the axial alignment is optimized; second, a more powerful sealing could result from topographically uncoupling both functions on the device.

Correlating these engineering reflexions with the obtained results leads to a device height of at least 22 to 23 mm with a possible optimum between 25 and 35 mm (21.5 ± 3.9 mm/22.3 ± 6.2 mm STJ height from the aortic valve). Also take into account, the longer the device, the more complex a future open procedure might become.

The proximal device diameter should measure at least 24 mm (aortic annulus transverse diameter 22.6 ± 2.0 mm/23.5 ± 3.3 mm) and considering the need for oversizing a proximal diameter of 25 to 26 mm becomes more appropriate. The distal device diameter increases as does the aortic root (26.0 ± 2.7 mm/28.2 ± 0.7). A distal diameter of more than 34 to 35 mm should allow for firm anchoring above the STJ where calcifications are less frequently encountered.

To allow a tight sealing, a synthetic or biological cuff at the annular stent level could be of use. The resulting increased device diameter in crimped state by the extra material might be overcome by choosing the transapical procedure allowing delivery device diameter of more than 33F (20) rather than the remote retrograde transfemoral approach requiring a highly flexible and tighter crimped device.

Motion and stress forces are known to be higher in the ascending aorta compared to the abdominal aorta segments (21). Previous reports have indicated diameter variations of the ascending aorta during the cardiac cycle ranging from 8% to 20%, which is in line with this. Such mechanical constraints may impact stent migration or paravalvular leaks (22), even more so in the presence of the remaining diseased aortic valve hindering an equal and smooth overlap between the stent and the aortic root wall. Because of the absence of aortic wall stiffening calcifications, coronary artery bypass patients showed typically a more important decrease of the ICSA compared to AVR patients during the heart cycle. This diminished wall compliance might be a favoring situation to decrease pulsatile-induced device migration. Additionally, on the device design side, two solutions might address this issue: first, radial oversizing by 10% to 20% above the aortic root diameters, a lesson learned from endovascular aneurysm stenting and from clinical experience with the current two aortic valved stent and second, memory-alloy–supported elastic radial expansion of the carrier stent to allow continual compliance with the vessel wall motion.

Reviewing device sizing four device diameters might provide sufficient support to fit 94% of the patients. An arbitrary classification of the 48 patients into device-adapted subgroups identified 45 patients (94%) being effectively treated with one of the four device sizes (Table 2).

Of greatest interest is the stent segment positioned within the sinus portion. One major challenge is providing continuity between suprasinusal and infrasinusal anchoring segments without interfering with the coronary flow but providing enough stability for long-term valve suspension. Linking struts might overcome this difficulty but are exposed to enormous pulsatile radial expansion stress in what might lead future to stent fractures. Another solution could be

TABLE 2 Arbitrary Patient Grouping Relating Two of the Smallest Number of Necessary Device Diameters to Fit the Greatest Patient Percentage Respecting the 10% to 20% Device Oversizing Rule

Aortic annular diameter	n	%	Device diameter	% Oversizing
<19 mm	1	2	none	
19–20 mm	6	6	22 mm	16–10
21–22 mm	11	23	24 mm	14–10
23–24 mm	20	42	27 mm	17–13
25–27 mm	8	17	30 mm	20–11
>27 mm	2	4	none	

to take advantage of the sinus portion to provide further support of the linking elements. Both attempts largely avoid direct overstenting of the coronaries—a probable troublemaker in the long run.

Finally, one question remains little explored—How does valved stent device interfere with coronary flow? In a previous work, the authors presented experimental results where no interference on the coronary flow pattern was identified using intracardiac echo Doppler for flow analysis (19). Of uppermost concern is the risk of coronary obstruction by remnants of the diseased valve. Reviewing the obtained data suggests the RC ostia originate approximately 10% above the RC-leaflet tip in both patient groups, a surprising result as one would believe that the leaflet excursion becomes typically reduced by the stenotic process. This implies that the stenotic disease does not reduce the risk for coronary occlusion by device compression of the valve leaflet against the aortic wall and the coronary ostia consecutively. To prevent device-related coronary occlusion, pre- and periprocedural assessments should include active measurements of the coronary ostia height as well as the leaflet mobility and length.

NORMATIVE VALUES OF THE ASCENDING AORTA FROM A CT PERSPECTIVE

Introduction

Historically, treatment of abdominal aortic aneurysms has been based on surgical repair until the 1990s (23–25). Since then, endovascular graft systems has been widely recognized and used for abdominal aortic aneurysms repair (EVAR) (26). The lack of off-the-shelf endografts warrants precise prepoperative imaging to define adequate device selection. Therefore, more and more importance has been placed on pre- and postoperative CT imaging protocols for the planning of endovascular abdominal aortic aneurysms (27).

With the advent of endovascular aneurysm repair and valve replacement, more focus is now turned to ascending aorta and aortic arch pathologies (28,29). Experience with endograft for ascending aortic disease is scarce because few groups are using such devices because of technological restriction. On one hand, the caseload being lesser for ascending aorta endoluminal procedures limits the device evolution, and on the other hand the large diameter and the curvature of ascending aorta and aortic arch render difficult the access to these vascular portions and the introduction, placement, tracking, and deployment of the graft, thus challenging device engineering. Blood flow in the coronary arteries and the supraaortic arteries should also be maintained by means of different fenestrated technologies and surgical bypasses depending on the graft landing zone (30,31). All these anatomical and technical constraints make precise knowledge of normal ascending aorta and aortic arch morphology mandatory.

Although normative thoracic aortic dimensions have already been determined by means of standard CT angiography (7,8,32,33), to the authors knowledge no exhaustive measurements have been established by means of ECG-gated CT angiography. Despite improvement in spatial and temporal resolutions (less than 150 ms) with fast-rotating multidetector CT technology, thoracic aorta remains a vascular segment difficult to analyze because of axial and transverse motions during the cardiac cycle, which is particularly true for ascending aorta (34–36). ECG assistance for aortic studies allows the synchronization of data acquisition to the heart cycle to obtain CT data during the diastolic phase when heart movement is minimal thus reducing motion artefact (37–39).

The purpose of this study is to provide an insight in normative values of the ascending aorta and its branches regarding endovascular procedures and devices by using ECG-gated multidetector CT technology.

The following study is in part reproduced with permission from Lu TL, Huber CH, et al. Ascending aorta measurements as assessed by ECG-gated multidetector CT: A pilot study to establish normative values for transcatheter therapies [published online ahead of print September 23, 2008]. Eur Radiol 2009; 19(3):664–669.

Method

Patients
Seventy-five patients were included in this retrospective study, with fifty-seven male patients and eighteen female patients. Their age ranged from 2 to 82 years. The mean and median ages were 49 and 50 years, respectively. The patients were addressed for coronary and abdominal pathologies. In 48 patients, data were available from the outflow tract up to the midascending aorta. Data were available up to the brachiocephalic artery in the remaining patients ($n = 27$).

CT Scan Protocol and Measurements
Data were acquired on 64 detectors GE Lightspeed VCT scanner (General Electric Medical Systems, Milwaukee, WI). Acquisitions were realized after an antecubital intravenous injection of 100 mL of nonionic contrast medium (Accupaque 350, GE Healthcare, Giles, UK) with 40 mL of water bolus at 5 mL/s. ECG-gated multiphase acquisitions were started during a single-held breath when sufficient contrast enhancement was present in the ascending aorta. Collimation was 0.625 mm with a table feed of 3.8 mm per rotation and a pitch of 3.8/40. Retrospective multiphase reconstructions were done with increments of 6% or 10% from 0% to 96% or 90% respectively.

Analysis of ascending aorta and aortic arch morphology was performed on a Hewlett-Packard xw8000 workstation running GE Advantage Windows version 4.3 software (GE Medical Systems). Two-dimensional multiplanar reformations and automatic segmentation were used and reviewed in consensus by two

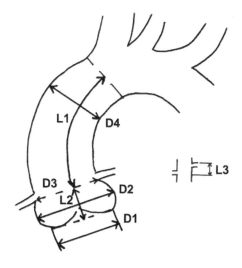

FIGURE 9 Diagram showing relevant measurements: (*D1*) outflow tract, (*D2*) coronary sinus, (*D3*) STJ, (*D4*) largest diameter of the ascending aorta, (*L1* + *L2*) distance from aortic valve to level of the right brachiocephalic artery, (*L2*) distance from aortic valve to proximal coronary ostium, (*L3*) distance between proximal and distal coronary ostia.

radiologists. Precision of measurements on this workstation is approximately 1 pixel. Image field of view was 512 × 512 pixels. Phantom studies showed that the difference between measurements with ECG-gated CT acquisitions and optical measurements is less than half a percent (40).

In close collaboration with cardiovascular surgeons, relevant measurements (Fig. 9) were identified as key parameters for development of future transcatheter cardiovascular therapies: aortic diameters perpendicular to aorta centerline axis at different levels (outflow tract, coronary sinus, STJ, and widest ascending aorta level); distances from the aortic valve to the right brachiocephalic artery, from the aortic valve to the proximal coronary ostium, and level difference between the most proximal and most distal limits of both coronary ostia; length of lesser curve of the ascending aorta from LC ostium to level of the right brachiocephalic artery; and length of the straight line between these two landmarks (Fig. 10). The aortic valve area was also measured. All these measurements were realized during diastole at 75% of the R-R phase when optimal image quality is achieved (41).

Dynamic analysis was done for measurement of the length of the nonmobile part of the anterior mitral leaflet in every patient. This nonmobile portion was identified on three-cavities view (Fig. 10) during cardiac cycle. Dynamic data were also used for measurement of the ascending aorta pulsatility. Pulsatility was defined as the percentage difference of minimal and maximal anteroposterior and lateromedial width of the ascending aorta at its largest diameter. Data were available in 54 patients.

Statistical Analysis
Mean, median, maximum, and minimum values were considered with standard deviations. Coefficients of variation were also computed. Data were not stratified by gender and age because of the limited number of patients.

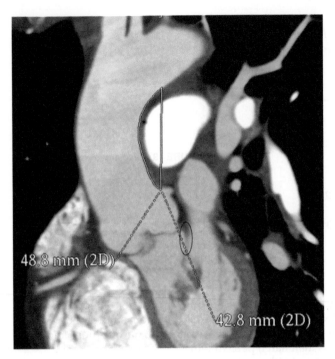

FIGURE 10 Lesser curve of the ascending aorta between the left coronary ostium and the level of the right brachiocephalic artery. Straight line between these two landmarks. (*In dark circle*) Nonmobile part of the anterior mitral leaflet visualized on the three-cavities view.

Results

Aortic Diameters at 75% of the R-R Phase (mm)

The mean diameter of outflow tract was 20.0 ± 3.6 with a coefficient of variation of 18%. The median was 19.8 and diameters ranged from 28.6 to 11.9. The mean diameter of coronary sinus was 32.9 ± 5.2 with a coefficient of variation of 16%. The median was 33.4 and maximum and minimum diameters were 45.4 and 17.4, respectively. The mean diameter of STJ was 28.7 ± 4.7 with a coefficient of variation of 16%. The median was 29.4 (14.1–37.8). The mean value of the maximal diameter of the ascending aorta was 31.1 ± 5.3 with a coefficient of variation of 17%. The median value was 31.6 and values ranged from 42.5 to 12.1.

Distances at 75% of the R-R Phase (mm)

The mean distance from the aortic valve to the right brachiocephalic artery was 89.3 ± 15.2 with a coefficient of variation of 17%. The median was 92.5 and maximum and minimum were respectively 119.9 and 45.6. The mean distance from the aortic valve to the proximal coronary artery was 11.7 ± 3.9 with a coefficient of variation of 33%. The median, maximum, and minimum were respectively 11.8, 25.6, and 2.9. The mean distance between both coronary ostia was 6.9 ± 3.0 with a coefficient of variation of 43%. The median distance was 6.3 with a maximum and minimal distance of 17.5 and 1.6 respectively.

Lengths at 75% of the R-R Phase (mm)

The mean length of the lesser curve of the ascending aorta from LC ostium to the level of the right brachiocephalic artery was 51.3 ± 10.6 with a coefficient of variation of 21%. The median length was 49.1. The length ranged from 32.7 to 78.0. The mean length of the straight line between these two landmarks was 44.4 ± 8.6. The coefficient of variation was 19%. The median was 43.3 with maximum and minimum lengths respectively 66.4 and 30.1.

Area of the Aortic Valve at 75% of the R-R Phase (mm²)

The mean area of the aortic valve was 563.0 ± 150.7 with a coefficient of variation of 27%. The median value was 568.5 with maximum and minimum values respectively 971.0 and 207.5.

Length of the Nonmobile Part of the Anterior Mitral Leaflet (mm)

The mean length of the nonmobile part of the medial mitral leaflet was 14.9 ± 3.6 with a coefficient of variation of 24%. The median, maximum, and minimum lengths were respectively 14.7, 26, and 7.2.

Variation of the Ascending Aorta Diameter During Cardiac Cycle, n = 54 Patients

The mean values of the ascending aorta diameter of anteroposterior and transverse diameters during the cardiac cycle varied from 33.0 to 29.7 mm and from 32.1 to 29.5 mm, respectively. The computed variations are respectively 10.0% and 8.1%.

Discussion

Transcatheter therapies of the aortic valve and of the ascending aorta will bring an innovative approach to the treatment of thoracic aorta pathologies. Nevertheless, indications for such type of minimal invasive procedure are still limited. The main restrictions are due to the size of the vascular access and the availability of dedicated devices. The latter are now being developed, but in the pursuit of the ideal ascending aorta endograft precise morphometric measurements of this vascular segment are needed. This study presents an insight into measurements of the ascending aorta by means of ECG-gated tomography. To the authors knowledge, few studies (21) are oriented to this topic and no study brings exhaustive morphometric measurements of the ascending aorta.

Other radiological modalities have already been used in the purpose to examine the ascending aorta. Nongated CT in adult subjects showed diameters of the aortic sinus between 29.8 and 36.2 mm and diameters of the ascending aorta between 30.9 and 35.1 mm (7,8). Morphometric measurements have also been done with transthoracic echocardiography. In children and young adults, aortic sinus and STJ diameters were measured between 17.5 and 27.5 mm for the former and between 14 and 22 mm for the latter (14). Normative data were also obtained by means of angiocardiographic acquisition. In children, ascending aorta diameters were measured between 7.5 and 27.5 mm (4,5). Magnetic resonance angiography experience for normative measurements was also described. However, few data are available (11).

The present results are in agreement with those studies. Nevertheless, comparison of agreement between those modalities and ECG-gated tomography is difficult, because measurement criteria are different for each study. Moreover, no study tested a specific modality against a gold standard technique or compared results to anatomopathological specimen. Based on the authors experience, ECG-gated tomography seems to be the imaging modality closest to a gold standard. As already mentioned, motion artifacts, particularly in the ascending aorta, can affect precision of measurements when tomography is not gated.

Although transthoracic echocardiography or even transesophageal echocardiography are readily available techniques and although gated ultrasound technologies offer even better temporal resolution compared to CT (42), image acquisition and interpretation are still operator-dependent (15). Interposition between the ascending aorta and the trachea makes visualization difficult and sometimes incomplete (43). It is also known that artifacts can appear in the ascending portion of the aorta because of reflection of ultrasound on the atrio–aortic interface and can cause false-positive findings, for example, in diagnosis of aortic dissection (16).

Cardiac magnetic resonance imaging is a promising technology. Nevertheless, reduced availability, cost, and patient discomfort are disadvantages compared to tomography. On a technical point of view, fast acquisition is required and sequences like echoplanar imaging are used. Such sequences offer a good ratio between duration of acquisition and image quality, but introduce geometric distortion and ghosting in the cardiac examination postprocessing and reconstruction (9). Multiple technical steps are needed to compensate these artifacts. Strong magnetic fields can also interfere with the ECG signal recording during magnetic resonance imaging scans, the so-called magnetohydrodynamic effect. Flowing blood-charged particles are deflected by the Lorentz force and create parasite potentials through blood vessels that are sufficient to increase the T wave. This larger T wave can be as high as the QRS complex and can induce false triggering (10).

As for angiocardiography, the technique is based on projectional views and summation images. Angle of x-rays incidence and structures overlapping can induce geometrical distortion (6). Considering that angiocardiography also requires an invasive procedure, it is not the most suitable technique to get aortic measurements.

Ideally, one standard endovascular device should fit any patient's anatomy. Experience with EVAR showed that it is practically impossible and selections of size, geometrical configuration, and anchoring options are needed depending on anatomical morphology and pathologies (44). The results confirmed that large interindividual variations exist. Distances between coronary ostia and the aortic valve and mean distances between both ostia showed coefficients of variation up to 43%. Variation of coronary anatomy is common (45) and becomes problematic when a fenestrated endograft is in scope (19). Although results were not stratified, differences exist through gender and age. Thus, a personalized approach might be required for every endograft procedure in ascending aorta pathologies. Motion and stress forces in the ascending aorta have been showed to be higher than in the abdominal aorta (21). It was showed that diameter change of the ascending aorta during cardiac cycle ranged between 8.3% and 19.6%, which is compatible with the present results. Such mechanical constraints may favor stent migration or endoleak (22), but more evidence is needed to correlate diameter change with endograft failure.

The aim of this study was to get an insight of normative values for the ascending aorta and the limitation is the quite low number of the studied population. To establish more solid normative tables, a larger population is needed. Besides, the results were not stratified for height and weight. Such normalization might be useful particularly in the pediatric population. Nevertheless, this study is a first step in establishing normative values. The authors think that ECG-gated CT is the most suitable and convenient way for such purpose. This study also proposes a potential checklist for preoperative examinations in the perspective of future endograft of the ascending aorta.

REFERENCES

1. Marty B, von Segesser LK, Schöpke W, et al. Die morphologie abdominaler aortenaneurysmata unter dem gesichtspunkt des endovaskulären gefässersatzes. Swiss Surg 1996; 2:219–222.
2. Schumacher H, Allenberg JR, Eckstein HH. Morphological classification of abdominal aortic aneurysm in selection of patients for endovascular grafting. Br J Surg 1996; 83(7):949–950.
3. Anderson RH. Clinical anatomy of the aortic root. Heart 2000; 84(6):670–673.
4. Trivedi KR, Pinzon JL, McCrindle BW, et al. Cineangiographic aortic dimensions in normal children. Cardiol Young 2002; 12(4):339–344.
5. Clarkson PM, Brandt PW. Aortic diameters in infants and young children: Normative angiographic data. Pediatr Cardiol 1985; 6(1):3–6.
6. Finet G, Masquet C, Eifferman A, et al. Can we optimize our angiographic views every time? Qualitative and quantitative evaluation of a new functionality. Invest Radiol 1996; 31(8):523–531.
7. Hager A, Kaemmerer H, Rapp-Bernhardt U, et al. Diameters of the thoracic aorta throughout life as measured with helical computed tomography. J Thorac Cardiovasc Surg 2002; 123(6):1060–1066.
8. Aronberg DJ, Glazer HS, Madsen K, et al. Normal thoracic aortic diameters by computed tomography. J Comput Assist Tomogr 1984; 8(2):247–250.
9. Kim YC, Nielsen JF, Nayak KS. Automatic correction of echo-planar imaging (EPI) ghosting artifacts in real-time interactive cardiac MRI using sensitivity encoding. J Magn Reson Imaging 2008; 27(1):239–245.
10. Tenforde TS. Magnetically induced electric fields and currents in the circulatory system. Prog Biophys Mol Biol 2005; 87(2–3):279–288.
11. Lorenz CH. The range of normal values of cardiovascular structures in infants, children, and adolescents measured by magnetic resonance imaging. Pediatr Cardiol 2000; 21(1):37–46.
12. Tamás E, Nylander E. Echocardiographic description of the anatomic relations within the normal aortic root. J Heart Valve Dis 2007; 16(3):240–246.
13. Vasan RS, Larson MG, Levy D. Determinants of echocardiographic aortic root size. The Framingham Heart Study. Circulation 1995; 91(3):734–740.
14. Poutanen T, Tikanoja T, Sairanen H, et al. Normal aortic dimensions and flow in 168 children and young adults. Clin Physiol Funct Imaging 2003; 23(4):224–229.
15. Van Dantzig JM. Echocardiography in the emergency department. Semin Cardiothorac Vasc Anesth 2006; 10(1):79–81.
16. Appelbe AF, Walker PG, Yeoh JK, et al. Clinical significance and origin of artifacts in transesophageal echocardiography of the thoracic aorta. J Am Coll Cardiol 1993; 21(3):754–760.
17. Berdajs D, Lajos P, Turina M. The anatomy of the aortic root. Cardiovasc Surg 2002; 10(4):320–327.

18. Roman MJ, Devereux RB, Kramer-Fox R, et al. Two-dimensional echocardiographic aortic root dimensions in normal children and adults. Am J Cardiol 1989; 64(8):507–512.

19. Huber CH, Tozzi P, Corno AF, et al. Do valved stents compromise coronary flow? Eur J Cardiothorac Surg 2004; 25(5):754–759.

20. Huber CH, Nasratulla M, Augstburger M, et al. Ultrasound navigation through the heart for off-pump aortic valved stent implantation: New tools for new goals. J Endovasc Ther 2004; 11(4):503–510.

21. van Prehn J, Vincken KL, Muhs BE, et al. Toward endografting of the ascending aorta: Insight into dynamics using dynamic cine-CTA. J Endovasc Ther 2007; 14(4):551–560.

22. Teutelink A, Muhs BE, Vincken KL, et al. Use of dynamic computed tomography to evaluate pre- and postoperative aortic changes in AAA patients undergoing endovascular aneurysm repair. J Endovasc Ther 2007; 14(1):44–49.

23. Dubost C, Allary M, Oeconomos N. Aneurysm of the abdominal aorta treated by resection and graft. Arch Mal Coeur Vaiss 1951; 44(9):848–851.

24. Dubost C, Allary M, Oeconomos N. Resection of an aneurysm of the abdominal aorta: Reestablishment of the continuity by a preserved human arterial graft, with result after five months. AMA Arch Surg 1952; 64(3):405–408.

25. Creech O Jr. Endo-aneurysmorrhaphy and treatment of aortic aneurysm. Ann Surg 1966; 164(6):935–946.

26. Parodi JC, Palmaz JC, Barone HD. Transfemoral intraluminal graft implantation for abdominal aortic aneurysms. Ann Vasc Surg 1991; 5(6):491–499.

27. Parker MV, O'Donnell SD, Chang AS, et al. What imaging studies are necessary for abdominal aortic endograft sizing? A prospective blinded study using conventional computed tomography, aortography, and three-dimensional computed tomography. J Vasc Surg 2005; 41(2):199–205.

28. Moon MC, Morales JP, Greenberg RK. The aortic arch and ascending aorta: Are they within the endovascular realm? Semin Vasc Surg 2007; 20(2):97–107.

29. Huber CH, von Segesser LK. Direct access valve replacement (DAVR)—Are we entering a new era in cardiac surgery? Eur J Cardiothorac Surg 2006; 29(3):380–385.

30. Ishimaru S. Endografting of the aortic arch. J Endovasc Ther 2004; 11(suppl 2):II62–II71.

31. Kasirajan K. Thoracic endografts: Procedural steps, technical pitfalls and how to avoid them. Semin Vasc Surg 2006; 19(1):3–10.

32. Pearce WH, Slaughter MS, LeMaire S, et al. Aortic diameter as a function of age, gender, and body surface area. Surgery 1993; 114(4):691–697.

33. Fitzgerald SW, Donaldson JS, Poznanski AK. Pediatric thoracic aorta: Normal measurements determined with CT. Radiology 1987; 165(3):667–669.

34. Rubin GD, Leung AN, Robertson VJ, et al. Thoracic spiral CT: Influence of subsecond gantry rotation on image quality. Radiology 1998; 208(3):771–776.

35. Qanadli SD, El Hajjam M, Mesurolle B, et al. Motion artifacts of the aorta simulating aortic dissection on spiral CT. J Comput Assist Tomogr 1999; 23(1):1–6.

36. Duvernoy O, Coulden R, Ytterberg C. Aortic motion: A potential pitfall in CT imaging of dissection in the ascending aorta. J Comput Assist Tomogr 1995; 19(4):569–572.

37. Marten K, Funke M, Rummeny EJ, et al. Electrocardiographic assistance in multidetector CT of thoracic disorders. Clin Radiol 2005; 60(1):8–21.

38. Roos JE, Willmann JK, Weishaupt D, et al. Thoracic aorta: Motion artifact reduction with retrospective and prospective electrocardiography-assisted multi-detector row CT. Radiology 2002; 222(1):271–277.

39. Schertler T, Glücker T, Wildermuth S, et al. Comparison of retrospectively ECG-gated and nongated MDCT of the chest in an emergency setting regarding workflow, image quality, and diagnostic certainty. Emerg Radiol 2005; 12(1–2):19–29.

40. Zhang J, Fletcher JG, Vrtiska TJ, et al. Large-vessel distensibility measurement with electrocardiographically gated multidetector CT: Phantom study and initial experience. Radiology 2007; 245(1):258–266.

41. Hoffmann U, Pena AJ, Cury RC, et al. Cardiac CT in emergency department patients with acute chest pain. Radiographics 2006; 26(4):963–978, discussion 979–980.
42. Smiseth OA, Stoylen A, Ihlen H. Tissue Doppler imaging for the diagnosis of coronary artery disease. Curr Opin Cardiol 2004; 19(5):421–429.
43. Erbel R, Mohr-Kahaly S, Oelert H, et al. Diagnostic goals in aortic dissection. Value of transthoracic and transesophageal echocardiography. Herz 1992; 17(6):321–337.
44. Wyers MC, Fillinger M, Schermerhorn M, et al. Endovascular repair of abdominal aortic aneurysm without preoperative arteriography. J Vasc Surg 2003; 38(4):730–738.
45. von Ludinghausen M. The clinical anatomy of coronary arteries. Adv Anat Embryol Cell Biol 2003; 167:III–VIII, 1–111.

8 Physiologic Response to Aortic Valved Stent with Emphasis on Coronary Flow

One of the main concerns of aortic transcatheter valve therapies (TCVT) is the risk of coronary flow impairment. Since the beginning of aortic valved stent implantation no study has specifically focused on coronary flow and flow disturbances caused by the device struts or aortic root geometrical distortion caused by the generally oversized device. The following study analyses preprocedural, per-procedural, and postprocedural coronary flow pattern by Doppler-enhanced intracardiac echocardiography.

The following study is in part reproduced from Huber CH et al. Do valved stent compromise coronary flow? Eur J Cardiothorac Surg 2004; 25:754–759.

DO VALVED STENT COMPROMISE CORONARY FLOW?

Introduction
Technical feasibility and clinical tolerance of remote access aortic valve implantation are clearly established in highly selected patients. However, in a percutaneous approach, severe limitations to aortic valve implantation remain. The access vessel diameter determines the maximal size of the device as well as the size of potential tools for removal of calcification and of the native valves. The precise positioning becomes more demanding because of the increased distance between the access and target site. Furthermore, the position of the coronary orifice and the close relationship with the anterior mitral leaflet considerably increase the technical difficulty, which means that the aortic valve region remains an important challenge.

Many pioneering studies presented supracoronary valve implantation to avoid the risk of coronary obstruction (1). Physiologically it is certainly preferable to implant the new valve in the orthotopic aorta, over the native valve, even if technically it is more demanding. Worldwide clinical experience shows that there is a justifiable risk of device-related coronary obstruction. Nevertheless, hardly any information on subclinical coronary flow impairment exists. Experiences and results from the ongoing research project on off-bypass pulmonary artery valve implantations (2) encouraged us to face the challenge of sutureless aortic valve implantation over the native leaflets using a specially designed self-expanding valved stent. This first prototype of an aortic valved stent is a cylindrical scaffold and a biological valve combined into one device (Fig. 1).

The honeycomb nitinol stent has a very low surface coverage and is self-anchoring. Despite the high radial expansion force, the stent can be collapsed when immerged into ice water. The valvular apparatus is derived from a clinically used equine pericardial valve, designed to be free of tissue between the

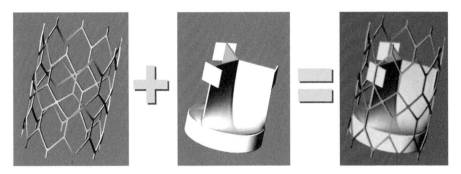

FIGURE 1 Valved stent—a combination of a nitinol scaffolding and valvular leaflets trimmed from equine pericardium.

commissures. Those special characteristics qualify the valved stent for aortic valve implantation without hindrance of the anterior mitral valve leaflet and very low risk of coronary orifice obstruction.

To avoid the initial difficulties previously reported with lamb and porcine experiments (3,4), the aortic valve implantation was performed in calves, known for their prominent residual aortic coronary sinus—a natural distance keeper in front of the coronary orifices as found also in the human heart (Chap. 7) (Fig. 2).

Method

A custom-made valved stent (Fig. 3) provided by former 3F Therapeutics, Inc., Lake Forest, CA, and its interference on coronary blood flow was evaluated for orthotopic sutureless aortic valve implantation over the native leaflets.

The self-expanding stent is made from nonthermosensitive memory nitinol. The honeycomb scaffold provides the necessary radial expansion force, yet it is flexible enough to be collapsed and folded. Spikes at both ends ensure safe autoanchoring. The valvular component is made from equine pericardium trimmed into leaflets and sutured by hand into the carrier stent. Special care is taken to leave the intercommissural space free of tissue. The outer radial diameter of the implanted device is 23 mm in full expansion and 10 mm in the folded status.

Before implantation, in vitro static and dynamic performance of all valved stents was evaluated. Leakage was determined by placing the valved stent inside a silicone tube and creating a water column of 61 cm (corresponding to 45 mm Hg) above the valvular level. A hydrodynamic pulsatile-flow mock loop circuit equipped with high fidelity tip-mounted Millar pressure transducer for gradient measurements and real-time intravascular ultrasound (IVUS) (12.5 MHz, 6F) (Clearview, Boston Scientific Corporation, Sunnyvale, CA) was used to assess valvular function over an observation period of 30 minutes. After qualifying for implantation, all valved stents were preserved in a 10% glutaraldehyde solution.

Acute in vivo evaluation was performed in six calves (mean body weight = 75.0 ± 2.5 kg; range = 70–78 kg). After premedication, general anesthesia, standard hemodynamic response to tracheal intubation, and respiratory and electrocardiographic monitoring, heparin was administered IV (300 IU/kg).

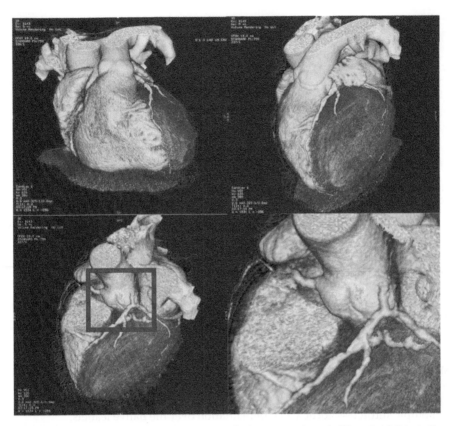

FIGURE 2 Three-dimensional reconstruction of a human aortic root. (*From top left to bottom right*): View of pulmonary artery; 90-degree clockwise rotation to provide a better view of the sinus portion of the aortic root; digital subtraction of the pulmonary truncus (*the red rectangle*) limits the zone of interest; magnification of the aortic root (note the coronary offspring at the upper-third of the sinus pouches).

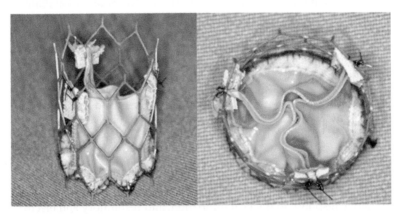

FIGURE 3 Illustration of the valved stent, prior to implantation, constructed from an outer honeycomb nitinol scaffold and a pericardial valve.

By intracardiac echocardiography (ICE), the aortic annulus was identified as target site and its diameter measured. The aortic root was screened paying special attention to the coronary orifice region for residual sinuses in front of the proper coronary arteries.

To ease delivery, a Teflon sheath was wrapped around the manually folded valved stent and held in the collapsed mode by a curved clamp. After arterial cannulation of the right carotid artery and the descending thoracic aorta as well as venous cannulation of the right atrium, the valved stents were delivered through a small transverse aortotomy at target site in four animals. In two calves, the valved stents were placed off-pump after induction of ventricular fibrillation and clamping of the distal ascending aorta. A longitudinal aortotomy was performed, and the valved stent delivered retrograde over the native aortic valve. To further shorten postdeployment clamping time, a tangential clamp was used for rapid closure of the aortotomy and the aortic clamp removed.

In vivo assessment was performed with the ICE and the IVUS including leaflet motion, planimetric valve orifice and transvalvular gradient, regurgitation, and paravalvular leaking in combination with continuous cardiac output measures.

The Residual Coronary Sinus Stent Index

In order to evaluate potential coronary flow impairment, a new echographic index, the residual coronary sinus stent index (RCSSI), was defined by calculating the distance between the stent and the aortic wall divided through the ostial coronary diameter of the left main coronary artery. This index compares the flow ratio between the native coronary flow and the blood flow required to pass through the valved stent after implantation. More specifically, the RCSSI is a comparison between the coronary cross-sectional surface area and the plane defined by the valved stent and the native aortic wall (Figs. 4 and 5). Coronary diameter was measured at the termination of the sinus portion. The residual stent aortic wall plane was measured at the level of the coronary orifice. All measurements were made using an ICE. To calculate the index value, the distance of the stent from the aortic wall (residual gap at the level of the aortic sinus portion) is divided by the coronary diameter. The index is based on the postulate that cardiopulmonary bypass (CBF) should not be impaired if the observed index value remains >1.

At the end of the experiments, the animals were sacrificed and macroscopic analysis was performed at necropsy. The protocol was approved by the institutional committee on animal research. All animals received human care in compliance with the principles of the Guide for the Care and Use of Laboratory Animals (5). All data are expressed as mean ± standard deviation.

Results

In vitro static leakage test showed full competence of the pericardial leaflets in all valved stents. In the hydrodynamic pulsatile-flow mock loop, all valved stents showed good valvular function. IVUS imaging demonstrated full opening and closing of the pericardial leaflets.

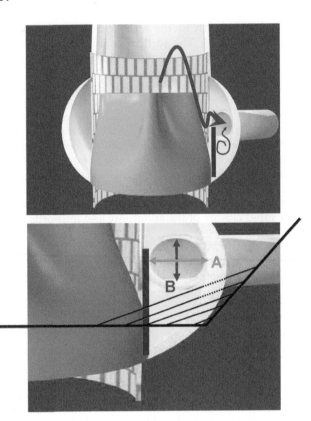

FIGURE 4 Residual coronary sinus stent index (RCSSI). The index is based on the asumption that CBF should not be impaired as long as the cross-sectional area defined by the stent and the residual sinus pouch opening is above the coronary orifice cross-sectionional area. (*Top*): Illustration of the modified flow path for coronary perfusion. (*Bottom*): Three-dimensional reconstructed illustration *Abbreviations*: A, distance from stent to aortic wall (sinus stent); B, diameter of main left coronary artery.

In Vivo Study

The mean aortic annular diameter measured with IVUS was 21.5 ± 0.8 mm. All valved stents were deployed correctly at the target site over the native aortic valves. Duration of delivery and deployment lasted about two minutes for on and off pump techniques.

Two-dimensional intracardiac ultrasound revealed good leaflet motion, with full valvular opening and closing in five of six valves. Planimetric valve orifice area was 1.75 ± 0.4 cm^2. The implanted valved stents showed a low transvalvular gradient of 5.3 ± 3.9 mm Hg (peak to peak) on invasive measurements and 4.7 ± 2.5 mm Hg in two-dimensional intracardiac ultrasound. ICE color Doppler investigation revealed laminar blood flow through five of six-valved stents. One of six valves showed mild-to-moderate regurgitation and one of six valves showed a moderate paravalvular leak due to size mismatch.

No signs of coronary flow impairments were found in the left main coronary artery. The RCSSI was 1.8 ± 1.2. The typical distances found between the

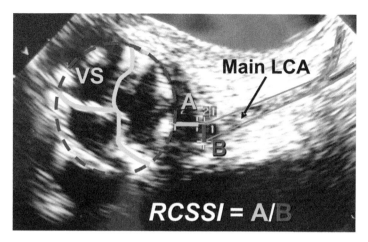

FIGURE 5 Example of the RCSSI calculation after implantation of a valved stent into the orthotopic aorta, over the native valve (RCSSI=A/B). *Abbreviations*: A, distance from stent to aortic wall (sinus stent); B, diameter of main left coronary artery; VS, valved stent; LCA, main left coronary artery.

stent scaffold and the proper left main coronary artery were 4 to 6 mm. Color Doppler and M-mode views showed normal coronary flow patterns in all animals having a RCSSI value greater than 1 (Figs. 6 and 7). No animal had a RCSSI value of the left main coronary artery less than 1.

The observation period was 1.9 ± 0.7 hours. Postmortem examination confirmed the correct position of the valved stents and excluded complete or partial

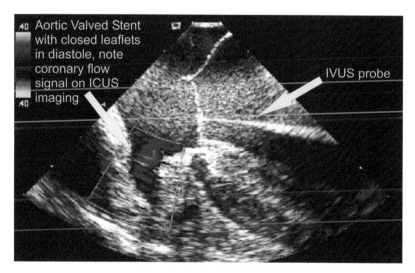

FIGURE 6 Two-dimensional intracardiac ultrasound illustrating diastolic main LCA flow after implantation of a valved stent in orthotopic position. *Abbreviations*: LCA, left coronary artery; IVUS, intravascular ultrasound.

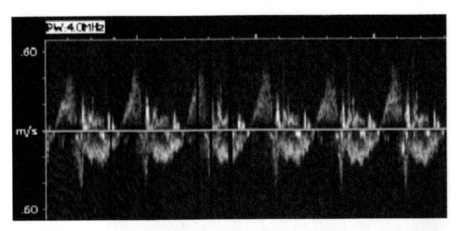

FIGURE 7 M-mode of the intracardiac echo showing flow characteristics in the main left coronary artery after orthotopic aortic valved stent implantation. (Note good diastolic flow curves.)

coronary orifice obstruction (Fig. 8). The self-anchoring mechanism safely hocked the stent into the aortic wall, and its high radial expansion property was shown by the stent "fingerprint" on the aortic intima (Fig. 9).

Methodical Considerations

The close proximity of the coronary orifice to the aortic valve leaflets and the continuity of the mitral valve annulus and the aortic annulus make remote access surgical sutureless aortic valve implantation a major challenge. Some previous experimental percutaneous techniques, placing valved stents in subaortic or supra-aortic position showed high complication rates (1). Previous experimental and clinical studies describe different devices, target sites, and access or delivery techniques (6–9) and interest in remote access or percutaneous orthotopic aortic

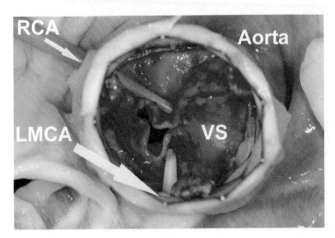

FIGURE 8 Top view of a valved stent in the orthotopic aorta implanted over the native valve. RCA and LCA *arrows* point toward coronary marker sticks. *Abbreviations*: RCA, right coronary artery; LCA, left coronary artery; VS, valved stent.

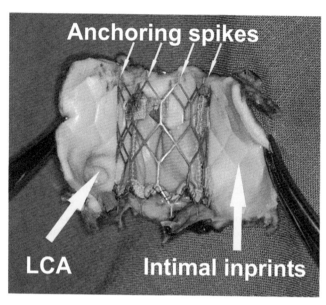

FIGURE 9 Self-anchoring mechanism of the valved stent with spikes at both ends and the stent fingerprint on the aortic intima. *Abbreviations*: LCA, main left coronary artery; RCA, right coronary artery.

valve replacement is greatly increasing (10). But further studies for the validation of other valved stent designs or new access locations, delivery, and deployment techniques are a necessity.

Recently a new self-expanding valved stent was developed in collaboration with the authors institution (University Hospital Lausanne, CHUV, Switzerland) and ATS Medical, Minneapolis, MN (previously 3f Therapeutics Inc.), specially designed for remote access surgical sutureless aortic valve implantation. A particularity of the design is that the native aortic wall keeps its natural function and is not lined with foreign tissue, for example, as after endoprostheses implantation. Furthermore, the stent has very little surface coverage and therefore minimizes the danger of coronary orifice obstruction because of rotational mispositioning. Before implanting in animals, we verified valvular function of all valved stents in vitro. Only devices presenting good valvular function and safe autoanchorage properties were implanted into the orthotopic aorta over the native valve leaflets.

The main concern after valved stent implantation in the orthotopic aorta is coronary flow impairment. The following are two potential dangers for impaired coronary flow or even complete occlusion of the coronary orifice and consecutive fatal myocardial infarction:

1. Obstruction by the native valve leaflets folded upward and being compressed against the coronary orifice.
2. Direct occlusion by parts of the valved stent. The investigator used per-procedural intracardiac and intravascular ultrasound to identify the

anatomical configuration of the aortic root and, in particular, to visualize the presence of a coronary sinus, serving as a natural distance keeper between the stent and the coronary artery.

The changes of coronary flow Doppler signal have to our knowledge not been analyzed yet. The use of an ICE considerably eliminates echocardiographic interferences and allows to get new insight into coronary flow patterns after valved stent deployment. In order to quantify potential interference of coronary flow dynamics, this study aimed at identifying a possible echocardiographic predictor for coronary flow impairment. Further investigations lead to the RCSSI as an indicator for potential coronary flow impairment. An index value greater than 1 was found to correlate in all animals with a normal left main coronary flow pattern and we concluded that the remaining flow in the cross-sectional area must be at least equal or bigger as the coronary orifice cross-section area, also see The Residual Coronary Sinus Stent Index above (Figs. 4 and 5). Of course the collected data is not sufficient yet, and further studies are presently underway at our institution to validate this new index. Nevertheless, precise preprocedural and per-procedural echocardiographic analysis of the aortic valve region is a prerequisite for successful valved stent implantation.

Another question arises in the context of coronary flow impairment: Should the native leaflets be removed prior to implantation? For example, in aortic insufficiency, native leaflets might be enlarged and could, therefore, increase the risk of coronary orifice obstruction. Removal would prevent this complication but, on the other hand, would strongly increase the regurgitation fraction and create a massive aortic insufficiency. Insertion of temporary catheter-mounted valves could solve this problem. Furthermore, after removal of the native leaflets, the rim caused by compressing the leaflets against the aortic wall would disappear and, therefore, loose its quality as natural distance keeper between the stent and the aortic wall. In aortic stenosis, keeping the heavily calcified valves after balloon valvuloplasty again creates a natural safety rim and keeps the stent from occluding the coronary orifice. But in so doing, the maximal diameter for the new aortic valve will further be reduced and an inherent risk of further spread of the calcification process onto the newly placed tissue valve might be of concern.

Considering the above-mentioned difficulties, new techniques, tools, and strategies for remote access surgical sutureless aortic valve replacement need to be developed. First, endoluminal utensils capable of remote decalcification and valve removal have to be designed. Currently, investigations are underway at the Christian-Albrechts-University of Kiel, Germany, for laser ablation of the human calcified aortic valves (11). Second, distal embolic protection devices have to be developed. Temporary filters, similar to those used in percutaneous carotid endarterectomy, might prevent from coronary or distal embolization. Third, temporary catheter mounted valves, as proposed in previous studies (12,13), could take over the native aortic valve function prior to the valved stent deployment. Finally, new self-orientating valved stents, similar to the stents proposed in a previous two-step strategy (14), with an additional capacity of being recollapsed after implantation have to be engineered.

Although a great deal of work remains to be done, valved stent implantation is feasible (1,2,4,7–9) and becomes a promising new technology for the treatment of aortic valve diseases. The advantage of our study is the implantation of the valved stent into the aortic annulus by using a self-expanding valved stent specifically designed for orthotopic implantation, showing no coronary flow restriction and no mitral valve hindrance. Nevertheless, one main limitation of this study is the short observation period in this acute setting. Medium- and long-term observation for device dislodgement and valve durability as well as aortic wall reaction and device thrombogenicity are planned in forthcoming studies.

In conclusion, this study shows feasibility of an acute surgical sutureless aortic valve implantation without compromising the coronary flow in properly placed and sized valved stents. The surgical approach allows for valved stents implantation of adult size with adequate valve function. A precise measure of the aortic valve region with specific attention to the coronary sinus dimension and the postdeployment coronary flow analysis is possible using intravascular or intracardiac ultrasound. The RCSSI values greater than 1 correlated in all animals with normal left main coronary artery flow pattern.

REFERENCES

1. Boudjemline Y, Bonhoeffer P. Percutaneous valve insertion: A new approach? J Thorac Cardiovasc Surg 2003; 125(3):741–742.
2. Zhou JQ, Corno AF, Huber CH, et al. Self-expandable valved stent of large size: Off-bypass implantation in pulmonary position. Eur J Cardiothorac Surg 2003; 24(2): 212–216.
3. Knudsen LL, Andersen HR, Hasenkam JM. Catheter-implanted prosthetic heart valves. Transluminal catheter implantation of a new expandable artificial heart valve in the descending thoracic aorta in isolated vessels and closed chest pigs. Int J Artif Organs 1993; 16(5):253–262.
4. Lutter G, Schwarzkopf J, Takahashi N, et al. Percutaneous transluminal implantation of an aortic valve in aortic position: A porcine study. J Thorac Cardiovasc Surg 2001; 49(suppl 1):67.
5. Guide for the Care and Use of Laboratory Animals. Institute of Laboratory Animal Research, Commission on Life Sciences, National Research Council. 140p. 1996.
6. Hufnagel CA, Harvey WP, Rabil PJ, et al. Surgical correction of aortic insufficiency. Surgery 1954; 35:673–680.
7. Sochman J, Peregrin JH, Pavcnik D, et al. Percutaneous transcatheter aortic disc valve prosthesis implantation: A feasibility study. Cardiovasc Intervent Radiol 2000; 23(5):384–388.
8. Moazami N, Bessler M, Argenziano M, et al. Transluminal aortic valve placement. A feasibility study with a newly designed collapsible aortic valve. ASAIO J 1996; 42(5):M381–M385.
9. Pavcnik D, Uchida BT, Timmermans HA, et al. Percutaneous bioprosthetic venous valve: A long-term study in sheep. J Vasc Surg 2002; 35(3):598–602.
10. van Herwerden LA, Serruys PW. Percutaneous valve implantation: Back to the future? Eur Heart J 2002; 23(18):1415–1416.
11. Lutter G, Ardehali R, Cremer J, et al. Percutaneous valve replacement: Current state and future prospects. Ann Thorac Surg 2004; 78(6):2199–2206.
12. Phillips SJ, Ciborski M, Freed PS, et al. A temporary catheter-tip aortic valve: Hemodynamic effects on experimental acute aortic insufficiency. Ann Thorac Surg 1976; 21(2):134–137.
13. Moulopoulos SD, Anthopoulos L, Stamatelopoulos S, et al. Catheter-mounted aortic valves. Ann Thorac Surg 1971; 11(5):423–430.
14. Boudjemline Y, Agnoletti G, Bonnet D, et al. Steps toward the percutaneous replacement of atrioventricular valves: An experimental study. J Am Coll Cardiol 2005; 46(2):360–365.

9 | Experimental Data

DEVICE CONSTRUCTION AND IN VITRO TESTING

The First-Generation Aortic Device

The first-generation aortic self-expanding stent is made from two components (Fig. 1): The first is a memory nitinol stent with honeycomb geometry. The scaffold provides the necessary radial expansion force, yet in the cooled stage it is flexible enough to be collapsed and folded. Spikes at both ends ensure safe autoanchoring. The second is the valvular component, which is made from equine pericardium trimmed into leaflets and sutured by hand into the carrier stent by six semicontinuous 4-0 Ethibond running sutures. Special care is taken to leave the intercommissural space free of tissue. The stent valve interface is realized by a polyester warp knit tube sutured first onto the stent and then the tissue valve leaflets are sutured within the in-stent polyester cuff. The outer radial diameter of the implanted device is 23 mm in full expansion and 10 mm in the folded status.

The Modified First-Generation Aortic Device

The same nitinol frame was used as scaffold carrier, but we modified the stent by manually removing two-thirds of the struts to lower the risk of coronary malperfusion or occlusion. The changed geometry was further developed in close collaboration with the providing company (formerly 3F Therapeutics Inc., Lake Forest, CA) and our design finally created the basic stent concept for the ATS 3f Enable Aortic Heart Valve (formerly 3f Therapeutics Enable Valved Stent; currently undergoing clinical trial) (Fig. 2).

In the modified first-generation aortic valved stent, the self-constructed tissue valve was replaced by a 3f Therapeutics Equine Pericardial Tissue Valve (currently ATS 3f Aortic Bioprosthesis) sutured directly to the carrier stent. The valve commissures were placed onto the remaining longitudinal struts. Before implantation, in vitro static and dynamic performances of all valved stents were evaluated. Leakage was determined by placing the valved stent inside a silicone tube and creating a water column of 61 cm (corresponding to 45 mm Hg) above the valvular level.

After qualifying for implantation, all valved stents were preserved in a 10% glutaraldehyde solution.

The Second-Generation Aortic Device Construction Concept

Because of the unavailability of a radially collapsible stent, we set out to develop a second-generation aortic device based on the pulmonary valved stent construction concept. The outer scaffold of the device is constructed by three linked nitinol Z-stents that form a cylindrical structure with minimal surface coverage. The self-expanding characteristics of this valved stent eliminate the need for balloon

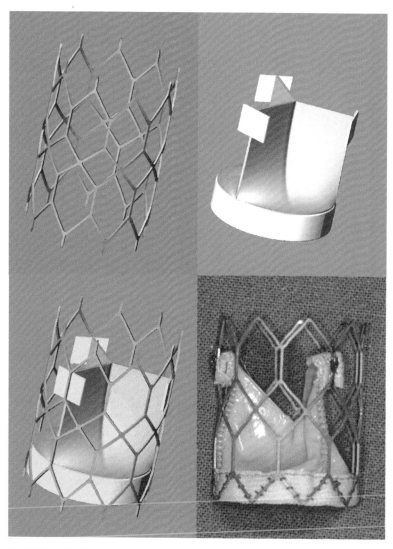

FIGURE 1 Modified first-generation aortic valved stent design based on the honeycomb nitinol stent concept.

expansion. A low-profile pericardial or porcine tissue valve is sutured into the stent scaffold (Fig. 3).

Before implantation in vivo, all valved stents undergo static and dynamic (30-minute) performance testing inside a pulsatile hydrodynamic mock loop circuit equipped with a high fidelity tip-mounted Millar pressure transducer (discussed later). Acute valve function is monitored in vitro with real-time intravascular ultrasound and invasive hemodynamic measures. Criteria determining the suitability for implantation include transvalvular gradient <8 mm Hg and regurgitation value less than 1+.

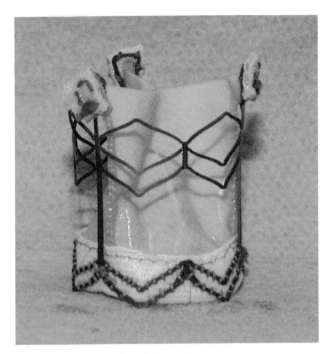

FIGURE 2 Aortic enable device developed in close collaboration with 3F Therapeutics. The device is now undergoing clinical studies by ATS Medical.

After construction, all devices were preserved and stored in a 10% glutaraldehyde solution.

The Delivery System

The off-pump valved stent was collapsed radially and then manually loaded into a standard endoprosthetic delivery device with a maximum diameter of 9.2 mm (Fig. 4).

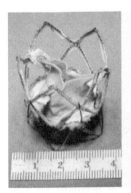 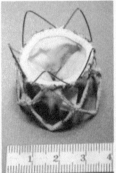 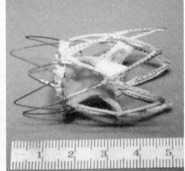

FIGURE 3 Second-generation self-expanding aortic valved stent design based on the nitinol Z-stent principle.

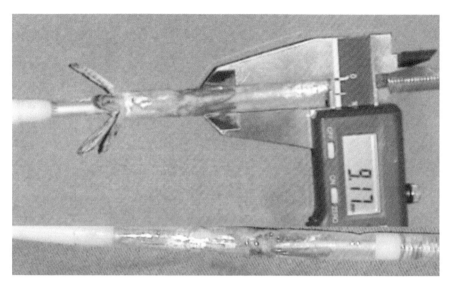

FIGURE 4 Delivery system modified from a commercially available Talent delivery system from Medtronic. Maximum diameter is 9.17 mm.

Tricuspid, Vena Cava, and First-Generation Pulmonary Valved Stent Construction

Remarks
The devices for tricuspid regurgitation are placed in the inferior and superior vena cava and are constructed the same way as the first-generation pulmonary valved stent. Therefore, the description of the devices has been merged.

Method
The following steps describe the construction concept for the tricuspid or vena cava and first-generation pulmonary valved stents.

A glutaraldehyde-preserved valved bovine jugular xenograft conduit (Contegra®) is trimmed 1.5 cm above the valve and 1 cm below the valve. Then the thick adventitia is partially trimmed off to thin down the conduit wall. Two self-expandable nonthermosensitive nitinol Z-stents are then taken down from an industrially made endovascular stent graft (Talent®) by sparing the original suture lines and a minimal rim of Dacron cloth in order to help enhance the friction coefficient of the device and consecutively diminish the risk for migration. The nitinol Z-stents' diameter measured 7 mm in the crimped state and expanded up to an internal diameter of 28 mm. The final device dimensions were 30.25 ± 0.15 mm for external diameter and 15.42 ± 0.34 mm for height.

With multiple running sutures of 7-0 prolene, the two self-expanding Z-stents are sewn in a parallel fashion about 5 to 10 mm apart onto the outside of the trimmed conduit. All precautions are taken so that the bovine valve is not sutured or damaged (Fig. 5).

Once the valved stent is prepared, device dimensions are measured prior to the glutaraldehyde preservation (Table 1).

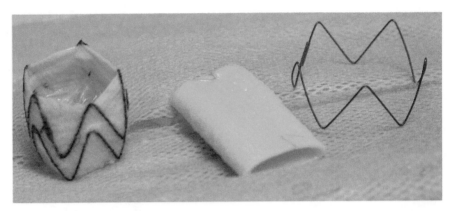

FIGURE 5 First-generation pulmonary valved stent construction concept used as well for the vena cava devices.

Static Device Testing for the Tricuspid, Vena Cava, and First-Generation Pulmonary Valved Stent

Valved stent regurgitation was assessed by pressurizing the device within a static water column. Assembly of the bench test included a water reservoir, a calibrated glass tube, a silicone tube with an inner diameter of 20 mm, and a measuring cylinder.

All valved stents were first crimped to a minimal diameter, loaded into the respective delivery device, and then reexpanded and deployed within the test chamber. In the next step, the devices were pressurized by a water column of 61 cm equivalent to 45 mm Hg by connecting the silicone tube with compliance characteristics to the water column (Fig. 6). Leakage is estimated by the tank and timer principle, measuring the amount of liquid recollected underneath the test column (Table 2).

Construction of the Second-Generation Pulmonary Valved Stent

Technique

The valved stent is constructed from two components—an endoprosthetic graft and a valved jugular vein conduit (Fig. 7). Both parts are chosen to approximate their respective diameters. On the basis of the experience gained from endoprosthetic therapies of aortic aneurysm as well as from the recent studies on aortic

TABLE 1 Examples of Measured Sizes of Seven Vena Cava Valved Stents

	Length (mm)	Inner diameter (mm)	Outer diameter (mm)
1	21.6	21.0	26.4
2	23.7	21.5	27.6
3	23.1	20.5	26.0
4	23.2	22.1	26.1
5	23.2	22.2	26.1
6	23.7	22.5	26.8
7	23.4	21.8	25.2
Mean	23.1 ± 0.7	21.6 ± 0.7	26.3 ± 0.7

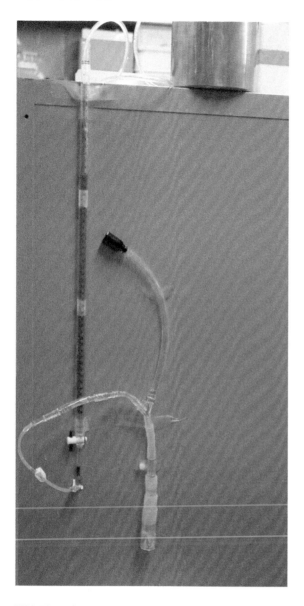

FIGURE 6 Static leakage test setup for the first-generation pulmonary devices.

TABLE 2 Examples of Seven Vena Cava Valved Stents Under In Vitro Static Performance Testing

Valved stent	1	2	3	4	5	6	7	Mean[a]
Leakage rate (mL/min)	35.3	47.6	18.1	28.9	50.1	23.8	23.6	32.5 ± 12.4

[a]Mean leakage rate was 32.5 ± 12.4 mL/min when subjected to a simulated afterload of 45 mm Hg. No valved stent showed migration.

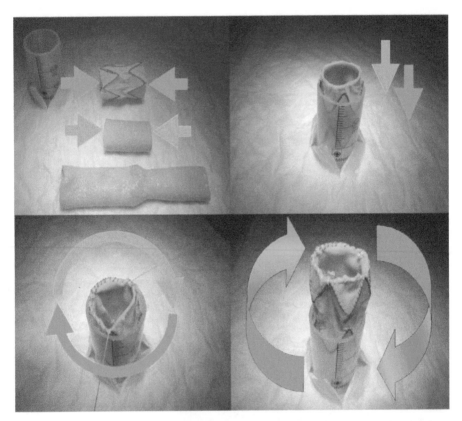

FIGURE 7 Second-generation pulmonary valved stent construction concept. (*Starting from top left to bottom right*): Shortening of the endoprosthetic graft and the valved conduit. Both components are placed within the stabilizer. Three Ti-Cron 2-0 sutures are placed at equidistance in a fashion to join the graft end and the valved segment. The three running sutures are completed. The obtained valved stent is removed, turned upside–down, and reinserted into the stabilizer to finalize the distal suture line with three more Ti-Cron 2-0 sutures.

valved stent implantation, it is generally advisable to slightly oversize the device by 15% to 20% of the target vessel diameter. Then the carrier stent is build by shortening the endoprosthetic graft to a certain length including two rows of Z-stents. It is recommended to leave a maximum of 1-mm cloth rim to allow for future suturing. Next the valved bovine jugular vein is trimmed down to fit the carrier stent taking care to position the valve portion within equal distance of the two suturing lines. This is done to keep the valve in the middle of the two future suture lines.

Before starting to suture, a stabilizer is prepared from a 60 mL syringe by cutting-off the tip at the 10 mL mark. Next the syringe is fixed on a plane working surface by double-sided sticky tape or fixed within the two blades of a sternal retractor. Then the carrier stent is inserted into the obtained stabilizer and finally the trimmed valve conduit is introduced into the graft. Both components are arranged to show congruent ends. Following this, three Ti-Cron 2-0 sutures (Tyco, Waltham, MA) are placed at equidistance on the presenting end of the future valved stent. Sutures are placed in a fashion to join the graft and the valved conduit. Each suture is tied down to prevent purse-string effect over the running suture line. Then, with each of the three Ti-Cron 2-0 a short running suture is started and tied with the next suture at each third of the circumference. The obtained double-walled cylinder is then removed, turned upside down, and reinserted into the stabilizer. Slight manual crimping might ease the insertion of the device. The suturing is now repeated in the same manner.

The finalized valved stent is removed from the stabilizer. Next, the valve is inspected visually and tested by filling with saline solution.

It is advisable to mark the future flow direction by drawing an arrow onto the outer wall of the valved stent before insertion into the delivery device.

The Delivery System

The delivery device for the transinfundibular insertion is easily constructed from a 5 mL syringe by removing its distal portion in a way to obtain an open cylinder (Fig. 8). Next the valved stent is loaded manually, facing the appropriate delivery direction for an antegrade approach. Loading can further be assisted by a heavy silk suture rapped around the stent and temporarily tightened by a second person until loaded into the delivery device. Now the system is ready for implantation. Delivery of the device is performed by pushing the piston and a slight pull back movement of the delivery tool during deployment to compensate for the forward shift.

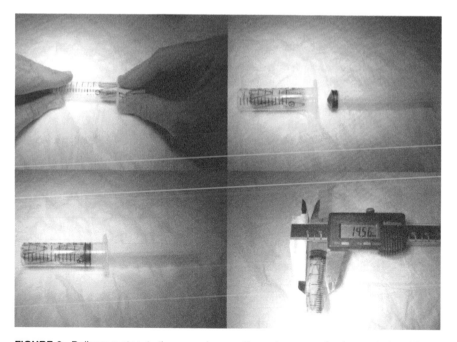

FIGURE 8 Delivery system to the second-generation pulmonary valved stent device. (*Starting from top left to bottom right*): Manual loading into the 5 mL delivery tool. The delivery device is then reassembled. The maximum outer diameter of 14.5 mm allows insertion via a small infundibular incision.

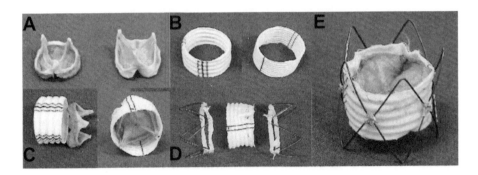

FIGURE 9 Multistep construction process of the mitral double-crowned valved stent.

Construction of the Mitral Double-Crowned Valved Stent

Stepwise description of the construction procedure for the mitral valved stents is as follows:

1. A glutaraldehyde-preserved aortic or pulmonary valvular homograft was trimmed to keep only the leaflets and the commissural leaflet suspension in place [Fig. 9(A)]. The diameter of the homograft was 20.46 ± 1.01 mm (Table 3).
2. A length of Dacron prosthesis was cut to fit the height of the trimmed homograft [Fig. 9(B)]. The diameter of the Dacron prosthesis was 23.80 ± 1.09 mm, and its height was 15.42 ± 0.77 mm (Table 3).
3. The aortic or pulmonary valvular homograft was mounted into the Dacron segment with a running suture of 6-0 prolene. The native geometry of the homograft was meticulously respected [Fig. 9(C)].
4. Two self-expanding nitinol Z-stents were dismantled from an endovascular stent graft-type Talent endovascular graft [Fig. 9(D)]. The diameter of the stents was 30 mm, while their height was 15 mm (Table 3).
5. Two self-expanding Z-stents were sutured at the centre of the mounted Dacron segment with 6-0 prolene, avoiding distortion of the valvular

TABLE 3 Measured Diameters and Heights of the Mitral Valved Stents

Valved stents	Homograft		Dacron		Z-stent	
	Diameter (mm)	Height (mm)	Diameter (mm)	Height (mm)	Diameter (mm)	Height (mm)
1	19.9	9.1	23.0	15.5	30.0	15.0
2	22.2	9.9	25.0	16.6	30.0	15.0
3	20.1	10.5	23.0	15.1	30.0	15.0
4	20.4	9.9	25.0	15.4	30.0	15.0
5	19.7	9.5	23.0	14.5	30.0	15.0
Mean	20.46	9.78	23.80	15.42	30.0	15.0
SD	1.01	0.52	1.09	0.77	0	0

TABLE 4 The Measured Sizes of the Constructed Valved Stents

Valved stent	Height (mm)	Inner diameter (mm)	Outer diameter (mm)
1	29.1	19.9	24.5
2	29.6	22.2	26.3
3	29.4	20.1	24.8
4	29.4	20.4	25.9
5	29.2	19.7	24.5
Mean	29.34	20.46	25.20
SD	0.19	1.00	0.84

homograft. It was the custom-made valved stent like double crowns [Fig. 9(E)] that gave the device its new name. The dimension of five-valved stents was measured (Table 4).

6. The completed devices (Fig. 10) were first measured and then preserved in a 10% glutaraldehyde solution and stored in a fully expanded state.

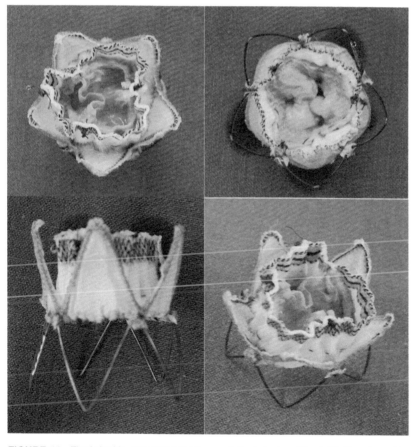

FIGURE 10 Final double-crowned mitral valved stent device. (*Top left*): Top view. (*Top right*): Upside down view. (*Lower left*): Side view. (*Lower right*): Oblique view.

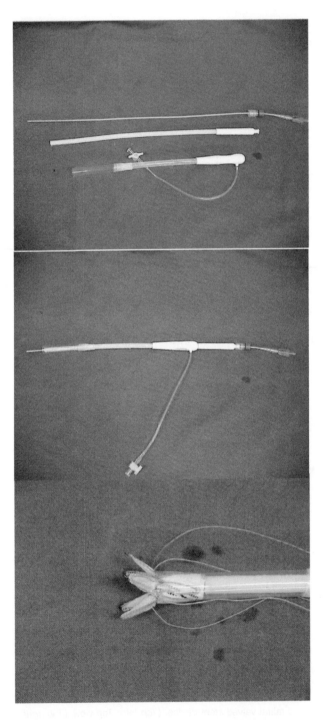

FIGURE 11 Mitral device delivery system. Note the sliding sling for controlled deployment.

Construction of the Mitral Device Delivery System

The delivery system consists of one guide wire sheath, an interior piston, and an exterior Teflon sheath (30F) as shown in Figure 11. All parts were trimmed to a length of 25 to 30 cm. Care was taken to keep the introducer tip short to prevent damage to the left ventricular structures. The valved stent was compressed to a small size and mounted inside the Teflon sheath. Deployment mechanism consisted of withdrawing the outside catheter while holding the inside piston in place. After deployment, the introducing system was withdrawn.

Static In Vitro Device Leakage Test for the Second-Generation Pulmonary and for the Mitral Valved Stents

Materials

5-Glutaraldehyde-preserved valved stents
One Dacron vessel prosthesis with an inner diameter of 26 mm
A water reservoir
A connecting tube
A clamp
A container and a measuring cylinder
A 1500 mm long measuring tape
An electronic timer

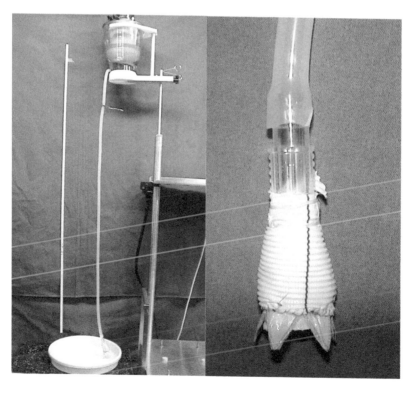

FIGURE 12 Static leakage test-column setup for the mitral device.

TABLE 5   The Leakage Test Under a 80 cm H_2O Water Column Pressure (Equivalent to 60 mm Hg)

Leakage (mL/min)	Valved stents					
	1	2	3	4	5	Mean ± SD
1	68.2	29.6	46.5	31.5	40.4	43.2 ± 15.5
2	53.4	33.4	55.2	41.1	28.8	42.4 ± 11.8
3	37.5	42.8	39.2	58.6	34.4	42.5 ± 9.5
4	30.8	54.7	36.8	42.1	35.6	40.0 ± 9.1
5	45.4	47.6	30.9	34.3	39.8	39.6 ± 7.1
Mean ± SD	47.1 ± 14.5	41.2 ± 10.2	41.7 ± 9.4	41.6 ± 10.6	35.8 ± 4.7	41.5 ± 10.1

Methods

The valved stent was tested for leakage by subjecting it to a pressure of 80 cm H_2O (or 60 mm Hg). It was then sutured into a Dacron prosthesis tube with a diameter of 26 mm at its center by a running suture and connected to the water column (Fig. 12). Leakage from the valved stent was confirmed by measuring the rate of water leakage below it. The rate of water filtered through the Dacron prosthesis was subtracted from the rate of water leaked through the Dacron prosthesis/stent in order to calculate the net leakage rate of valved stent (Table 5).

10 Preclinical Valved Stent Device Testing*

UNDERSTANDING DURABILITY, FATIGUE LIFE TESTING, AND FAILURE ANALYSIS

Introduction

Replacement heart valve device design and physician use have advanced over the past 50 years from the first implant of the Hufnagel valve in the descending thoracic aorta without cardiopulmonary bypass in 1952 (1) to recent clinical use of transcatheter implantation or replacement heart valves (2–6). Along with the evolution of heart valve designs and materials, the preclinical testing of devices has also improved over the past quarter-century, providing data critical to the initiation of clinical investigations. During this time, test method development for replacement heart valves has progressed because of advances in measurement techniques and systems, lessons learned from previous clinical device failures (7), unanticipated clinical complications not discovered during preclinical testing (8), and the introduction of new types of replacement heart valves, such as stentless bioprostheses (9). Preclinical evaluation of transcatheter heart valves will again necessitate the development of testing methods based on specific design and intended use.

In many ways, transcatheter heart valves offer unique challenges in preclinical and clinical evaluation. However, for preclinical testing, viewing current transcatheter heart valve designs as stented valve conduits delivered by nontraditional methods could provide an initial roadmap with regard to performance evaluation. A first-pass in evaluation of transcatheter valves may be covered by the existing preclinical test methodologies outlined in the International Standards Organization (ISO) and U.S. Food and Drug Administration (FDA) documents developed in the 1980s and revised during the 1990s (10,11). The standards and guidance documents will necessarily need to be updated to cover transcatheter valves, mainly for the various delivery methods and final device configurations when implanted in a nonuniform manner. The collapsible–expandable supporting structure used to deliver and secure the valve to the implant site necessitates additional testing for evaluation and characterization of these features. For preclinical testing, the delivery of these devices (i.e., collapsed to a small diameter for navigating the vasculature and then expanded into position) requires special steps for deployment prior to testing and the development of new fixtures to hold the device in test systems that simulate the intended clinical implant environment, especially for evaluation of migration potential.

The existing standards and guidance documents can provide a starting point for preclinical testing of transcatheter heart valves. The documents that cover replacement heart valve's reference can develop methods for valve

---

*This chapter contributed by Jack D. Lemmon, PhD, R&D Manager, Cardiovascular Division, St. Jude Medical, St. Paul, Minnesota, U.S.A.

functional evaluation that are based on an extensive clinical history and provide a general outline for the areas that should be considered in testing transcatheter heart valve designs. Other standards from the area of vascular stents and balloon catheters (12) can provide starting points for areas of investigation that are not addressed in heart valve guidance documents. These guidelines can provide a reference for device evaluation, but the valve and delivery system should be assessed in relation to the outcome of risk management activities (13), depending on device design and intended use.

The preclinical testing performed on replacement heart valves is guided by project risk management activities. The risk management activities allow for the identification of clinical complications, severity of identified hazards, potential failure modes, effects on device and patient, methods to detect failure modes, and controls to mitigate the risks associated with identified hazards. These activities examine the failure modes and effects associated with both device design and manufacturing processes and potential failure modes induced by the operator. Preclinical testing is one of the methods used for risk mitigation in evaluating the identified failure modes. Risk assessment for the product and its intended use is updated continuously during the product development cycle, adding information to the analysis as it is gathered from preclinical and clinical evaluation.

Preclinical testing of transcatheter heart valve substitutes includes component and device-level testing. Many of the replacement heart valve test methodologies are available in the published literature and can provide valuable information on lessons learned for test setup and data gathering/interpretation. Preclinical testing of transcatheter heart valve substitutes can be separated into three main areas: evaluation of device hydrodynamic function, device durability/life cycle, and device biocompatibility/host response.

Hydrodynamics

Hydrodynamics testing is used to evaluate the function of replacement heart valves under a range of physiologic conditions. It uses a mock circulatory loop (14,15) that can be operated over a range of heart rates (typically 45–150 beats/min) and cardiac outputs (typically 2–10 L/min). The replacement heart valve is placed in the mock circulatory loop in a configuration intended to simulate the implant environment. The mock circulatory loop is operated over a range of flow conditions by changes in heart rate and cardiac output to obtain measurements of pressure drop, effective orifice area, and regurgitant flow volume (Figs. 1–3). The valves can also be evaluated for regurgitant flow and susceptibility to migration under increasing systematic pressure and simulating conditions ranging from normal to hypersensitive.

Measurements of flow rate, pressure drop, and effective orifice area give an overall view of valve function by measuring bulk flow properties. Other measurement techniques are needed to determine more precisely the flow field patterns and level of fluid velocity through the valve. This additional information can provide assessment of laminar and turbulent flow regions as well as identifying areas of stagnant flow that could lead to complications such as thrombus formation. Flow visualization studies in a pulsatile flow system can be performed using a laser light sheet illumination, a test solution seeded with small glass or plastic particles (16). This test provides excellent reconstruction of flow patterns through the valve by using particles that are neutrally buoyant so that

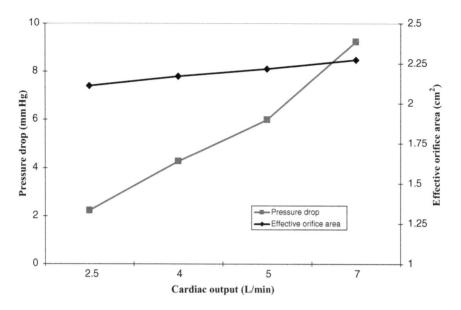

FIGURE 1   Pressure drop and effective orifice versus flow rate.

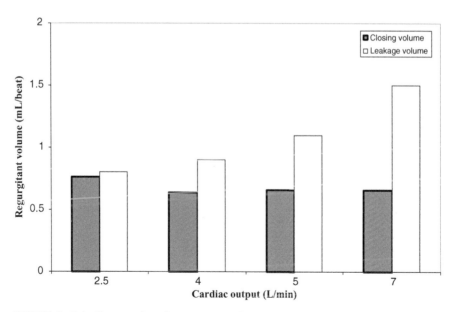

FIGURE 2   Pulsatile regurgitant flow versus cardiac output. Regurgitant volume is separated into the closing volume and leakage volume through the valve.

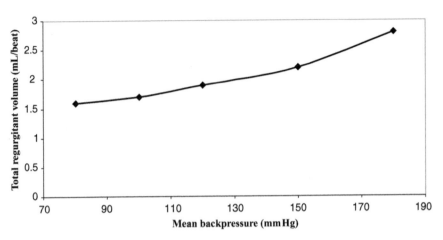

FIGURE 3 Pulsatile regurgitant leakage volume as a function of mean systemic back pressure.

they outline the pulsatile flow fields when illuminated by the laser light sheet. Recording these flow patterns via video or still images provides visualization of streaklines that detail how the flow passes through the valve. More quantitative data can be obtained via other measurement techniques for evaluating velocity, turbulence, and time-dependent flow structures (Fig. 4) (17–19).

Hydrodynamic test methods are also used for verification of clinical measurement techniques for replacement heart valves. Since Doppler ultrasound is primarily used during patient follow-up, verification of the Bernoulli relationship to measure pressure drops can be performed in a pulse duplicator system (20). For this evaluation, the peak velocity of the flow through the replacement heart valve is measured by continuous-wave Doppler ultrasound, and this velocity is used to calculate the pressure drop via the Bernoulli equation ($\Delta p = 4v^2$). For comparison, the pressure drop is measured directly using pressure transducers. These measurements are compared in order to find out whether the Bernoulli relationship used to calculate pressure drop using continuous-wave velocity measurements and the coefficient 4 in the equation is accurate. This determines how accurate the Bernoulli relationship is for calculating pressure drop measurements by clinical methods but caution is warranted in the clinical setting, since other factors may influence this measurement during follow-up examinations.

Test Setups

Device Durability

Evaluation of the structural integrity of the transcatheter heart valve must give consideration to the potential damage induced during operation, ultimate failure modes of the device, and the fatigue life of the materials used. Each piece of the information feeds into the overall assessment of the structural performance of the transcatheter heart valve, ensuring proper function of the device under the intended operating conditions. Areas of testing can include failure mode analysis, accelerated wear, stent evaluation, computational analysis, stent

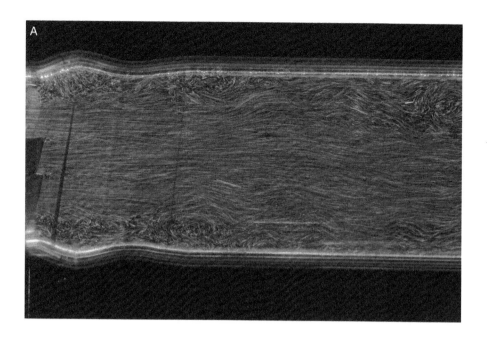

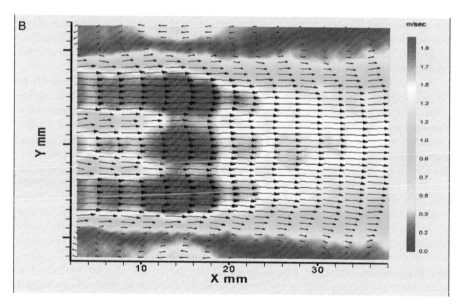

FIGURE 4 (**A**) Qualitative streaklines and (**B**) quantitative velocity measurements of flow through the valve from flow visualization and particle image velocimetry studies, respectively. The data provides information on the general flow patterns and if the flow field is turbulent.

fatigue testing, and fatigue lifetime analysis. Although every implant configuration cannot be evaluated, worst-case implant conditions such as nonuniform deployment and over expansions should be considered in the analysis along with nominal conditions.

Failure Mode Analysis

Failure mode analysis is a test methodology that examines the exact nature of how the transcatheter valve fails during operation. Its purpose is to determine if the failure mode is catastrophic or degenerative. Failure modes can be induced by acceleration of the cycle rate and/or elevation of the loading to which the device is subjected. A change in operation variables is required, since real-time observation of failures is neither reasonable nor expected in the time frame of a product development cycle. An increase in cycle rate will apply a great number of cycles to the materials in a short period of time to produce damage on the valve, but may not produce ultimate failure. Testing replacement valves under elevated loads will produce device failures by overloading the device in order to determine the weakest components. Valves might fail due to valve incompetence via leaflet abrasion, stent migration, and stent fracture. The identification of failure modes along with accelerated wear findings provided details of greatest damage during operation.

Accelerated Wear Testing

As previously noted, real-time testing to determine the damage induced during the operational life of a transcatheter heart valve is not feasible during a product development cycle. Historically, accelerated wear testing of heart valves has produced adequate information to indicate which regions of the device exhibit contact and how that contact induces damage to the device (21–24).

Accelerated wear testing is performed under conditions that are 10 to 20 times the physiologic cycle rates, allowing the equivalent number of cycles seen clinically in five years to be achieved in five to six months in the laboratory. For this testing, the valves are cycled under normal pressures based on the intended implant site. The acceleration of the device cycling allows for evaluation of the wear patterns on either the tissue or the stent, if performed properly. To obtain meaningful results from this type of test, two main requirements are that the opening and closing of the leaflets should be full and complete and that a sustained pressure should be developed upon closing to hold the leaflets closed for a portion of the cycle. These conditions should be monitored periodically during testing to ensure that valve opening and closing are properly maintained throughout the duration of the test. The devices are also removed from the test and examined periodically for damage to record its type, location, and progression over time. The function of the device can also be evaluated at time intervals during testing by hydrodynamic evaluation methods to record any changes over time.

For biological valves, guidance documents indicate evaluation of the device for 200 million cycles representing five years of clinical implantation. The testing duration may be shorter if the implant is not intended as a permanent replacement and/or the duration meets the needs outlined in the risk analysis. Accelerated wear testing provides information about the progressive nature of damage that can occur to the transcatheter heart valve during years of clinical service.

Stent Testing

Failure mode analysis and accelerated wear testing target device-level evaluation and in particular concentrate on the valve leaflets, since they are typically the weakest components of the replacement heart valve. This testing does provide some information about the frame to which the valve leaflets are attached, but specific component testing is better suited for complete evaluation of these elements. Currently, manufacturers have utilized metal stents for the delivery of the transcatheter heart valves so that is the type of frame discussed here. There is some history of metal sent testing methodologies, and regulatory bodies have outlined recommended testing and evaluation for preclinical assessment of intravascular stents (9). The testing and analysis called for in the documents covering intravascular stents overlap with the testing described in the heart valve guidance, because test analysis methodologies for a stented heart valve replacement are covered in the heart valve guidance.

Stent testing is required to address hazards outlined during the risk analysis activities. In general, the stent must be characterized for mechanical properties, radial strength, recoil, foreshortening, deployment uniformity, and stent-to-balloon pressure dimensional verification. These elements identify general characteristic of the stents prior to rigorous testing under normal and worst-case use conditions. Since the stents provide the structure to the device, it is essential that fatigue testing and analysis be utilized in addition to the accelerated wear testing to ensure that no failures will occur over the life cycle of the device. The fatigue analysis should include computational analysis, structural fatigue life testing, and fatigue lifetime analysis.

Computational Analysis

In order to perform a fatigue analysis for the device, the stresses on the structural components must be calculated based on the loading conditions that will be experienced in its intended use. Finite element analysis provides a means to calculate these stresses for comparison with the material and fatigue properties. The analysis should consider the steps involved in manufacturing, handling of the device during implant, and intended operating conditions to calculate induced stresses on the device during each step. In the case of the transcatheter valve, consideration must also be given to the loading of the stent by the closed leaflets. The loading to be considered should be the worst-case conditions for the intended implant configuration. This type of analysis can be used to evaluate the range of worst-case conditions that the frame configuration may take upon implantation.

For the analysis, either assumptions of physiologic parameters (pressure or deflection) based on implant site conditions or experimentally measured data from the laboratory are employed in the analysis to supply the loading conditions for the model to calculate the maximum stress. Several different loading conditions may need to be considered for the analysis, depending on the totality of clinically relevant loading conditions. As will be discussed later in this chapter, the peak stresses are used in the fatigue life analysis to determine whether the device design is robust enough to function in the intended implant environment.

Fatigue Life Testing

While accelerated wear testing does apply loads to the stent for a prescribed number of cycles, the fatigue life testing is carried out under normal pressure levels. To ensure that the stent does not fail catastrophically over the life of the implant, fatigue testing of the stent is performed under more rigorous conditions and for a higher number of cycles. The loading conditions of the stent used in the fatigue testing can come from several sources, including the aforementioned finite element analysis. One approach is to use the finite element analysis results under hypertensive conditions to provide the strain on the device during loading and to use that strain level to control the testing of the device for fatigue life. Once the loading levels have been determined, testing can be performed using pulsatile pressure in a mock circulatory system with the stent deployed to a maximum size. At the end of the test, the stents are examined visually to determine if any types of failures have occurred, for example, strut fractures or cracks on the stent because of cyclic loading.

Fatigue Life Analysis

Although the fatigue testing previously described provides a pass/fail test for the stent, a conservative fatigue analysis is needed in order to predict the expected fatigue life of the device. What the pass/fail testing does not provide is a factor of safety determination for the device design operating under worst-case loading conditions. The fatigue analysis can be performed in several ways, including methodologies that fall under stress/life principles or damage tolerance analysis (25,26). For stents, the traditional stress/life analysis (Sn) has been used to experimentally obtain the endurance limit of the device (Fig. 5). Experiments are performed loading devices at different alternating stress levels to determine the number of cycles to failure, evaluating both low-cycle and high-cycle fatigue.

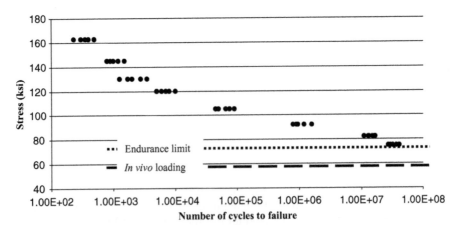

FIGURE 5 Example of stress versus number of cycles to failure of test samples to determine endurance limit of the device. Estimated in vivo loading is provided for comparison to estimate safety factors.

Durability Analysis

The assessment of device durability combines the results from the failure mode analysis, accelerated wear testing, computational analysis, fatigue life testing, and fatigue life analysis to determine if the design is robust enough for the intended application. No single test from this list can be used to determine device durability. The failure mode and accelerated wear testing provide data on the weakest components and areas of contact during device operation. The computational results and fatigue life analysis provide quantitative data on the level of operating stresses for the device and where that level is related to the inherent fatigue properties of the device. The durability testing of the individual structural components provides a pass/fail examination of the device when functioning under worst-case in vivo conditions. In total, the durability test and analysis provide the data to evaluate valve performance in the proposed fatigue environment.

Biological Testing

The testing discussed above provides the in vitro evaluation of the device and its components. Preclinical animal studies provide the final verification testing prior to clinical trials to determine the host response to the implant. This testing evaluates the transcatheter heart valve for biocompatibility and chronic implantation (27). Biocompatibility testing provides data on inflammation, cytotoxicity, sensitization, irritation, thrombogenicity, and pyrogenicity of the device. Chronic animal studies are used to test the host response at the implant site, the device histology, and the hemodynamic function of the valve. These studies provide the final piece of data to address potential failure modes prior to start of a clinical trail.

Summary

During the product development cycle, preclinical tests are utilized to help understand how the transcatheter heart valve may operate clinically. Preclinical in vitro testing allows for accurate assessment under controlled conditions to determine the functionality and durability of the device. Preclinical in vivo testing provides a biological environment for device evaluation to provide further proof that the device will perform as intended. In total, the preclinical testing is used to address the risks indentified with regard to implantation and operation of the device during clinical use. A well-designed, controlled clinical trial provides the ultimate evaluation of the device in the intended implant population and for treatment of the indicated pathologies.

PRECLINICAL BENCH TESTING—THE DYNAMIC MOCK LOOP SETUP

Introduction

The aim was to evaluate valved stent performance in a simulated dynamic circulation. The bench test was constructed from a pulsatile pump (Biventricular support system 5000, Oberdorfstrasse, Baar ZG, Switzerland), two compliance chambers made from latex gloves to simulate the elastic resistance of blood vessels, a compliant silicone tube with an inner diameter of 18 mm serving as target vessel equivalent, a reservoir, an intravascular ultrasound (IVUS) (Clearview, Boston Scientific Corporation, Sunnyvale, CA), two 5F Millar pressure

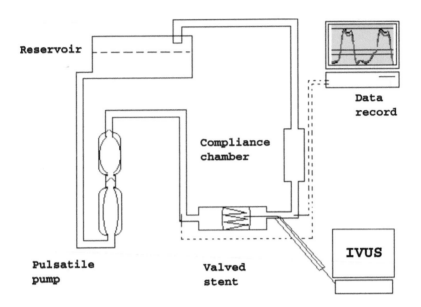

Reservoir

Data record

Compliance chamber

IVUS

Pulsatile pump

Valved stent

FIGURE 6 Schematic mock loop setup.

transducer catheters (MPC-500, Millar Instruments, Inc., Houston, TX), a data recording system, and several connecting tubes Ø 1/2 (Figs. 6 and 7).

The mock loop generated flow rates from 2 to 5 L/min, building up systolic pressures between 80 and 150 mm Hg. Rapid cycling ranged from 30 to 180 beats/min.

The device was loaded into the circuit via a "Y" connector on the 18 mm silicon tubing and deployed with a 24F delivery system. After complete withdrawal of the delivery catheter, the IVUS probe was inserted via a hemostatic valve mounted on the Y connection. Finally the setup was supplemented by the Millar catheters to measure transvalvular gradient. The valved stent was loaded into the 24F introducing catheter by hand crimping.

The introducing catheter now containing the valved stent was inserted into the silicone tube via the plastic tube. Once the introducer was in position, the valved stent was released by withdrawing the outside catheter while holding the inside piston in place. After deployment, the introducing system was withdrawn. The distal end of the plastic tube was connected to a hemostatic valve permitting the IVUS catheter to go in from here.

Typical Measurements for the Second-Generation Pulmonary Valved Stent Device

The Millar catheter was used to measure the pressure on both sides of the valve for estimation of valve gradient. The IVUS catheter was inserted from the hemostatic valve to the valved stent to measure valvular function.

Dynamic mock loop results of the second-generation pulmonary valved stent device are as follows: The peak systolic gradient across the valve was 6.42

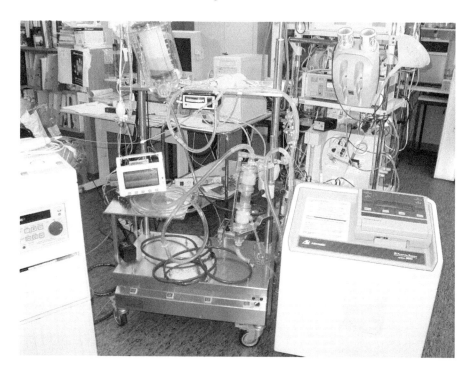

FIGURE 7 Overview of the mock loop setup for dynamic valved stent testing.

± 2.75 mm Hg at a mean flow rate of 4.32 ± 0.97 L/min. In Figure 8, the graph shows the gradient and results from the difference between the two curves.

At the sonographic assessment of the valve function, the open area of the valved stent was measured to be 204.8 ± 10.5 mm^2 and the closed area presented a residual opening of 7.2 mm^2 (Fig. 9). From the IVUS images, the two leaflets of the valve were seen to open and close completely. The valve was well-fixed in the silicone tube and showed no signs of migration.

In summary, the competence of the valved stent (as judged by its opening and closure) tested favorably under our mock loop system as evident from the IVUS and Miller catheter findings.

Setup of a Novel Ex Vivo Mock Loop System for Dynamic Mitral Valved Stent Testing

Introduction

Previous preclinical bench test (28,29) for prosthetic heart valves were mainly to assess aortic devices (Fig. 10) mostly made of silicone tubing or Perspex but hardly any, if at all, biological components were used (30–33). Only a few studies describe in vitro testing in the mitral position (34,35), while no studies can be found describing a mock loop system using an explanted heart for ex vivo testing.

The novel ex vivo bench test concept aims at simulating anatomical structures and tissue compliance most realistically. The devices were to be released in

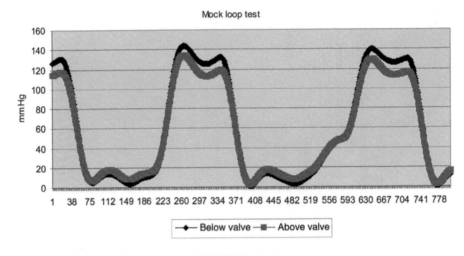

FIGURE 8 Computer aided dynamic pressure curve recording.

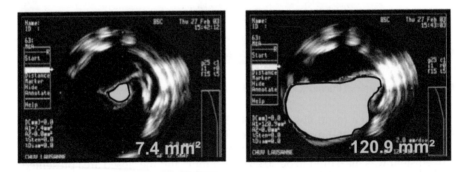

FIGURE 9 IVUS views of the valve in closed (*left*) and opened (*right*) state.

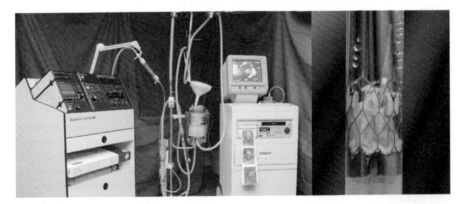

FIGURE 10 Aortic valved stent device mock loop bench test setup including a pulsatile flow generator, an expansion reservoir, a valve chamber, and an intravascular assessment unit.

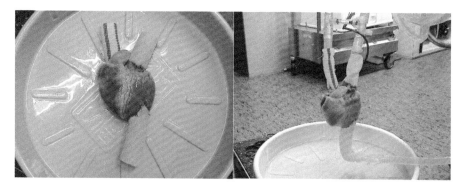

FIGURE 11 Construction of the ex vivo setup. Dacron prostheses are sewn to the left atrium, the aorta, and the apex of the explanted pig's heart to allow connection to the cardiopulmonary bypass (CPB) circuit.

the mitral position of a freshly explanted pig's heart, which was connected to the mock loop system. All measurements and recordings were taken by endoscopy, an IVUS probe, and invasive Millar pressure transducer catheters.

Setup of the Mock Loop System
The pig's heart were connected to the mock loop by anastomosing a 25 mm Dacron tubing to the ascending aorta, another Dacron prosthesis to the left atrium, and a third tube to the left ventricular apex in order to facilitate further connection with the silicone circuit (Fig. 11).

In order to simulate the characteristics of the left heart most realistically, the test circuit was setup according to Figure 12 (note that the following numbers in bold refer to the numbers in Fig. 12). The system was powered by a ventricular assist device (Datascope System 83) **1**. The pneumatic pump **15** was pulsatile and the pulse rate, flow, and systolic pressure could easily be regulated. The diastolic pressures were changed by the height of two water reservoirs **8** and **9**. Recording and analysis was computer aided (sampling rate, 50 Hz), **12** and **14**. For further details, see Figure 13.

Deployment of the Valved Stent
The mitral valved stent was deployed into the mitral annulus under endoscopic guidance. Then the anastomosis between the left atrium and the Dacron tubing was finalized. Construction of the custom-made valved stent and the delivery process has been extensively reported (36–38).

Measurements
Three Millar catheters (5F Millar pressure transducer catheters, MPC-500, Millar Instruments, Inc., Houston, TX) were used to measure the pressure in the aorta, left atrium, and left ventricle.

An IVUS (Clearview, Boston Scientific Corporation, Sunnyvale, CA) catheter was inserted through the hemostatic valve to the valved stent in order to measure valvular function.

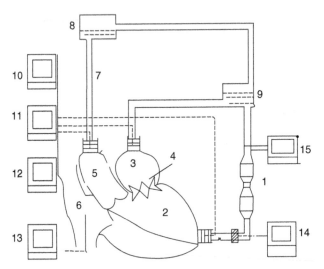

FIGURE 12 Schematic mock loop including **1**, pulsatile flow generator; **2**, left ventricle; **3**, left atrium; **4**, valved stent; **5**, aorta; **6**, right atrium; **7**, silicone tubing; **8**, water reservoir A (90 cm in height); **9**, water reservoir B (20 cm in height); **10**, endoscope; **11**, intravascular ultrasound (IVUS); **12**, computer and pressure recording system; **13**, intracardiac ultrasound (ICUS); **14**, flow recording system; **15**, pulsatile flow generator (Datascope System 83).

An endoscope (KARL STORZ GmbH & Co. KG, Tuttlingen, Germany) was used to show intracardiac structures on video. The endoscope probe was inserted through the Dacron tube controlled by two purse-string sutures.

Results
1. During the experiment, pressures of LV and LA both before and after implantation were measured (Fig. 14). The diastolic pressure gradient across the valved stent (mitral position) was close to zero (0.48 mm Hg) at a mean flow rate of 2.81 ± 0.26 L/min. There was no pre- and postimplantation difference.

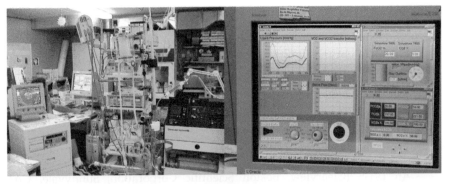

FIGURE 13 Mock loop overview including an IVUS and ICUS, pulse generator, hemodynamic measurement unit, and a computer aided flow analysis station.

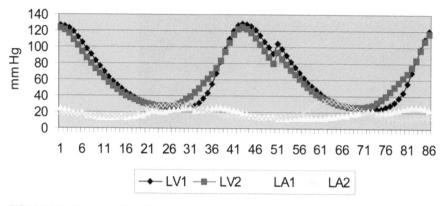

FIGURE 14 The computer aided pressure curve recordings. *Abbreviations:* LV1, left ventricle pressure before implantation; LV2, left ventricle pressure after implantation; LA1, left atrium pressure before implantation; LA2, left atrium pressure after implantation.

2. The IVUS showed complete valve closure and opening. The open area of the valved stent was 254.8 ± 10.5 mm^2 with an open diameter of 19.6 ± 1.4 mm (Fig. 15).
3. Endoscopic imaging showed complete valve closure and opening (Fig. 16). The device was safely anchored in the mitral annulus. No signs of migrations were observed.

Methodical Considerations

A complete and detailed in vitro testing is mandatory in order to perform an animal or clinical trial of a new prosthesis valve (10,11). The type of in vitro evaluation is limited to valves placed in the aortic and pulmonary position (39). However, for the mitral position, an increased valve area should be considered and evaluated under a diastolic pressure rather than systolic pressure gradient. The interaction between prosthesis valve and native valves and the subvalvular apparatus should be taken into account, as the anatomy and the flow dynamics as well as the annular motion are very unique to the mitral valve. Therefore, we

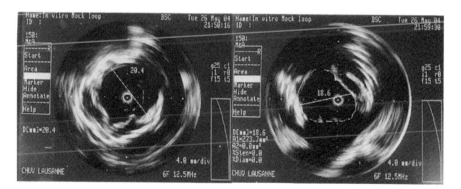

FIGURE 15 IVUS findings of the valved stent during mock loop cycling.

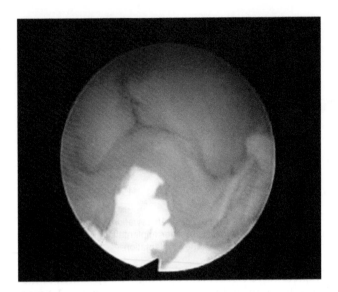

FIGURE 16 Endoscopic view showing complete valve closure of the device.

developed a new left heart ex vivo (in vitro) mock loop system for most realistic testing of either mitral or aortic valve.

The proposed mock loop model differed from others in three ways: (1) the tested valves were mounted in a fresh ex vivo pig's heart, (2) direct optical assessment became possible using an endoscope, and (3) functional and visual sonographic analysis was performed with IVUS.

The preservation of the native valvular and subvalvular apparatus is essential for left ventricular geometry and consequently to the physiological functioning and ventricular contractility. Preservation of the mitral valve apparatus allows to most reliably simulate in situ conditions.

However, the evaluated valved stents, designed for off-bypass implantation, present a higher profile (length 29.34 ± 0.19 mm) that could interfere with the native valves and the left ventricle outflow tract. Therefore, not only the valved stents devices but also their interaction with surrounding structures should be considered and tested in vitro before animal experimentation.

The fluid used in this closed circuit was distilled water supplemented with a fluidity enhancer to increase viscosity to a similar level as blood viscosity. In so doing, endoscopic viewing was facilitated greatly. Intracardiac structure and motion of valves as well as adequacy of fixation of the implanted valved stent could be viewed directly with the endoscope from both the left atrial and left ventricular side. The good direct visibility showed the well-coapting and fully opening valve leaflets of the fully deployed valved stent.

The important role of an IVUS in off-bypass implantation of valved stent in vena cava and pulmonary position has been already reported (40). Using an IVUS, we not only measured the size of annulus and inspected the motion of leaflets but also accumulated much experience of cardiac leaflets and annulus measurement, which was beneficial to our animal experiment.

REFERENCES

1. Hufnagel CA, Harvey WP. Aortic plastic valvular prosthesis. Bull Georgetown Univ Med Center 1952; 4:1.
2. Bonhoeffer P, Boudjemline Y, Saliba Z, et al. Percutaneous replacement of pulmonary valve in a right-ventricle to pulmonary-artery prosthetic conduit with valve dysfunction. Lancet 2000; 356:1403–1405.
3. Cribier A, Eltchaninoff H, Bash A, et al. Percutaneous transcatheter implantation of an aortic valve prosthesis for calcific aortic stenosis: First human case description. Circulation 2002; 106:3006–3008.
4. Piazza N, Grube E, Gerckens U, et al. Procedural and 30-day outcomes following transcatheter aortic valve implantation using the third generation (18 Fr) CoreValve Revalving System: Results from the multicentre, expanded evaluation registry 1-year following CE mark approval. EuroIntervention 2008; 4(2):242–249.
5. Ye J, Cheung A, Lichtenstein SV, et al. Six-month outcome of transapical transcatheter aortic valve implantation in the initial seven patients. Eur J Cardiothorac Surg 2007; 31(1):16–21.
6. Leon MB, Kodali S, Williams M, et al. Transcatheter aortic valve replacement in patients with critical aortic stenosis: Rationale, device descriptions, early clinical experiences, and perspectives. Semin Thorac Cardiovasc Surg 2006; 18(2):165–174.
7. Kumar N, Balasundaram S, Rickard M, et al. Leaflet embolisation from Duromedics valves: A report of two cases. Thorac Cardiovasc Surg 1991; 39:382–383.
8. Bodnar E. The Medtronic parallel valve and the lessons learned. J Heart Valve Dis 1996; 5:572–573.
9. Yoganathan AP, Eberhardt CE, Walker PG. Hydrodynamic performance of the Medtronic freestyle aortic root bioprosthesis. J Heart Valve Dis 1994; 3:571–580.
10. ISO 5840:2005. Cardiovascular implants—cardiac valve prostheses. March 1, 2005.
11. U.S. Department of Human Health Service, Public Health Service, Food and Drug Administration. Draft replacement heart valve guidance. October 14, 1994.
12. U.S. Department of Human Health Service, Food and Drug Administration, Center for Devices and Radiological Health. Guidance for industry and FDA staff: Non-clinical tests and recommended labeling for intravascular stents and associated delivery systems. January 13, 2005.
13. ISO 14971:2000. Medical devices—application of risk management to medical devices. March 23, 2001.
14. Yoganathan AP, Woo YR, Sung HW, et al. In vitro hemodynamic characteristics of tissue bioprostheses in the aortic position. J Thorac Cardiovasc Surg 1986; 92:198–209.
15. Scotten LN, Walker DK. New laboratory technique measures projected dynamic area of prosthetic heart valves. J Heart Valve Dis 2004; 13:120–132.
16. Gross JM, Shermer CD, Hwang NH. Vortex shedding in bileaflet heart valve prostheses. ASAIO Trans 1988; 34:845–850.
17. Hasenkam JM, Westphal D, Reul H, et al. Three-dimensional visualization of axial velocity profiles downstream of six different mechanical aortic valve prostheses, measured with a hot-film anemometer in a steady state flow model. J Biomech 1987; 20:353–364.
18. Lim WL, Chew YT, Chew TC, et al. Particle image velocimetry in the investigation of flow past artificial heart valves. Ann Biomed Eng 1994; 22:307–318.
19. Woo YR, Yoganathan AP. Two-component laser Doppler anemometer for measurement of velocity and turbulent shear stress near prosthetic heart valves. Med Instrum 1985; 19:224–231.
20. Stewart SF, Nast EP, Arabia FA, et al. Errors in pressure gradient measurement by continuous wave Doppler ultrasound: Type, size and age effects in bioprosthetic aortic valves. J Am Coll Cardiol 1991; 18:769–779.
21. Reul H, Potthast K. Durability/wear testing of heart valve substitutes. J Heart Valve Dis 1998; 7:151–157.
22. Campbell A, Baldwin T, Peterson G, et al. Pitfalls and outcomes from accelerated wear testing of mechanical heart valves. J Heart Valve Dis 1996; 5(suppl 1):S124–S132.

23. Hasenkam JM, Pasquino E, Stacchino C, et al. Wear patterns in the Sorin biocarbon mechanical heart valve: A clinical explant study. J Heart Valve Dis 1997; 6:105–114.
24. More RB, Chang BC, Hong YS, et al. Wear analysis of retrieved mitral bileaflet mechanical heart valve explants [abstract]. In: Proceedings of Society for Heart Valve Disease. First Biennial Meeting; London, UK; 2001:284 (abst).
25. Ritchie RO, Lubock P. Fatigue life estimation procedures for the endurance of a cardiac valve prosthesis: Stress/life and damage-tolerant analyses. J Biomech Eng 1986; 108:153–160.
26. Ryder JK. Cao H. Structural integrity assessment of heart valve prostheses: A damage tolerance analysis of the CarboMedics prosthetic heart valve. J Heart Valve Dis 1996; 5(suppl 1):S86–S96.
27. ISO 10993-1:2003. Biological evaluation of medical devices—Part 1: Evaluation and testing. August 1, 2003.
28. Eichinger W, Däbritz S, Lange R. Update of the European standards for inactive surgical implants in the area of heart valve prostheses. Eur J Cardiothorac Surg 2007; 32:690–695.
29. Gerosa G, di Marco F, Casarotto D, et al. Searching for a correct method of evaluation for valve prosthesis performance. J Heart Valve Dis 2004; 13(suppl 1):S1–S3.
30. Chambers J, Ely JL. Early postoperative echocardiographic hemodynamic performance of the On-X prosthetic heart valve: A multicenter study. J Heart Valve Dis 1998; 7:569–573.
31. Fraund S, Pethig K, Wahlers T, et al. ON-X bileaflet valve in aortic position—early experience shows an improved hemodynamic profile. Thorac Cardiovasc Surg 1998; 46:293–297.
32. Chambers J, Ely J. A comparison of the classical and modified forms of the continuity equation in the On-X prosthetic heart valve in the aortic position. J Heart Valve Dis 2000; 9:299–301; Discussion 301–302.
33. Hwang NH, Reul H, Reinhard P. In vitro evaluation of the long-body On-X bileaflet valve. J Heart Valve Dis 1998; 7:561–568.
34. Verdonck P, Van Nooten G, Van Belleghem Y. Pulse duplicator hydrodynamics of four different bileaflet valves in the mitral position. Cardiovasc Surg 1997; 5:593–603.
35. Verdonck P, Dumont K, Segers P, et al. Mock loop testing of On-X prosthetic mitral valve with Doppler echocardiography. Artif Organs 2002; 26(10):872–878.
36. Huber CH, Cohn LH, von Segesser LK. Direct-access valve replacement a novel approach for off-pump valve implantation using valved stents. J Am Coll Cardiol 2005; 46(2):366–370.
37. Huber CH, Nasratulla M, Augstburger M, et al. Ultrasound navigation through the heart for off-pump aortic valved stent implantation: New tools for new goals. J Endovasc Ther 2004; 11:503–510.
38. Huber CH, Marty B, von Segesser LK. Acceptance and introduction of disruptive technologies—simple steps to build a fully functional pulmonary valved stent. Interact Cardiovasc Thorac Surg 2007; 6(4):430–432.
39. Robert CA Jr, Daniel JG, David D, et al. Development of an intraluminal device for the treatment of aortic regurgitation: Prototype and in vitro testing system. J Thorac Cardiovasc Surg 1996; 112:979–983.
40. Zhou JQ, Corno AF, Huber CH, et al. Self-expandable valved stent of large size:Off-bypass implantation in pulmonary position. Eur J Cardiothorac Surg 2003; 24:212–216.

TRANSCATHETER VENA CAVA VALVE IMPLANTATION FOR TRICUSPID REGURGITATION

The following study is in part reproduced from Corno AF et al. Off-bypass implantation of a self-expandable valved stent between inferior vena cava and right atrium. Interact Cardiovasc Thorac Surg 2003; 2(2):166–169.

Introduction

Tricuspid regurgitation might be an underdiagnosed and underestimated disease. After the reported experimental studies with percutaneous valve replacement in pulmonary (1) and aortic (2,3) position and the introduction of percutaneous insertion of a biological valve in pulmonary position in the clinical practice (4,5), this experimental study has been designed to evaluate the feasibility of the off-bypass implantation of a self-expanding valved stent in inferior vena cava.

Materials and Methods

A glutaraldehyde-preserved valved bovine jugular xenograft, with proved results for surgical repair of complex congenital heart defects (6), was mounted in two rings of nonthermosensitive nitinol Z-stents expanding from 7 to 28 mm of internal diameter (Fig. 1). In vitro static performance was tested in five valved stents with a column of water developing a pressure of 45 mm Hg. Dynamic test evaluation of the valve regurgitation was performed with a mock loop including a pulsatile pump. Valve function was assessed with flow and pressure drop measurements as well as intravascular ultrasound (IVUS) (Boston Scientific Corporation, Sunnyvale, CA) with a 6F and 12.5 MHz transducer in real time.

The self-expanding valved stent was crimped into a Teflon sheath stent-graft delivery system with an overall diameter of 8.0 mm (=24F) (Fig. 2).

Acute in vivo evaluation was performed in five adult pigs (mean body weight = 80.5 ± 5.0 kg; range = 74–85 kg). After general anesthesia, tracheal intubation, and mechanical ventilation with continuous monitoring of electrocardiogram, arterial pressure, and oxygen saturation, heparin was administered IV (1 mg/kg).

The internal diameter and length of the inferior vena cava was been measured with an IVUS, with access via the right iliac vein through retroperitoneal approach. The self-expanding valved stent was introduced off-bypass into the inferior vena cava by the same retroperitoneal approach, positioned at the target level between hepatic veins and cavo–atrial junction and then unloaded; mean duration of deployment was eight minutes.

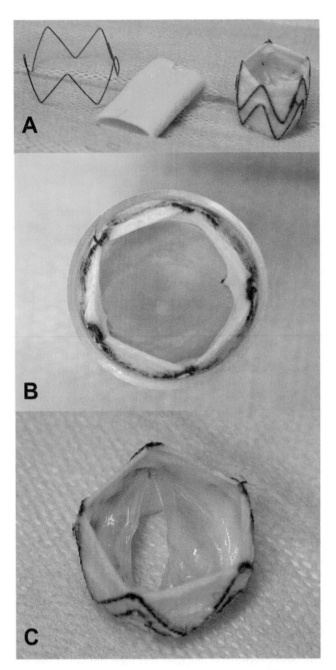

FIGURE 1 (**A**) Self-expanding nitinol Z-stent, bovine valved jugular vein, and expanding valved stent with mounted valve. (**B**) Valved stent with valve in open position. (**C**) Valved stent with valve leaflets in an intermediate state.

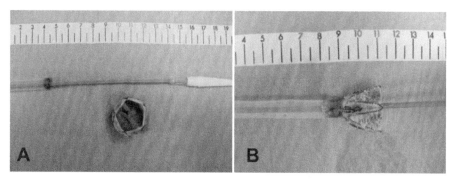

FIGURE 2 Self-expanding valved stent before (**A**) and after (**B**) loading on a Teflon sheath stent-graft delivery system.

A high fidelity tip-mounted Millar pressure transducer system was used to measure the pressure, proximal and distal to the valve, and an IVUS was used to assess the valve function.

At the end of the study, after a mean observation period of four hours, the animals were electively sacrificed to check the adequate positioning of the self-expanding valved stent as well as its deployment and anchorage and the presence of any valve deformation.

All animals received human care in compliance with the principles of the Guide for the Care and Use of Laboratory Animals (7). The protocol was approved by the institutional committee on animal research.

Results

The mean length of the valved stent was 22.80 ± 1.06 mm, the mean internal diameter was 20.97 ± 0.5 mm, and the mean external diameter was 26.67 ± 0.9 mm.

In vitro static performance testing of the valved stent showed a mean leakage rate of 32.5 ± 12.3 mL/min for an afterload of 45 mm Hg. The valve leakage rate under pressure was not statistically different from the results obtained with the original valved xenograft before mounting in the stent. The dynamic mock loop evaluation showed a peak-to-peak pressure gradient of 6.4 ± 2.7 mm Hg through the valve at 4.30 ± 0.97 L/min of pulsatile flow.

The IVUS showed a mean length of the inferior vena cava between the heart and the liver of 79 ± 2 mm (range = 75–84 mm) and the internal diameter of the inferior vena cava was 20.4 ± 1.6 mm (range = 18.71–22.56 mm). The mean pressure gradient recorded across the valved stent implanted in the inferior vena cava was 1.0 ± 0.5 mm Hg (range = 0–2 mm Hg).

The IVUS showed partial opening and closing of the valve, with a mean area reduction from 148.5 to 81.5 mm^2; almost complete valve closure occurred only during deep breaths in these healthy animals.

In all animals, autopsy confirmed the adequate position of the valved stent at about 2 cm proximal to the right atrial junction without any deformation of the valved stent.

Discussion

Previous experimental studies demonstrated the feasibility of implantation of a valved stent in the aortic position, which was reached from the abdominal aorta via a retroperitoneal access (8) or from the surgically isolated right common carotid artery (9,10), while another experimental study tested the deployment of a stented valved bovine jugular vein in the inferior vena cava or in the external iliac vein as a potential treatment for venous insufficiency (11).

The first goal of this study was to evaluate the feasibility of biological valve implantation within a self-expanding stent. Both the in vitro tests and the in vivo acute animal studies demonstrated the adequacy of this home-made self-expanding valved stent. The self-expanding device design might represent an advantage on the currently available biological platinum–iridium stent–mounted balloon-expanding valved stents (1,4,5).

The most important goal of this study was to demonstrate the feasibility of transcatheter off-bypass implantation of the self-expanding valved stent between the inferior vena cava and the right atrium. With regard to the mismatch between the size of the vena cava and the self-expanding valved stent, the study demonstrated that the internal diameter and the length of the inferior vena cava are suitable for implantation of the valved stents. Our measurements of the inferior vena cava by an IVUS provided results in agreement with the values reported with computerized tomography scans on human beings between 2 and 19 years of age, where the mean diameter of the inferior vena cava varied from 13.8 mm (range = 6.1–21.6 mm) at two years of age to a mean diameter of 28.4 mm (range = 20.5–36.4 mm) at 19 years of age, while the length of the inferior vena cava (measured from the confluence of the iliac veins to the diaphragm) varied from 116 mm (range = 71–162 mm) at two years of age to a mean length of 225 mm (range = 179–272 mm) at 19 years of age (12).

The retroperitoneal approach allowed for an easy and reproducible valved stent introduction via the right iliac vein as well as its positioning between the inferior vena cava and the right atrium. Special characteristics of the device design allow harboring a 22 mm internal diameter of tissue valves. This size is validated in clinical practice to be adequate for handling the entire systemic venous return when implanted in pulmonary position in patients of very large size and body weight up to 91 kg (6).

This might represent a potential clinical advantage over the currently available designs inserted from the femoral vein with limited valve size up to an internal diameter of 18 mm (5). In absence of right heart failure and systemic venous hypertension, the study demonstrated complete opening of the valve but also identified only partial closure of the valve leaflets, which almost completely closed only during deep breaths because of missing regurgitation volume to allow for full valve closure. Finally, both the implantation and the postimplantation device assessment were performed with intracardiac echo and plain fluoroscopy, avoiding contrast medium–associated angiography (13).

In summary, the in vitro and in vivo experiments confirmed (a) the feasibility of transcatheter off-bypass self-expanding valved stent implantation into the inferior vena cava and (b) the intracardiac echo (ICE) guidance being sufficient without the need of angiography for delivery monitoring and postimplantation device assessment.

SELF-EXPANDING FIRST-GENERATION VALVED STENT
FOR TCVT OF THE PULMONARY VALVE

Introduction

After previous experimental studies with percutaneous valve replacement in pulmonary (1) and aortic (2,3) position, the percutaneous insertion of a biological valve in pulmonary position has been introduced in the clinical practice (4,5). Insertion of a valve in pulmonary position is indicated mainly in two situations: (a) pulmonary valve regurgitation, generally after surgical repair for tetralogy of Fallot (14–22) and (b) dysfunction of the biological valved conduit previously implanted to establish the continuity between the right ventricle and the pulmonary artery during repair of complex congenital heart defects (23,24).

So far the conventional treatment for the above situations consisted of pulmonary valve replacement and replacement of the biological valved conduit (23–25), even with uncertainty about the adequate timing for pulmonary valve insertion in order to prevent or reduce the incidence of sudden death, arrhythmias, and right ventricular dysfunction (5,14–22).

Several alternative strategies, particularly in the presence of a dysfunction of a biological valved conduit, have been considered within the last years, including other types of biological valved conduits (6,26,27) or endovascular stent implantation to dilate and delay the surgical replacement of the obstructed conduit (28–30).

The main limit in the use of endovascular stents to dilate an obstructed biological conduit implanted between the right ventricle and the pulmonary artery is that, even if the obstruction is relieved or substantially reduced without requiring a reoperation on cardiopulmonary bypass, the patient remains with a pulmonary valve regurgitation, frequently worse than before. The subsequent right ventricular volume overload can cause irreversible myocardial damages with the known incidence of sudden death, arrhythmias, and right ventricular dysfunction (5,14–22,31).

The advantages of the percutaneous insertion of the pulmonary valve over the conventional surgical techniques are quite evident in terms of avoiding an operation on cardiopulmonary bypass and at the same time in the ability of implanting a functioning valve therefore reducing or abolishing both the pressure and the volume overload on the right ventricle (1,4,5). The major limit of this recently reported technique is the mismatch between the size of the venous access and the size of the introducer (at least 18 Fr), restricting the use of this strategy to older children and the size of the valve to an 18-mm internal diameter biological valve (5).

Because of the above problems, an experimental study was initiated to evaluate about alternative strategies aiming at the off-bypass transcatheter implantation of a self-expanding valved stent of large size in pulmonary position from right ventricular approach.

The following study is in part reproduced from Zhou JQ, Corno AF, Huber CH, et al. Self-expandable valved stent of large size: Off-bypass implantation in pulmonary position. Eur J Cardiothorac Surg 2003; 24(2):212–216.

Materials and Methods

A glutaraldehyde-preserved valved bovine jugular xenograft with internal diameter of 22 mm was mounted in two rings of nonthermosensitive nitinol Z-stents, expanding from 7 to 24 mm of internal diameter. In vitro static performance and dynamic test evaluation of this valved stent have been already reported (32). The self-expanding valved stent was prepared with a Teflon sheath stent-graft delivery system with an overall diameter of 8.0 mm (=24 F).

Acute in vivo evaluation was performed in six adult pigs having a mean body weight of 55.6 kg (range = 47–67 kg). After general anesthesia, tracheal intubation, and mechanical ventilation with continuous monitoring of electrocardiogram, arterial and central venous pressure, and oxygen saturation, the chest was opened through a conventional median sternotomy. Heparin was administered IV (1 mg/kg). After a short incision (4 mm) on the anterior aspect of the right ventricle, controlled by a purse string on 4-0 polypropylene suture, through the sheath stent-graft delivery system the valved stent was implanted off-bypass in pulmonary valve position by transventricular approach (Fig. 3). The correct positioning of the valved stent was evaluated and confirmed before definitive deployment by the IVUS technique.

Valve function was assessed with color Doppler echocardiography, flow and pressure drop measurements with Swan–Ganz Oximetry (Baxter-Edwards, Irvine, CA) catheter as well as IVUS (Boston Scientific Corporation, Sunnyvale, CA) with a 6F, 12.5 MHz transducer, and intracardiac ultrasound (ICUS) (Acuson Corporation, Mountain View, CA) with 10F, 7.5 MHz transducer in real time.

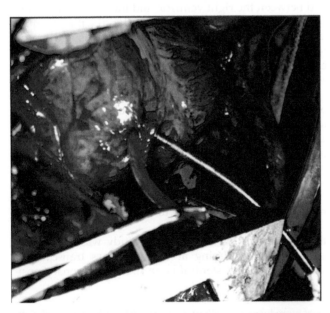

FIGURE 3 After a short incision (4 mm) on the anterior aspect of the right ventricle, controlled by a purse string on 4-0 polypropylene suture, through the sheath stent-graft delivery system the valved stent has been implanted off-bypass in pulmonary valve position by the transapical procedure.

A high fidelity tip-mounted Millar pressure transducer system was used to invasively measure the pressure, proximal and distal to the valve.

At the end of the study, the animals were electively sacrificed to check the adequate position of the valved stent as well as its deployment and anchorage and the presence of any deformation of the valve.

All animals received human care in compliance with the *Principles of Laboratory Animals* formulated by the National Society of Medical Research and the *Guide for the Care and Use of Laboratory Animals* prepared by the Institute of Laboratory Animal Resources and published by the National Institutes of Health (7). The protocol was approved by the institutional committee on animal research.

Statistical analysis: the Student *t* test was utilized and all data were expressed as mean ± standard deviation.

Results

The mean diameter of the main pulmonary artery measured with an IVUS was 21.7 ± 1.6 mm. The mean length of the valved stent was 23.1 ± 0.7 mm, the mean internal diameter was 21.6 ± 0.7 mm, and the mean external diameter was 26.3 ± 0.7 mm.

The mean peak pressure gradient recorded across the valve was 6.33 ± 2.8 mm Hg (range = 4.5–9.6 mm Hg) at Doppler echocardiography and 4.5 ± 3.1 mm Hg (range = 0–7 mm Hg) at invasive measurement, with a mean pulmonary blood flow of 3.03 ± 0.05 L/min.

The IVUS showed complete opening and closure of the valve (mean area reduction from 315.08 ± 54.13 to 0 mm^2) (Fig. 4). In all animals, Doppler echocardiography confirmed the absence of any valve regurgitation as well as paravalvular leak (Fig. 5).

No significant changes were recorded in electrocardiogram, arterial and central venous pressure, and oxygen saturation after self-expanding valved stent implantation.

Postmortem examination confirmed the adequate position of the valved stent in pulmonary position (Fig. 6) as well as ruled out any valve deformation or thrombus (Fig. 7).

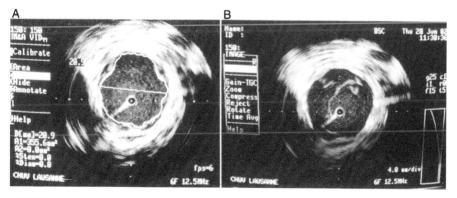

FIGURE 4 Intravascular ultrasound showing complete opening (**A**) and closure (**B**) of the valve.

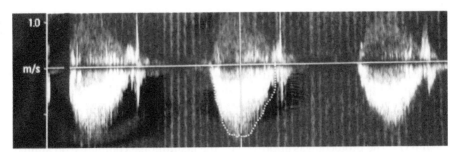

FIGURE 5 Doppler echocardiography confirming the absence of any valve regurgitation as well as paravalvular leak.

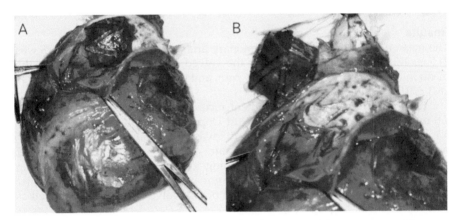

FIGURE 6 Postmortem examination confirming the adequate position of the valved stent in pulmonary position (**A**) and showing the fingerprint of the Z-stent on the pulmonary artery wall (**B**).

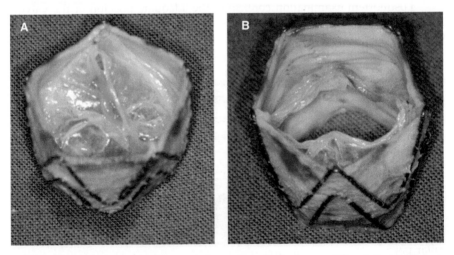

FIGURE 7 Postmortem examination with the explanted valve in open (**A**) and closed (**B**) position, excluding any valve deformation or thrombus.

Discussion

The implant of a valve in pulmonary position has the ideal purpose of abolishing the pulmonary valve regurgitation to prevent or reduce the incidence of sudden death, arrhythmias, and right ventricular dysfunction (5,14–22) with the lowest possible surgical risk.

Because of the difficult balance between costs (risks) and benefits (competent pulmonary valve), timing and type of management so far have not reached a general agreement (31).

The percutaneous insertion of a pulmonary valve, recently introduced in the clinical practice (4,5), presents the advantages of avoiding an operation on cardiopulmonary bypass and at the same time the possibility of implanting a functioning valve therefore reducing or abolishing both the pressure and the volume overload on the right ventricle (1,4,5). The major current limit of this technique is the mismatch between the size of the venous access and the size of the introducer (at least 18 Fr), restricting its use to older children (>25 kg of body weight) and the size of the valve to an 18 mm internal diameter biological valve (5).

This experimental study proposes an alternative strategy allowing the off-bypass implantation of a self-expanding valved stent of large size (internal diameter, 22 mm) in pulmonary position from right ventricular approach without cardiopulmonary bypass.

The implant of a functioning pulmonary valve can therefore be accomplished, overcoming the limits of the currently available techniques, with the only additional risks of a limited chest opening. In this initial experimental study, a median sternotomy was used to evaluate feasibility of this new technique. On the basis of this first experience, the implant of the valved stent in pulmonary position can be accomplished through a limited left anterior thoracotomy, particularly advantageous in clinical practice in the presence of a previous median sternotomy.

With regard to the size of the valved stent, the mean external diameter of 26.3 ± 0.7 mm should allow adequate implant even in patients with dilated right ventricular outflow tract because of severe pulmonary valve regurgitation like the situation encountered years after repair of tetralogy of Fallot with transannular patch. With regard to larger-sized tissue valves, the internal diameter of the 22 mm bovine jugular vein conduit presents an excellent hemodynamic performance without pressure gradient in patients up to 91 kg of body weight (33).

Overall, this study showed feasibility of off-bypass implantation of self-expanding valved stent in pulmonary position and in the context of a surgical approach to allow for valved stent implantation of adult size with adequate hemodynamic functioning.

SECOND-GENERATION VALVED STENT DEVICE FOR TRANSAPICAL PULMONARY VALVE REPLACEMENT

Introduction

Reoperative pulmonary valve replacement becomes necessary in two particular situations: firstly, pulmonary valve regurgitation generally after surgical transannular patch repair in tetralogy of Fallot patients (14,16,19,34,35); secondly, dysfunction of the biological valved conduit previously implanted to establish the continuity between the right ventricle and the pulmonary artery during repair of complex congenital heart defects (24). Current practice consists of pulmonary valve replacement or replacement of the failing conduit. The ideal timing for reintervention on the failing pulmonary valve aiming toward reduction of sudden death, arrhythmias, and right ventricular dysfunction (34,36,37) remains a matter of debate. The trend seems to go toward earlier reoperation.

Several alternative strategies, particularly in the presence of dysfunction of the biological valved conduit, have been considered within the last years, which include new biological valved conduits (6,25,27) and endovascular procedures to delay the surgical replacement of the obstructed conduit (1,4,28–30) and allow implanting a bigger-sized valve considering the patient's age and growth potential.

Endovascular stenting of stenosed right ventricular conduits is limited by the resulting pulmonary regurgitation and the subsequent right ventricular volume overload resulting in increased incidence of sudden death, ventricular arrhythmias, and ventricular dysfunction (28,29).

There is no doubt about the many advantages of valved stent implantation for both stenotic and dilated conduits. Unfortunately, there is a size restriction due to the maximum size of the valves harvested from bovine jugular veins up to 22 mm. Furthermore, the currently available pulmonary valved stent can only be implanted for a small percentage of patients (13%) because of the very variable morphology of the aneurysmal conduits (38,39). A further challenging limitation is the size mismatch between the venous access vessel and the introducer size. The 18F introducer allows implantation only in older children (5).

This study addresses the mentioned shortcomings by focusing on approaching the failing conduit by a direct access valve replacement (DAVR) strategy via the right ventricular apex in the so called transapical procedure (TAP). A new device allowing per-procedural construction was designed and tested in vivo. Further, the proposed valved stent concept was validated by random participants at two consecutive medical technology events in Switzerland (40).

The following study is partially reproduced with permission from Huber CH et al. Valved stents for transapical pulmonary valve replacement—preventing reoperation for postoperative pulmonary regurgitation. J Thorac Cardiovasc Surg. In print.

Methods
On the basis of our previous experience on pulmonary valved stents, a second-generation device allowing per-procedural construction was implanted in eight pigs (48.5 ± 6.0 kg). Performing direct access valve replacement (DAVR) via the transapical procedure (TAP) through a subxyphoidal incision permitted for off-pump implantation.

Valved Stent and Delivery Device Construction
The valved stent is build from two components: a valved bovine jugular vein conduit (Contegra®Pulmonary Valved Conduit, Medtronic International Trading SARL, Tolochenaz, Switzerland) and a size-matched endoprosthetic graft (Valiant™ Thoracic Stent Graft, Medtronic International Trading SARL, Tolochenaz) (Fig. 8). The scaffold is constructed by shortening the endoprosthetic

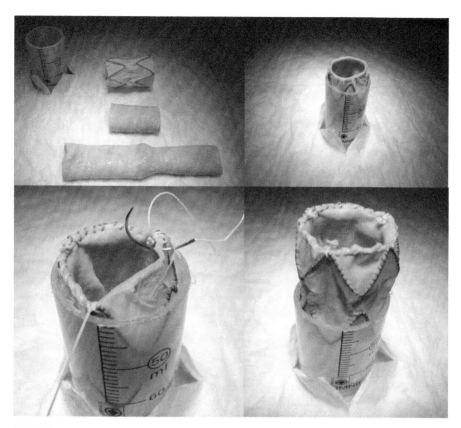

FIGURE 8 Display of four stages of device construction (*from top left to bottom right*). The Contegra Pulmonary Valved Conduit and the shortened Valiant endograft segment. Both the obtained cylinders are combined in a two-layer fashion and placed into a modified 60-mL syringe. The distal and the proximal ends are each sewn in semicontinuous fashion with three Ti-Cron 2-0 sutures (Tyco Healthcare, Waltham, MA).

graft down to a two-segment length including two rows of Z-stents. The valved conduit is then cut to approximate the stent graft length. The trimmed valve conduit is introduced into the stent graft and two suture lines are started at each end to safely secure the two-layer composite device.

The delivery device consists of a large 25F endograft delivery system (XCelerant® Delivery System, Medtronic International Trading SARL, Tolochenaz) (Fig. 9) to accommodate for the manually crimped and loaded valved stent. Delivery is performed by counter-clock turning of the rotational handle or by a quick release mechanism resulting in a pullback motion of the delivery sheath. A more detailed description of the device assembly has been reported previously (40).

All devices (Fig. 8) underwent in vitro testing prior to experimental in vivo implantation. Static leakage testing and dynamic pulsatile mock loop assessment was performed. Real time IVUS (12.5 MHz, 6F, Clearview, Boston Scientific Corporation, Sunnyvale, CA) was used to assess the correct functioning of the valved

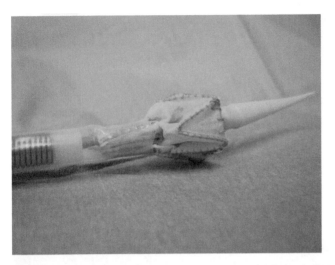

FIGURE 9 The valved stent manually crimped and partially loaded into the 25F Valiant delivery system.

stent over an observation period of 30 minutes. Both tests have been described previously (41,42).

Surgical Access
For tracheal intubation and mechanical ventilation, general anesthesia was induced by ketamine (22 mg/kg), atropine (0.8 mg/kg) was administered intramuscularly, thiopental (15 mg/kg) was administered intravenously, and maintained by isoflurane (2.5%). Continuous monitoring of electrocardiogram, arterial pressure (from a catheter in the right carotid artery), central venous pressure, and oxygen saturation was performed. Additional IV access was gained via the superficial vein of the left ear.

After bilateral preparation of the carotid arteries and the jugular veins, a Swan–Ganz catheter for continuous cardiac output measurements was temporarily inserted via the right jugular vein and a second IV line was placed on the left jugular vein. Then the arterial pressure line was inserted into the left carotid artery. Access for the ICUS was obtained by exposing the proximal right femoral vein and insertion of an 11F introducer (B Braun Medical, Inc., Bethlehem, PA).

Next, the endoscope was introduced into the right lower hemithorax to identify the preferred primary access for device insertion. Frequently the location was sub- to paraxyphoidal.

Then a 2 to 4 cm incision was performed. A Xylocaine (1.5 mg/kg) drip was started to minimize arrhythmias before mobilization of the pericardium. Two Teflon felt reinforced prolene (4-0) orthogonal U-stitches were placed on the right ventricular apex. Following heparinization (300 IU/kg), the 10F ICUS probe with the bidirectionally steering tip (Sequoia, operating frequencies 4.0 to 10.0 MHz, 90 cm insertion length; Acuson Corporation, Mountain View, CA) was inserted in order to visualize the delivery process as well as to measure the right ventricular outflow tract (RVOT) dimensions and the native pulmonary valve including annular diameter, valvular surface, and morphology of the pulmonary root.

Off-Pump Pulmonary Valved Stent Implantation

The valved stent was hand crimped onto the delivery system (Fig. 9). Next the prepared right ventricular apex was punctured and an over the needle 8F introducer system (Arrow International, Inc., Reading, PA) inserted. Under fluoroscopic guidance, a soft tip 0.035 in guidewire was first advanced into the right pulmonary artery and then the transcatheter was exchanged for an ultra-stiff backup Meier wire (0.035 in; 185 cm; Boston Scientific Meditech, Watertown, MA) (Fig. 10). Then the monorail wire-guided disposable IVUS 6F catheter transducer (Sonicath Ultra 6, 12.5 MHz Imaging Catheter, Meditech, Watertown, MA) providing a cross-sectional view with 80 mm of diameter was inserted. Simultaneous tracking of the IVUS probe with fluoroscopy allowed for identification and marking of the desired landing zone. Two radiopaque markers were placed on the body surface (13,43) in order to temporarily define the target zone: one at the fluoroscopic level of the pulmonary annulus and the second at the level of the pulmonary bifurcation.

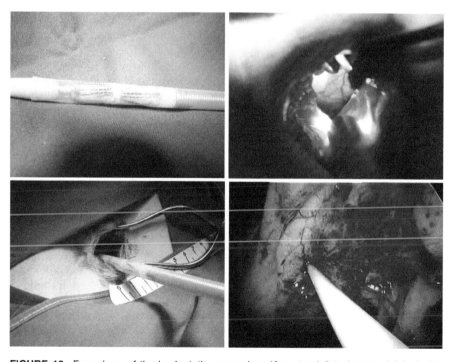

FIGURE 10 Four views of the implantation procedure (*from top left to bottom right*): device loaded onto delivery system, endoscopic assessment of the ideal TAP access location, 2 to 4 cm para- or subxyphoidal incision, and insertion of the delivery system tip into the right ventricular apex.

Per-Procedural Valved Stent Position Assessment with ICUS and Fluoroscopy
The IVUS probe and the 8F introducer were removed. The loaded and flushed valved stent delivery system was inserted over the guidewire under fluoroscopy and simultaneous ICUS guidance. After fluoroscopic and sonographic target site were congruent, the valved stent was deployed orthotopically over the native valves in a two-step procedure. First the distal and if the location stayed unchanged, the proximal end was released. In order to accommodate for minor position corrections, the valved stent initial landing site was chosen slightly above the prior identified target site. Therefore, after opening the first row of Z-stent, the whole device could be pulled back until landing and target site matched fluoroscopic and sonographic assessments. No contrast medium was used throughout the procedure.

Outcome Assessment
After Device deployment, the 6F IVUS transducer was reintroduced through the valve. Further measures were taken by the Doppler supporting 8F ICE probe positioned in the right atrium. Finally a 5F catheter (Cook, Inc. Bloomington, IN) was inserted over the guidewire to assess for transvalvular gradient, and the 7.5F Swan–Ganz catheter was advanced into the pulmonary artery and cardiac output was measured. Observation period was of six hours.

Acute in vivo assessment included length and diameter of pulmonary trunk preimplant, device position, leaflet motion, planimetric valve orifice, transvalvular gradient, regurgitation, and paravalvular leaking. At the end of the experiments, the animals were sacrificed and macroscopic analysis was performed at necropsy.

The institutional committee on animal research approved the protocol and all animals received human care in compliance with the *Principles of Laboratory Animals* formulated by the National Society of Medical Research and the *Guide for the Care and Use of Laboratory Animals* prepared by the Institute of Laboratory Animal Resources and published by the National Institutes of Health (7). All data are expressed as mean ± standard deviation.

Results
Procedural success was 100% (eight out of eight pigs) at the first attempt. Mean procedure time was 75 ± 15 minutes. All valved stents were delivered at the target site over the native pulmonary valve with good acute valve function. No valved stents dislodged into either the right ventricle or the pulmonary trunk.

No significant hemodynamic differences between mean carotid arterial pressure and oxygen saturated central venous pressure, before and after the implantation, were identified (P1 = 0.45, P2 = 0.57, P3 = 0.64); during implantation in two cases, temporary supraventricular tachycardia was experienced. Continuous cardiac output remained stable throughout the procedure 4.20 ± 1.35 L/min.

Peak-to-peak transvalvular pressure gradient ranged from 5.7 ± 3.1 mm Hg (range = 4.2–10.4 mm Hg) at Doppler echocardiography to 4.9 ± 2.4 mm Hg (range = 1–7 mm Hg) on invasive measurements.

The native pulmonary artery diameter at the valve level was 19.4 ± 1.6 mm (~2.9 cm^2). Length of the pulmonary trunk measured 4.2 ± 0.4 cm. On ICE, no animal had significant regurgitation or paravalvular leaking following implantation. The IVUS demonstrated the complete opening and closure of the valve with a planimetric valve orifice of 2.85 ± 0.32 cm^2.

No damage to the pulmonary artery or structural defects of the valved stents was found at necropsy. Macroscopic analysis confirmed the adequate positioning within the defined landing zone. Neither thrombus formation nor leaflet damage or structural device failure was identified on gross visual examination.

Discussion

Transcatheter pulmonary valve replacement harbors many benefits even more so in the setting of reoperation for dilated conduits or progressive pulmonary incompetence after a nonvalved RVOT enlargement strategy. Purpose of the valve replacement is to restore physiologic hemodynamic conditions and to prevent or reduce the incidence of sudden death, arrhythmias, and right ventricular dysfunction (14,16,17,19–21) with the lowest possible surgical risk.

Reoperations become necessary in at least 10% of all patients after primary correction of tetralogy of Fallot. Indications typically are RVOT enlargement and progressive pulmonary regurgitation after patch repair (34). Peri- and postoperative mortality of surgical pulmonary valve replacement is close to zero (19). Nevertheless, timing of reintervention negotiates between the risks and benefits balance and has not reached a general agreement. A trend toward earlier and more aggressive restoration of pulmonary competency might become identifiable (19,31,34). Postoperative results are excellent with marked clinical improvements due to right ventricular end-diastolic volume regression as seen on recent MRI studies (36).

Transvenous remote insertion percutaneous pulmonary valve replacement remains restricted to a small percentage (38) of patients. The Melody™ Transcatheter Pulmonary Valve (Medtronic B.V., PJ Heerlen) has twofold limitations: first by a very defined morphology of the failing right ventricular conduit and second by the size of the access vessel allowing insertion of the 18F delivery system only in bigger-sized femoral veins or children over 25 kg of weight. Overall, the Melody device is not suitable in most native RVOT lesions.

This experimental study presents an alternative off-pump approach. The direct access valve replacement (DAVR) via the TAP through the right ventricular apex allows for "bigger-sized" device implantation regardless of the patient age and vascular tree allowing implant also in grown-up patients (33). Increased device dimensions rationalize implantation also in patients with worsening dilatation of the RVOT after previous patch enlargement. In a previous porcine study with heavier adult animals, mean external device diameter was measured at 26.3 ± 0.7 mm (44).

The present study focused on reproducing condition of a more pediatric patient population. As the device is self-expanding, it might be able to adapt to the growing pulmonary artery and further device dilatation might be supplemented by balloon dilatation. Further, the device design might make it more suitable for native RVOT.

Valved stent construction is believed to be simple and safe enough when handled by trained and experienced hands. The per-procedural patient-adapted construction concept was further validated in two consecutive medical technology meetings with over 70 random participants and a 92% successful device construction and implantation (40).

Biotolerance, functionality, and approval of both the components are expected to face no major resistance because the bovine jugular vein conduit as well as the endograft is approved for clinical use. The first for RVOT reconstruction in congenital patients with failing conduits and the second in endoluminal grafting of aortic aneurysm. The valve has also shown its validity in percutaneous procedures in over 300 patients with the commercially available Melody device (45).

A similar device Shelhigh Injectable Pulmonic Valve (Shelhigh, Inc. Union, NJ) (46) showed very promising results (47,48) and confirmed clinical feasibility of intraoperative implantation for pulmonary regurgitation. Six patients (9–27 years) with primary total correction of tetralogy of Fallot at 4.2 ± 4.0 years of age received the injectable porcine pulmonary valved stent. No major adverse event was reported and all except one implantation were successful and the 6 to 12 months follow-up data was very encouraging. The one device requiring surgical reintervention presented a major paravalvular leak.

The presented preliminary experimental data are limited to acute experimental observation but harbor essential conditions for clinical implementation in the near future. Of course the concept requires further validation in chronic studies.

In summary, off-bypass transapical implantation of a self-expanding valved stent is feasible over the native pulmonary valve. Intravascular and intracardiac ultrasound combined with fluoroscopy makes implantation and evaluation easy and reproducible; there is no need for angiography. The off-bypass transapical approach allows for valved stent implantation of any size, including the adult size, with adequate hemodynamic functioning regardless of the size of the access vessel.

MITRAL TRANSCATHETER VALVE THERAPIES WITH THE DOUBLE-CROWNED MITRAL DEVICE

Introduction
The following study explores the possibility of transcatheter mitral valve replacement.

Previous experiences of the transcatheter valve therapies (TCVT) program for pulmonary (44), tricuspid, (32) and aortic valve replacement (49,43) encouraged to design a mitral valved stent for orthotopic off-pump implantation. This study presents description and preliminary results of the first self-expanding mitral valved stent.

The following study is partially reproduced with permission from Ma L, Tozzi P, Huber CH, et al. Double-crowned valved stents for off-pump mitral valve replacement. Eur J Cardiothorac Surg 2005; 28(2):194–198.

Materials and Methods
The self-expanding valved stent is specially designed for atrioventricular valve implantation taking into account the very particular anatomy of the mitral valve. The fundamental design principle is based upon a double opposing crown with a

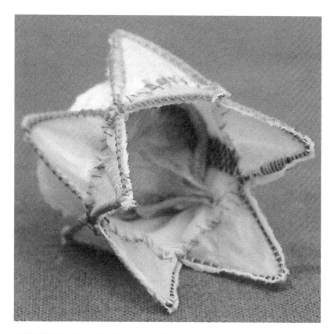

FIGURE 11 The double-crowned valved stent. A porcine pulmonary valve sutured into a Dacron conduit. The two self-expanding nitinol Z-stents were linked on the external surface of the prosthesis in a fashion to create two self-expanding anchoring crowns.

central circumferential narrowing. This groove between the two crowns is placed at the level of the mitral annulus and aims at securely anchoring and centering the device within the mitral valve annulus (Fig. 11). The valved stent was then loaded into a custom-made Teflon sheath stent-graft delivery system with an overall diameter of 10 mm (Fig. 12).

Endpoint of the study is to validate device design and to assess feasibility of transcatheter mitral valve replacement with regard to deployment, anchoring, valve performance, and hemodynamic tolerance in the off-pump setting.

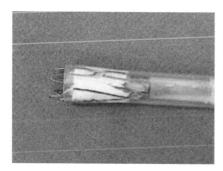
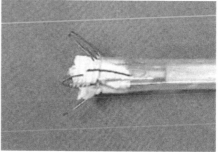

FIGURE 12 The self-expanding valved stent fully loaded and half-deployed in a Teflon sheath stent graft delivery system.

Study Design

Acute in vivo evaluation was done in eight pigs with a mean body weight of 46.0 ± 4.3 kg (range = 43–56 kg). Under general anesthesia, ECG, and blood pressure monitoring, both the internal jugular veins were exposed for volume resuscitation and introduction of the Swan–Ganz catheter. ECG, heart rate, mean blood pressure, cardiac output, and pulmonary artery pressure were recorded before and 30 minutes after the device deployment. The left femoral vein was exposed for insertion of the ICE probe.

A left posterolateral thoracotomy in the fourth intercostal space was performed and the pericardium was incised to reach the left atrium. The atrioventricular groove was marked with three to four radiopaque clips to define the targeted implantation site in the mitral annulus over the native valve.

Heparin (100 IU/kg) was administered intravenously. The ICE probe was advanced into the right atrium in order to precisely identify target location and to visualize delivery process as well as postimplantation valve function. Intracardiac echo guidance was enhanced by fluoroscopic visualization, matching the marked target location with the sonographically identified landing zone.

Next, two purse-string sutures were placed with 6-0 polypropylene thread on the left atrium. The atrium was then punctured with a needle and a guidewire inserted in analogy with the TAP. A 9F sheath was then introduced to allow insertion of the 6F IVUS probe (12.5MHz, 6F, Clearview, Boston Scientific Corporation, Sunnyvale, CA). Extensive measures including the diameter and area of the mitral valve were taken by the IVUS and the ICE. In the following step, the IVUS was removed to allow introducing the previously loaded delivery system.

Additionally, the left atrial wall was incised within the purse-string defined location to prevent uncontrolled rupture of the thin atrial wall during delivery device insertion. Then the delivery system was introduced and forwarded into the desired target location defined as mid portion of the device reaching the mitral annulus at the level of the previously placed markers. For release, the sheath was pulled back while the piston was held in place and the ventricular side of the valved stent deployed. A gentle pull on the delivery system ensured that distal fixation was kept during deployment of the atrial side (Fig. 13).

Valve competence and function was confirmed by ICE. The pressure gradient between left atrium and ventricle (proximal and distal to the valved stent) was directly measured with a needle.

The double-crowned valved stent function was assessed for at least one hour and after the deployment for up to three hours. Then, animals were sacrificed in order to check for adequate device positioning and anchoring.

All the pigs received care in compliance with the *Principles of Laboratory Animals* formulated by the National Society of Medical Research and the *Guide for the Care and Use of Laboratory Animals* prepared by the Institute of Laboratory Animal Resources and published by the National Institute of Health (7). The protocol was approved by the institutional committee on animal research.

Results

The mean height of the valved stents was 29.4 ± 0.2 mm, with an internal diameter of 20.4 ± 1.0 mm, and an external diameter of 25.5 ± 0.8 mm. The procedure was successfully completed in all animals. Mean procedure time was 18 ± 8 minutes and all valves were deployed in less than 30 seconds. Hemodynamic data

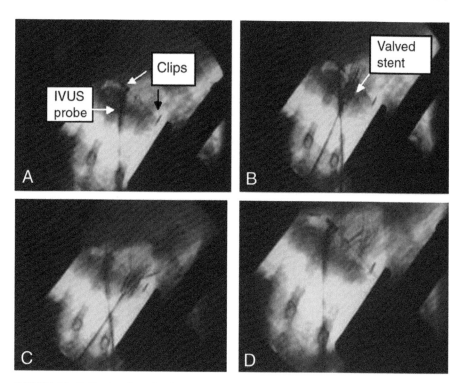

FIGURE 13 Delivering the valved stent under the guidance of fluoroscopy. The custom-made delivery introducer loaded with the valved stent was pushed along the guidewire, until the middle of the valved stent reached the mitral annulus previously marked with metallic clips. The sheath was pulled back while the piston was held in place, and the ventricular side of the valved stent was deployed. Continuous gentle traction on the introducer ensured fixation of the valved stent before deploying the atrial side.

before and 30 minutes after valve deployment are reported in Table 1. In vivo evaluation showed a native mitral annulus diameter of 24.9 ± 0.6 mm, and a mean mitral valve area of 421.4 ± 17.5 mm². Comparatively, the diameter and area of double-crowned valved stents were 19.8 ± 0.4 mm and 238.5 ± 15.2 mm², respectively, after implantation. Intracardiac echo confirmed complete valve opening and closure of the valved stents (Fig. 14) and showed mild paravalvular regurgitation in three out of eight animals. In these animals, there was the highest

TABLE 1 Hemodynamic Data Before and 30 Minutes After the Valved Stent Deployment

	Valved stent deployment	
	Before	After 30 min
ECG	Sinus rhythm	Sinus rhythm
HR (beats/min)	80 ± 12	83 ± 11
MAP (mm Hg)	66 ± 8	69 ± 8
CO (L/min per m²)	3.96 ± 0.8	3.86 ± 0.6
PAP (mm Hg)	20 ± 1	20 ± 1

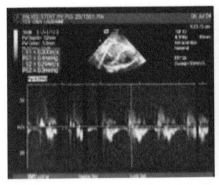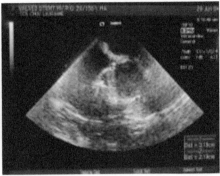

FIGURE 14   ICE showed a good fixation of the valved stent in the mitral position.

degree of size mismatch between the native mitral annulus and the device: The
annulus diameter was more than 20% bigger than the valved stent diameter.

Mean pressure gradient across the valved stent was 2.6 ± 3.1 mm Hg
(range = 0–8 mm Hg). Mean pressure gradient across the left ventricular
outflow tract (LVOT) was 6.6 ± 5.2 mm Hg (range = 1–15 mm Hg). The mean
survival time was 97.5 ± 56.3 minutes (survival time range was 40–180 minutes). One animal died due to the valve displacement 40 minutes after the
valve deployment. Mean blood loss during the procedure was 55 ± 25 cm³.
Postmortem evaluation confirmed that the native mitral annulus was in between
the two crowned stents in seven out of eight animals. In one animal, the valved
stents migrated into the ventricle causing the complete occlusion of the LVOT.
No atrial or ventricular lesions due to the valved stents were found (Fig. 15).
Detailed results are reported in Tables 2 and 3.

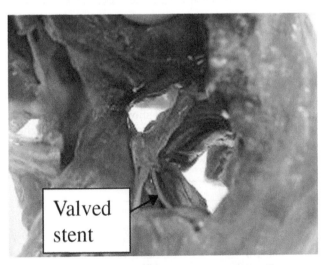

FIGURE 15   Postmortem evaluation confirmed good positioning of valved stents in the mitral
position and no left ventricle outflow tract obstruction.

TABLE 2 Summary of Procedural Data

Procedure successfully completed	8 out of 8 animals
Mean procedure time	18 ± 8 min
Valve deployment time	<30 sec
Native mitral annulus diameter	24.9 ± 0.6 mm
Native mitral valve area	421.4 ± 17 mm^2
Double-crowned valved stents diameter	19.8 ± 4 mm
Double-crowned valved stents area	238.5 ± 15.2 mm^2
Blood loss during procedure	55 ± 25 cm^3
Complication	One late valve displacement

TABLE 3 Echocardiography Assessment of Double-Crowned Valved Stents in Mitral Position

Pressure gradient across the valve	2.6 ± 3.1 mm Hg
Pressure gradient across the LVOT	6.6 ± 5.2 mm Hg
Mild mitral regurgitation	3 out of 8 animals

Discussion

The special anatomy of mitral valves requires very specific device specifications. To accommodate for this larger atrioventricular valve, the valved stent is made up of a three-layered construction: the first is the most internal part the valve, the second is the most outer component the anchoring part, and the third is the linking portion between the outer and the inner element preventing paravalvular leaking. The ventricular stent guarantees the fixation of the device to the mitral annulus, while the atrial stent holds in place the homograft sutured on the prosthesis. The two stents are connected in the center of the device to avoid mutual interference and in such a way to squeeze the mitral annulus in a sandwich-like technique. The porcine aortic or pulmonary homograft valves are easily sutured into a 20 mm diameter Dacron tube graft. The graft acts like an external support to the homograft, preventing its collapse during manipulation and after deployment.

The valve in its crimped state presents a profile of 10 mm but sheath diameter was not concerned regarding the external diameter while using a direct access strategy. The introducer was trimmed to 25 to 30 cm in length for easy manipulation, and its tip was kept short (<2 cm) because of space restriction in the left ventricle.

The valved stents were unloaded from the introducer system following a two-stage procedure. The ventricular stent was deployed first under fluoroscopic and ICE control by pulling the delivery sheath against the internal pistol. During this phase the device could be readjusted so as to orient the valved stents' groove to fit the marked mitral valve annulus. Then the atrial side was deployed under continuous traction. This approach increased the successful rate of deployments.

The duration of deployment was about 15 to 20 seconds, and no significant hemodynamic changes were noted probably because the deployment was quick enough not to impair the left ventricular function. All the implanted valves worked properly without significant hemodynamic changes after successful deployment (Table 1). However, in three animals a mild paravalvular leak was identified most likely because of the mismatch between native annulus and valve size. The annulus diameter was more than 20% bigger than the valved stent diameter. This problem was difficult to overcome because only a limited number of homograft was available for this study.

A more important choice of device diameter might better accommodate for mitral annular variability and decrease the risk for paravalvular leaks. In one animal, valve displacement occurred 40 minutes after its deployment causing sudden occlusion of the LVOT and the death of the animal. The dislodgment of the device occurred because it was undersized in respect of the annulus diameter preventing it from stable anchoring. Postmortem evaluation confirmed the good positioning of seven out of eight valved stents in the mitral position with the mitral annulus "sandwiched" in between the atrial and the ventricular stents.

This study presents the first mitral valved stent design and shows feasibility of off-pump transcatheter mitral valve implantation. As such, this novel technique might become a promising less invasive therapy for mitral valve replacement. Valved stents implantation may protect the left ventricular function from severe regurgitation, even temporarily, for example, a bridge to surgery in younger patients or allow intervention at earlier disease stage to interrupt disease progression and associated cardiac changes. Another most interesting situation is prevention of reoperations after previous biological mitral valve replacement in the valve-in-valve concept.

Study Limitations

The LVOT obstruction is one of the main drawbacks of this technique even if, in this study, the gradient across the LVOT was quite low, thanks to the particular geometry of the pig's left ventricle, mitral and aortic valves lie almost on the same plane. In the human hearts, the ventricular portion of the valved stents might protrude into the left ventricle in such a way to push the anterior leaflet of the mitral valve toward the LVOT, miming systolic anterior movement. Moreover, the subvalvular apparatus is displaced as well and can significantly contribute to the LVOT obstruction. In order to prevent this potential complication, a second-generation low profile valved stent needs to be designed.

REFERENCES

1. Bonhoeffer P, Boudjemline Y, Saliba Z, et al. Transcatheter implantation of a bovine valve in pulmonary position: A lamb study. Circulation 2000; 102:813–816.
2. Boudjemline Y, Bonhoeffer P. Steps toward percutaneous aortic valve replacement. Circulation 2002; 105:775–778.
3. Lutter G, Kuklinski D, Berg G, et al. Percutaneous aortic valve replacement: An experimental study. I. Studies on implantation. J Thorac Cardiovasc Surg 2002; 123:768–776.
4. Bonhoeffer P, Boudjemline Y, Saliba Z, et al. Percutaneous replacement of pulmonary valve in a right-ventricle to pulmonary-artery prosthetic conduit with valve dysfunction. Lancet 2000; 356:1403–1405.
5. Bonhoeffer P, Boudjemine Y, Qureshi SA, et al. Percutaneous insertion of the pulmonary valve. J Am Coll Cardiol 2002; 39:1664–1669.
6. Corno AF, Hurni M, Griffin H, et al. Bovine jugular vein as right ventricle-to-pulmonary artery valved conduit. J Heart Valve Dis 2002; 11:242–247.
7. Guide for the Care and Use of Laboratory Animals. Institute of Laboratory Animal Research, Commission on Life Sciences, National Research Council. 140p. 1996.
8. Andersen HR, Knudsen LL, Hasenkam JM. Transluminal implantation of artificial heart valves. Description of a new expandable aortic valve and initial results with implantation by catheter technique in closed chest pigs. Eur Heart J 1992; 13:704–708.

9. Pavcnik D, Wright KC, Wallace S. Development and initial experimental evaluation of a prosthetic aortic valve for transcatheter placement. Radiology 1992; 183:151–154.
10. Sochman J, Peregrin JH, Pavcnik D, et al. Percutaneous transcatheter aortic disc valve prosthesis implantation: A feasibility study. Cardiovasc Intervent Radiol 2000; 23:384–388.
11. Gomez-Jorge J, Venbrux AC, Magee C. Percutaneous deployment of a valved bovine jugular vein in the swine venous system: A potential treatment for venous insufficieny. J Vasc Interv Radiol 2000; 11:931–936.
12. Steinberg C, Weinstock DJ, Gold JP, et al. Measurements of central blood vessels in infants and children: Normal values. Catheter Cardiovasc Interv 1992; 27:197–201.
13. von Segesser LK, Marty B, Ruchat P, et al. Routine use of intravascular ultrasound for endovascular aneurysm repair: Angiography is not necessary. Eur J Vasc Endovasc Surg 2002; 23:537–542.
14. Rocchini A.P., Rosenthal A., Freed M. Chronic congestive heart failure after repair of tetralogy of Fallot. Circulation 1977; 56:305–310.
15. Bove EL, Kavey REW, Byrum CJ, et al. Improved right ventricular function following late pulmonary valve replacement for residual pulmonary insufficiency or stenosis. J Thorac Cardiovasc Surg 1985; 90:50–55.
16. Warner KB, Anderson JE, Fulton DR, et al. Restoration of the pulmonary valve reduces right ventricular volume overload after previous repair of tetralogy of Fallot. Circulation 1993; 88(suppl 2):189–197.
17. Dietl CA, Cazzaniga ME, Dubner SJ, et al. Life threatening arrhythmias and RV dysfunction after surgical repair of tetralogy of Fallot. Circulation 1994; 90:7–12.
18. Yemets IM, Williams WG, Webb GD, et al. Pulmonary valve replacement late after repair of tetralogy of Fallot. Ann Thorac Surg 1997; 64:526–530.
19. Therrien J, Siu SC, McLaughlin PR, et al. Pulmonary valve replacement in adults after repair of tetralogy of Fallot: Are we operating too late? J Am Coll Cardiol 2000; 36:1670–1675.
20. Discigil B., Dearani JA, Puga FJ, et al. Late pulmonary valve replacement after repair of tetralogy of Fallot. J Thorac Cardiovasc Surg 2001; 121:344–351.
21. de Ruijter FTH, Weenink I, Hitchcock FJ, et al. Right ventricular dysfunction and pulmonary valve replacement after correction of tetralogy of Fallot. Ann Thorac Surg 2002; 73:1794–1800.
22. Kanter KR, Budde JM, Parks J, et al. One hundred pulmonary valve replacements in children after relief of right ventricular outflow tract obstruction. Ann Thorac Surg 2002; 73:1801–1807.
23. Corno AF, Giamberti A, Giannico S, et al. Long-term results after extracardiac valved conduits implanted for complex congenital heart disease. J Card Surg 1988; 3:495–500.
24. Stark J, Bull C, Stajevic M, et al. Fate of subpulmonary homograft conduits: Determinants of late homograft failure. J Thorac Cardiovasc Surg 1998; 115:506–516.
25. Homann M, Haehnel JC, Mendler N, et al. Reconstruction of the RVOT with valved biological conduits: 25 Years experience with allografts and xenografts. Eur J Cardiothorac Surg 2000; 17:624–630.
26. Stock UA, Nagashima M, Khalil PN, et al. Tissue-engineered valved conduits in the pulmonary circulation. J Thorac Cardiovasc Surg 2000; 119:732–740.
27. Hoerstrup SP, Kadner A, Breymann C, et al. Living, autologous pulmonary artery conduits tissue engineered from human umbilical cord cells. Ann Thorac Surg 2002; 74:46–52.
28. Powell AJ, Lock JE, Keane JF, et al. Prolongation of RV-PA conduit life span by percutaneous stent implantation. Intermediate-term results. Circulation 1995; 92:282–288.
29. Saliba Z, Bonhoeffer P, Aggoun Y, et al. Treatment of obstruction of prosthetic conduits by percutaneous implantation of stents. Arch Mal Coeur Vaiss 1999; 92:591–596.
30. Pedra CA, Justino H, Nykanen DG, et al. Percutaneous stent implantation to stenotic bioprosthetic valves in the pulmonary position. J Thorac Cardiovasc Surg 2002; 124:82–87.

31. Hanley FL. Management of the congenitally abnormal right ventricular outflow tract—what is the right approach? J Thorac Cardiovasc Surg 2000; 119:1–3.
32. Corno AF, Zhou J, Tozzi P, et al. Off-bypass implantation of a self-expandable valved stent between inferior vena cava and right atrium. Interact Cardiovasc Thorac Surg 2003; 2:166–169.
33. Corno AF, Hurni M, Griffin H, et al. Glutaraldehyde-fixed bovine jugular vein as a substitute for the pulmonary valve in the Ross operation. J Thorac Cardiovasc Surg 2001; 122:493–494.
34. Oechslin EN, Harrison DA, Harris L, et al. Reoperation in adult with repair of tetralogy of Fallot: Indications and outcomes. J Thorac Cardiovasc Surg 1999, 118(2): 245–251.
35. van Huysduynen BH, van Straten A, Swenne CA, et al. Reduction of QRS duration after pulmonary valve replacement in adult Fallot patients is related to reduction of right ventricular volume. Eur Heart J 2005; 26:928–932.
36. van Straten A, Vliegen HW, Lamb HJ, et al. Time course of diastolic and systolic function improvement after pulmonary valve replacement in adult patients with tetralogy of Fallot. J Am Coll Cardiol 2005; 46(8):1559–1564.
37. Therrien J, Provost Y, Merchant N, et al. Optimal timing for pulmonary valve replacement in adults after tetralogy of Fallot repair. Am J Cardiol 2005; 95:779–782.
38. Schievano S, Coats L, Migliavacca F, et al. Variations in right ventricular outflow tract morphology following repair of congenital heart disease: Implications for percutaneous pulmonary valve implantation. J Cardiovasc Magn Reson 2007; 9(4):687–695.
39. Nordmeyer J, Coats L, Bonhoeffer P. Current experience with percutaneous pulmonary valve implantation. Semin Thorac Cardiovasc Surg 2006; 18:122–125.
40. Huber CH, Marty B, von Segesser LK. Acceptance and introduction of disruptive technologies—simple steps to build a fully functional pulmonary valved stent. Interact Cardiovasc Thorac Surg 2007; 6(4):430–432.
41. Ma L, Tozzi P, Huber CH, et al. Setup of a new in vitro mock loop system and testing of a valved stent in mitral position. Swiss Perfusion 2007; 20:4–7.
42. Huber CH, Zhou JQ, La L, et al. Bench test construction for valved stent assessment. Interact Cardiovasc Thorac Surg. In press.
43. Huber CH, Nasratulla M, Augstburger M, et al. New tools for new goals: Ultrasound navigation through the heart for off pump aortic valved stent implantation. J Endovasc Ther 2004: 11(4):503–510.
44. Zhou JQ, Corno AF, Huber CH, et al. Self-expandable valved stent of large size: Off-bypass implantation in pulmonary position. Eur J Cardiothorac Surg 2003; 24(2):212–216.
45. Bonhoeffer P. Oral communications, Boston, MA, 2004.
46. U.S. Food and Drug Administration. FDA request recall of all Shelhigh medical devices. FDA News Communication. May 2007; P07-78.
47. Berdat PA, Schönhoff F, Pavlovic M, et al. Cardiology in the Young. Abstract book. May 2006; O-39:15.
48. Schreiber C, Hörer J, Vogt M, et al. A new treatment option for pulmonary valve insufficiency: First experiences with implantation of a self-expanding stented valve without use of cardiopulmonary bypass. Eur J Cardiothorac Surg 2007; 31:26–30.
49. Huber CH, Tozzi P, Corno AF, et al. Do valved stents compromise coronary flow? Eur J Cardiothorac Surg 2004; 25(5):754–759.

INTRODUCTION

Surgical aortic valve replacement (SAVR) is the only validated therapy for aortic stenosis (AS) and represents the current standard of care. Aortic valve replacement (AVR) is the most frequently performed operation for acquired structural heart disease. In the United States, more than 56,000 underwent SAVR in 2005 alone (1), and with an aging population in Western countries this number is expected to rise considerably (Chap. 3). It is estimated that up to 33% of patients with severe aortic valve stenosis and related age and left ventricular dysfunction risk factors do not benefit from surgical therapy (2). There are two main reasons for the lack of surgical treatment of AS. First, the patients who meet the current treatment criteria are simply not referred to their surgical colleagues (approximately 45% of all U.S. AS patients). Second, the patients who meet the treatment criteria are perceived to be not eligible for surgery because they might appear to be "too sick" or "too old" for a reasonably safe intervention (approximately 22% of all U.S. AS patients). Therefore, only 33% of the patients with AS do meet the treatment criteria and are eligible for AVR surgery (3).

Similar numbers have been reported by the European Heart Survey on Valvular Heart Disease (4). In a 2001 prospective survey of 5001 patients with valvular heart disease from 92 hospitals in 25 countries in Europe, 32% of patients did not receive treatment according to the established guidelines (5), despite New York Heart Association (NYHA) class III/IV symptoms. In June 2006, the revised guidelines for the treatment of aortic valve stenosis were issued by the ACC/AHA task force. The indications for surgery are listed in Table 1.

Why Are Patients Not Referred to Surgery?

AVR is a simple and safe routine operation for experienced cardiac surgeons. Medical device companies provide excellent mechanical or tissue heart valve prostheses with increasing device durability. The patients tolerate surgery very well and outcomes have been reported to be excellent even in elderly patients (6). Nevertheless, results do vary from center to center and from surgeon to surgeon, and with the increasing number of patient comorbidities there can also be a rise in patient mortality. Reported mortality for conventional AVR can range between 2.7% (4) and 6.5% (7) and is highly dependent on the selection of surgical candidates as well as of the surgeons' caseload and has been described as high as, for example, 29% for cardiopulmonary bypass runs of more than 124 minutes or 23% for patients with body surface area of less than 1.82 m^2 (Table 2).

There is unfortunately a widespread false belief in the medical community that a surgical option should only be chosen late in the disease state. This belief receives further support if the patient responds favorably to medical therapy. In fact, a delay in adequate management of stenotic aortic valve disease results in

TABLE 1 Indication for Aortic Valve Replacement

Symptomatic patients with severe aortic stenosis (class I-B)
Patients with severe aortic stenosis undergoing CABG (class I-C)
Patients with severe aortic stenosis undergoing cardiac valvular surgery (class I-C)
Patients with severe aortic stenosis and LV systolic dysfunction, EF < 50% (class I-C)
Patients with moderate aortic stenosis undergoing CABG or aortic or other heart valve surgery
  (class IIa-b)

Abbreviations: CABG, coronary artery bypass graft; EF, ejection fraction; LV, left ventricle.
Source: From Ref. 5.

TABLE 2 Review of Literature of Operative Mortality After AVR Surgery—High-Risk Series

Paper	$N =$	Operative Mortality	Comorbidities
Ambler et al. (8)	32,839	6.4%	All comers
Bloomstein et al. (9)	180	16.7%	70-/80-yr-old patients
		23.2%	BSA < 1.82 m^2
		8.1%	BSA > 1.82 m^2
		8.9%	CPB < 100 min
		10.2%	CPB > 100–124 min
		29.6%	CPB > 124 min
Chiappini et al. (10)	115	8.5%	Mean age 82.3 yr
Collart et al. (11)	200	7%	Mean age 83 yr, EuroSCORE 9.1
Collart et al. (12)	215	8.8%	Mean age 83 yr, mean additive EuroSCORE 9.5%, mean logistic EuroSCORE 15.1%
Craver et al. (13)	601	9.1%	< 80 yr
Edwards et al. (14)	49,073	4%	STS database
		7.64%	Previous cardiac surgery
		17.07%	Dialysis
		10.09%	3-vessel disease
		7.03%	Peripheral vascular disease
Rankin et al. (15)	409,904	9.4%	70 yr
		11.3%	Reoperation
		8.4%	Female patients
		5.5%, 6.4%, 8.1%, 10.5%	1, 2, 3, or 4 comorbidities
		5.4%	Isolated aortic (overall)
Nowicki et al. (16)	5793	6.8%	Female patients
		8.9%	Diabetic patients
		7.9%	History CHF
		5.3%, 11.4%	NYHA III/IV
		9.4%	BSA <1.7 m^2
		12.8%, 4.6%	Serum cr. > 1.3, serum cr. < 1.3
Jamieson et al. (17)	86,580	5.3%	Age 70–79 yr
		8.5%	Age 80–89 yr
		14.5%	Age 90–99 yr
Sundt et al. (18)	133	11%	Age > 80 yr

progressive cardiac failure with a dilated left ventricle that can negatively impact the procedural outcome.

Even when honoring all the merits of heart valve surgery, cardiac surgery with the support of cardiopulmonary bypass remains an important trauma for patients triggering a significant inflammatory response. The healing process of the sternotomy requires a prolonged recovery period allowing the patients to return to work only after two to three months. To reduce the effects of the surgical procedure, several less invasive approaches have been proposed, including hemisternotomy (19,20), right anterior thoracotomy (21–23), parasternal approach (24,25), and transverse sternotomy access (26–28). Except for the hemisternotomy, none of the remaining techniques has gained wide popularity or represents a significant milestone compared to the standard technique in relation to patient morbidity or mortality.

In contrast to the above-mentioned surgical modification, the concept of a transcatheter AVR represents a very exciting and promising novel technique and yields to bridge the gap of an unmet clinical need. But what are the patients to benefit from this approach.

Patients Selection Criteria for Transcatheter Aortic Valve Therapies

In the beginning, TCVT may be beneficial to patients in high-risk groups, such as, extreme age, previous thoracic surgery, combined cardiac operations, or extended comorbidities. Patient data from the various ongoing clinical trials of TCVT for AVR reflect similar characteristics: elderly patients, reoperations, and important comorbidities. But with broader clinical experience, more user-friendly devices, and extended patient outcome data, the indication will expand to younger patients with less surgical risk.

Significant improvements have been seen from the early days of surgical AVR until today. Initially, only patients in the final stages of the disease were allowed to undergo surgery, and even though the procedural outcomes were poor they were promising enough to encourage improved techniques and devices. At the same time, wider knowledge on disease progression has been gained which will lead to earlier interventions and finally to improved outcomes. The same development can be observed with TCVT for acquired structural heart disease. The novel technique and line of therapy is at an early stage; most of the devices are in their second generation; and clinical experience is limited to a small number of centers, surgeons, and patients worldwide. The next step is a feedback-coupled learning process resulting in major technical and device-related modifications and improvements. In parallel, the introduction of teaching tools will popularize the intervention and facilitate overall acceptance (Chap. 5, Introduction of New Technologies). The following data have been verified and approved by the respective companies prior to publication.

EDWARDS LIFESCIENCES REMOTE ACCESS ANTE- AND RETROGRADE CLINICAL DATA

Encouraged by the excellent experimental animal results (29,30), Alain Cribier and his team pioneered the field of clinical aortic TCV implantation (31,32). The early balloon-expandable valved stent devices were constructed by Percutaneous Valve Technologies, Inc., acquired by Edwards Lifesciences, Inc., (Irvine, CA) (Chap. 13, Company Overview) in 2004 and 3F Therapeutics, Inc., acquired by

ATS, Inc., (Minneapolis, MN) in 2006. The device height measured 14.5 mm. Only a 23-mm device was available initially that could accommodate a 21- to 23-mm annulus. The delivery system required a 24F access sheath that could be introduced into either the femoral vein for the antegrade transseptal approach or the femoral artery for the remote retrograde access (Chap. 6, Access to the Aortic Valves).

The first implant was performed on April 16, 2002, by Cribier in Rouen, France (20) (Chap. 2, Historical Background). The first study, called Initial Registry of EndoVascular Implantation of Valves in Europe (I-REVIVE), a single-center pilot study, was started in August 2003 and was later expanded and renamed the Registry of Endovascular Critical Aortic Stenosis Treatment (RECAST). Cribier published the midterm outcomes of 36 patients enrolled at the Charles Nicolle Hospital, University of Rouen, France (33). Inclusion criteria required severe aortic valve stenosis (≤ 0.7 cm^2), associated symptoms with NYHA $\geq$ IV, denied by two cardiac surgeons for surgical replacement on the basis of increased surgical risk, but be expected to benefit from a prospective aortic valve implantation. Exclusion criteria included vascular disease precluding access, chest deformation, intracardiac thrombus or unprotected left main coronary artery stenosis not amendable to PCI, myocardial infarction (MI) within seven days, existing prosthetic heart valves, active infections, leukopenia coagulopathy, or active bleeding or acute anemia. Patients with aortic annular sizes of more than 24 mm or less than 19 mm of diameter were also excluded. All implants were performed under mild sedation and local anesthesia. Of the 36 enrolled patients (34) who underwent the procedure, 1 patient died while awaiting the intervention, 1 patient arrested during predilatation, and 1 patient was cancelled because of balloon aortic annulus size mismatch. In the remaining 33 patients, 26 patients benefited from an antegrade transseptal approach and the procedure was performed successfully in 22 of those patients; 2 of the remaining 4 patients did not tolerate the mitral valve crossing and the 2 others experienced device migration.

Using the retrograde approach resulted in four successful implantations in a total of seven enrolled patients. In one patient, implant failure resulted from material limitations and in two patients the retrograde aortic valve crossing was impossible. Early (24 hours) echocardiographic results showed a significant aortic valve area (AVA) increase from 0.60 ± 0.09 cm^2 to 1.70 ± 0.11 cm^2. This increase remained stable over the next 24 months. The mean aortic valve gradient decreased from 37 ± 13 mm Hg to 9 ± 2 mm Hg and showed no significant change over time. Paravalvular regurgitation was the only source of identifiable aortic regurgitation. In 10 patients, the regurgitation was quantified as mild, in another 10 patients as moderate, and in 5 patients as moderate to severe. Of the total of 27 patients with successful implantation, 2 died because of pericardial tamponade; 1 patient died from urosepsis. Irreversible brain damage resulted after complete heart block and pacing lead loss in one patient and another patient expired following a stroke during retrograde valve crossing of secondary multiple organ failure. Finally, another death was attributed to uncontrollable hypertension after sheath removal from his femoral artery.

The remaining 21 patients from the 36 enrolled ones experienced remarkable improvement in symptoms and functional class. By December 2005, 11 patients were alive including 3 patients from the I-REVIVE trial and 8 patients from the RECAST registry. Obviously, these numbers have to be placed in the context of the first in-man implantation in end-stage disease patients with impressive surgical risks and comorbidities. Nevertheless, those numbers also very well illustrate the fragility of this patient population and any aortic intervention might be of only marginal value regarding life expectancy and quality of life in the long run.

Following the Edwards Lifesciences, Inc., acquisition of Percutaneous Valve Technologies, Inc., in 2004, a formal transfer of their percutaneous heart valve studies was accepted by the U.S. Food and Drug Administration. In 2005, feasibility investigations were initiated in U.S. clinical sites under the *R*andomization of *EndoV*ascular *I*mplantation of *VALv*es (REVIVAL I) and Pe*R*cutaneous *EndoV*ascular *I*mplantation of *VALv*es (REVIVAL II) trial protocols for the 23-mm valve model. The 26-mm model was first used in the REVIVAL II trial. In these protocols, enrollment was conducted for transcatheter implantation in symptomatic patients with severe to critical senile degenerative calcific AS who required aortic AVR, but who were not good candidates for open chest surgery because of extremely high operative risk or comorbid conditions. The first trial allowed both the antegrade transseptal and retrograde transfemoral implantations. Seven patients were enrolled and implanted in this study all with the antegrade transseptal approach. Because of the greater degree of technical complexity associated with this approach and observed serious adverse events, the retrograde approach using the Edwards retrograde delivery system was chosen for the REVIVAL II study. The first implant in the REVIVAL II trial with the transfemoral RetroFlex™ delivery system was in late 2005. In fall 2006, the protocol was amended to allow the enrollment of patients employing the transapical approach with the Ascendra™ delivery system. The REVIVAL II feasibility trial closed enrollment in February 2008 with a total of 95 patients [55 transfemoral procedures in 55 patients and 40 transapical procedures (TAP) in 40 patients] in four U.S. institutions in Detroit, Cleveland, New York City, and Dallas.

John Webb and colleagues in Vancouver, Canada, refined the transfemoral retrograde approach, and in 2006 they reported the results of 18 patients deemed to be excessive surgical risk because of their comorbidities that underwent the modified procedure. Implantation was successful in 14 patients and AVA increased from 0.6 ± 0.2 cm^2 to 1.6 ± 0.4 cm^2. Mortality at 30 days was 11% in this group whose mean age was 82 years. Iliac artery injury occurred in the first two patients, but did not recur following improvements in screening and access site management.

In a follow-up publication in 2007 on 50 patients, Webb reported an improvement in procedural success from 76% in the first 25 patients to 96% in the second 25 ($p = 0.10$) and a decrease in 30-day mortality from 16% to 8% ($p = 0.67$). Successful valve implantation was associated with an increase in echocardiographic AVA from 0.6 ± 0.2 cm^2 to 1.7 ± 0.4 cm^2 (35). These patients were implanted under the Canadian Special Access compassionate use regulation.

During enrollment for the REVIVAL II trial in the United States, a similar transfemoral feasibility trial was being conducted in Europe. The REVIVE I and II trials are prospective multicenter nonrandomized trials designed to involve a total of 90 symptomatic adult subjects who require AVR due to severe senile degenerative AS and who are very high-risk candidates for AVR surgery at the time of study enrollment. The goal of this study was to determine if transcatheter prosthetic aortic valve implantation is safe and effective in this patient population. The protocol initially allowed for percutaneous delivery of the transcatheter valve via the femoral veins (antegrade transseptal approach) as the REVIVE I trial or via the femoral arteries (retrograde approach) renamed REVIVE II; however, as was the case in the REVIVAL trial, the use of the antegrade transseptal approach was subsequently discontinued. The REVIVE II trial was conducted in nine European centers in France, Germany, Spain, Denmark, and also included patients from Vancouver, Canada.

Inclusion criteria for both the REVIVAL and REVIVE trials included severe symptomatic AS, age > 70 years, and high surgical risk (EuroSCORE ≥ 20) or a documented refusal from the surgeon to perform surgery. Both trials are 100% monitored and adjudicated with use of the same echo, ECG, quality of life and vascular Corelabs, Clinical Event Committee, and Data Safety Monitoring Board. Postimplantation follow-up was planned at discharge, 30 days, 3 months, 6 months, and 1 year. The interim data have been presented at the Euro PCR in May 2008. Table 3 shows the patient demographics and risk score assessments in both trials. Mean age is 83.9 and 83.7 years respectively for the REVIVE II and REVIVAL II trials. Age ranged between 66 and 96 years and between 69 and 95 years with 70.5% of the REVIVE II and 69.4% of the REVIVAL II patients being in their 90th decade. The majority of patients in both trials are women—for the REVIVE II trial 51.4% and for the REVIVAL II trial 54.5%. The NYHA functional

TABLE 3   REVIVE II and REVIVAL II Transfemoral Baseline Demographics

	REVIVE II ($N = 106$)	REVIVAL II ($N = 55$)
Age (yr)	$N = 105$	$N = 55$
Mean + SD	83.9 ± 5.4	83.7 ± 5.2
Range (min–max)	66–96	69–95
< 70 yr	2 (1.9%)	1 (1.8%)
70–79 yr	17 (16.2%)	19 (34.6%)
80–89 yr	74 (70.5%)	25 (69.4%)
> 90 yr	12 (11.4%)	11 (20.0%)
Gender	$N = 105$	$N = 55$
Female	54 (51.4%)	30 (54.6%)
Male	51 (48.6%)	25 (45.5%)
NYHA classification	$N = 97$	$N = 55$
Class I	1 (1.0%)	0 (0%)
Class II	6 (6.19%)	7 (12.7%)
Class III	58 (59.8%)	29 (52.7%)
Class IV	32 (32.9%)	19 (34.6%)
Logistic EuroSCORE	$N = 105$	$N = 55$
Mean + SD	$29.9 \pm 13.2\%$	34.1 ± 18.0
Range (min–max)	16–43	8–83
STS risk score		$N = 55$
Mean + SD	Not collected	13.1 ± 7.2
Range (min–max)	Not collected	4–31
AVA	$N = 33$	$N = 43$
Mean + SD	0.56 ± 0.04 cm^2	0.57 ± 0.04 cm^2
Range (min–max)	0.3–0.8 cm^2	0.3–0.9 cm^2
Mean gradient	$N = 34$	$N = 46$
Mean + SD	45.2 ± 6.74 mm Hg	44.7 ± 4.83 mm Hg
Range (min–max)	22–119 mm Hg	13–74 mm Hg

Abbreviations: AVA, aortic valve area; NYHA, New York Heart Association.

classification shows the majority of patients in both studies to be in classes III and IV at 92.7% and 87.3%. The logistic EuroSCORE in both cohorts is sufficiently above the inclusion criteria of 20 with the REVIVAL patient group score being higher at 34.1 ± 18.0% than the European group which was at 29.9 ± 13.2%. The mean AVA was 0.56 ± 0.04 cm^2 in the REVIVE II cohort and 0.57 ± 0.04 cm^2 in the REVIVAL II patients. Available baseline mean gradients were measured as 45.2 ± 6.74 mm Hg for REVIVE II patients and 44.7 ± 4.83 mm Hg for REVIVAL II patients. STS risk scores were only calculated in the United States with a mean score of 13.1 ± 7.2 ranging between 4 and 31.

In addition to meeting the inclusion and exclusion criteria, many of these patients had additional "high-risk conditions" that are not necessarily part of the risk scoring systems, such as, porcelain aorta, sterna radiation therapy, severe pulmonary disease, chest deformities, and surgical refusal that influenced the decision to include the patients in the trials. The presence of these high-risk conditions in addition to the high-risk score explains the gravity of the disease state in this patient population.

Review of the 30-day clinical events in both groups demonstrated a 13.2% early mortality rate in the REVIVE II cohort while in the REVIVAL II group a lower mortality of 7.3% was seen. Other early events that were calculated included MI, emergency cardiac events, neurological events, and vascular and vascular access complications. In the REVIVAL II group, 16.4% of patients were reported with having had a MI. It should be noted that in this study, MI was defined as a creatinin kinase (CK) enzyme elevation of more than two times normal with an elevated creatinin kinase MB fraction (CKMB). Seven of the nine reported patients had CK elevations without clinical evidence of the event. In the REVIVE II group, 8.5% of patients had an MI. Neurological events were also fewer in the REVIVE II trial at 2.8%. In the REVIVAL II trial, 14.5% of patients had a neurological event including stroke, transient ischemic attack (TIA), extremity weakness, aphasia, and seizures. Vascular complications including access-related events were comparable in both trials at 12.3% in REVIVE II patients and 12.7% in REVIVAL II patients. These events are shown in Table 4.

Hemodynamic improvement in both trials is demonstrated over the follow-up periods by significant improvements in mean gradients and effective orifice areas (EOAs) which remain stable over time. Gradients drop over 30 mm Hg from a mean of 44.9 ± 3.9 mm Hg in both groups to 10.4 ± 0.8 mm Hg at the discharge interval and remain stable until 18 months with 10.3 ± 2.4 mm Hg. Figures 1 and 2 show the pooled results of these parameters. Similarly, the EOA improves significantly from a baseline calculation of 0.56 ± 0.03 cm^2 to 1.53 ± 0.09 cm^2 at discharge and 1.53 ± 0.10 cm^2 at one year. In addition progressive increases in left ventricular ejection fraction were also observed.

TABLE 4   REVIVE II and REVIVAL II 30-Day Clinical Events

	REVIVE II ($n = 106$)	REVIVAL II ($n = 55$)
30-day mortality	14 (13.2%)	4 (7.3%)
Myocardial infarction	9 (8.5%)	9 (16.4%)
Emergency cardiac events	1 (0.9%)	1 (1.8%)
Neurologic events	3 (2.8%)	8 (14.5%)
Vascular/access complications	13 (12.3%)	7 (12.7%)

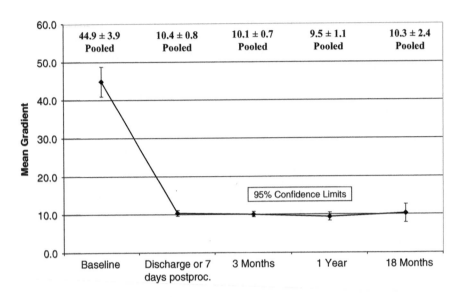

FIGURE 1 REVIVE II and REVIVAL II pooled mean gradients (mm Hg).

The combined baseline ejection fraction was $49.9 \pm 3.9\%$ and improved progressively to $55.4 \pm 3.4\%$ at discharge to $59.1 \pm 3.8\%$ at one year. Figures 3 and 4 show the pooled results of this parameter. Overall survival from all-cause mortality for the transfemoral patient population was calculated on the available follow-ups for the two study cohorts at one year. In the REVIVE II trial, the freedom from

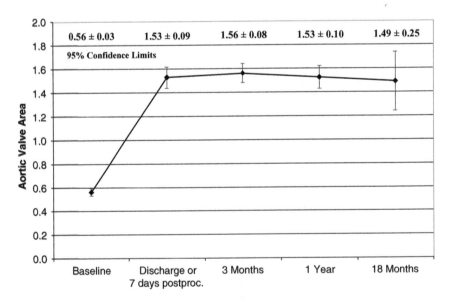

FIGURE 2 REVIVE II and REVIVAL II pooled effective orifice area (cm^2).

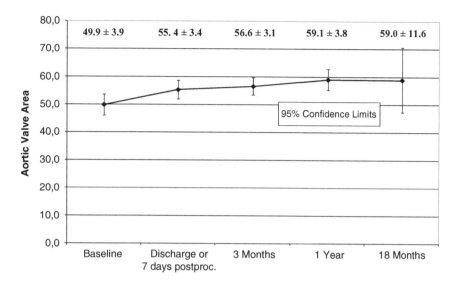

FIGURE 3   REVIVE II and REVIVAL II pooled ejection fraction (%).

death at six months and one year was 78.3 ± 0.04% and 71.4 ± 0.05% and in the
REVIVAL II trial was 83.4 ± 0.05% and 75.8 ± 0.05%.

CLINICAL EXPERIENCE AND RESULTS OF THE REMOTE ACCESS
RETROGRADE COREVALVE DEVICE
In contrast to the former balloon-expandable device design, a self-expanding
valved frame was developed by CoreValve, Inc., from 2001 onward. Preclinical
testing was completed by 2004 and a first in-man feasibility study initiated in
July 2004 (36) enrolling 14 patients at three centers (Germany, India, Venezuela)

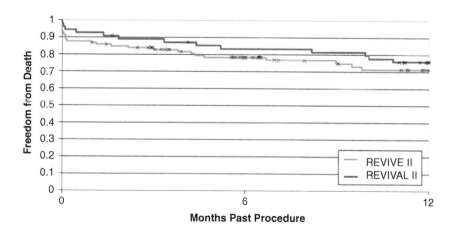

FIGURE 4   REVIVE II and REVIVAL II overall survival (%).

with the first-generation 25F device. Consecutively, Eberhard Grube reported the Siegburg experience (34), Germany, including 25 patients undergoing implantation of the self-expanding aortic valved frame from CoreValve from February to November 2005 for severe AS, including 17% of patients with concomitant aortic regurgitation. All devices were delivered retrograde including the first- (25F delivery sheath) and the second-generation devices (21F delivery sheath). Access was gained via the iliac artery in 9 patients, via the subclavian artery in 3 patients and via the common femoral artery in 13 patients. All interventions were performed under general anesthesia and extracorporeal circulation. Acute procedural success was reported in 21 of the 25 patients undergoing the intervention; 2 patients experienced significant aortic regurgitation because of device mispositioning and both patients underwent urgent rescue cardiac surgery with device removal and successful SAVR by a mechanical prosthetic valve.

Altogether the term "inoperable patient" might have to be reconsidered or might not apply to parts of the selected populations after all, as in all above-mentioned studies patients were selected on a too-high-risk-for-surgery basis—with other wards being denied surgery by external cardiac surgeons as reflected by the more than 20% mortality prediction by logistic EuroSCORE population. Nevertheless, some of those patients requiring emergent conversion to open heart surgery tolerated the more aggressive nature of surgery well and recovered even facing an iatrogenically aggravated disease by a complication of the initial TCVT attempt.

Following up on the Siegburg study, one patient underwent isolated aortic balloon dilatation because of failure to cross the stenosed aortic valve and died 12 hours later. A second patient expired from cardiac tamponade on the second postoperative day. Hemodynamic performance was assessed by transvalvular peak and mean pressure gradient. The study does not mention any increase in valve area. The peak pressure dropped from 69.9 ± 22.9 mm Hg to 21.3 ± 5.1 mm Hg after implantation and was measured at 22.1 ± 3.61 mm Hg at 30 days' follow-up. The mean pressure gradient of 44.2 ± 10.8 mm Hg decreased to 12.4 ± 3.0 mm Hg and to 11.8 ± 3.4 mm Hg at 30 days respectively. Four of the twenty-one patients presented aortic regurgitation degree 2+ decreasing over time and remaining present only in one patient at one-month follow-up. Also at follow-up, eight patients showed 1+ aortic regurgitation and nine patients were free of regurgitation. Of the 25 patients included, four periprocedural adverse events were reported as described earlier. Three additional deaths occurred caused by progressive hemodynamic failure in one, as a consequence of coagulopathy in another one, and finally because of sepsis in the third. Hospital mortality was 20%. No device dislodgement or thrombosis was reported but 1 patient suffered minor stroke, and major bleeding occurred in 5 of 10 patients with the first-generation device (24F delivery sheath) and 1 of 15 patients being treated by the second-generation device (21F). Of the 18 discharged patients with successful CoreValve implantation, none had an adverse event within the 30-day follow-up interval.

A first safety and efficacy study that enrolled 65 patients with the second-generation 21F device was conducted between August 2005 and August 2006 at seven sites distributed over Belgium, Canada, Germany, and Netherlands. This study was later supplemented with another safety and efficacy study enrolling

112 patients benefiting from implantation of the third-generation (18F delivery sheath) device. This study was conducted between October 2006 and June 2007 at nine sites in Canada, Germany, Netherlands, and United Kingdom. The inclusion criteria for both studies were as follows: severe AS with AVA of less than 1 cm² or AVAI ≤ 0.6 cm²/m² in patients older than 80 years or with logistic EuroSCORE ≥ 20% for the 21F group and age ≥ 75 years or a logistic EuroSCORE ≥ 15% for the 18F group or older than 65 years with multiple defined comorbidities. The exclusion criteria included sepsis, active endocarditis, allergy to any study medication, excessive access vessel calcification or tortuosity, aortic aneurysm, recent MI or stroke, coagulopathy, intracardiac thrombus or mitral or tricuspid regurgitation, prosthetic valves, pregnancy or creatinine clearance less than 20 mL/min, and finally less than a one-year life expectancy. The study endpoints considered procedural success, morbidity and mortality, as well as 30-day and long-term outcomes.

Preliminary analysis by August 8, 2007, of the 177 patients enrolled in the combined safety and efficacy studies (21F + 18F) were presented at ESC 2007 (Vienna, Austria) by Raoul Bonan of the Montreal Heart Institute (37). The combined mean theoretical surgical risk level was estimated by logistic EuroSCORE at 24%, with a mean age 82 years, and mean preprocedural AVA of 0.61 cm² and a mean gradient of 44.3 mm Hg. Approximately, one-quarter of patients were deemed totally inoperable. Gender distribution was 60% female patients and 79% of patients were in NYHA class III/IV. Procedural success was 92%, and 91% of patients were discharged with a CoreValve device. The mean gradient decreased to 7.9 mm Hg and AVA increased to 1.62 cm², with 86% of patients in NYHA class I/II. Procedural and procedure-related mortality were < 1% and 8%, respectively. Total 30-day mortality was 15% and the mean follow-up to 9 months (range 1 to 23 months) 23% of none-valve related mortality among these octogenarians. At last follow-up, substantially improved quality of life was documented for 77% of patients with a mean gradient at 11 mm Hg and an ejection fraction of 56% and 88% of patients in NYHA class I/II. No valve dysfunction or migration was observed either postprocedurally or at long-term follow-up. In 66% of patients, the aortic regurgitation was unchanged or even improved compared to 20% presenting an augmented grade 2+ aortic regurgitation and from 0 to grade 1+ in 14% of patients. At 30-day follow-up, no significant change in aortic regurgitation grade was observed with an equal number of patients presenting worsening (from 1+ to 2+) and improved (from 2+ to 1+ or 0) aortic regurgitation of close to 6%.

In December 2007, baseline echographic Corelab data were available in 88 patients. Existing aortic regurgitation improved significantly after percutaneous aortic valve replacement (PAVR). PAVR was associated with mild paraprosthetic aortic regurgitation (mostly due to low implantation of the prosthesis) and remained stable up to 6 months. There was no migration of the prosthesis throughout follow-up. The results are shown in Table 5.

The CoreValve 18F device gained CE mark during 2007, but the product was not immediately market released. Instead, the company initiated an expanded clinical evaluation registry in a limited number of sites in Europe (38). On February 15, 2008, this registry had enrolled 478 patients with demographics very similar to those of the safety and efficacy studies. The mean age was

TABLE 5 Echographic Corelab Data at Baseline, Discharge, 3 and 6 Months, December 2007

Variable	Baseline $n = 88$	Discharge $n = 62$	3 Months $n = 45$	6 Months $n = 39$	P
Heart rate, bpm	72 (65–81)	75 (65–85)	74 (63–80)	75 (65–82)	NS
LA diam., mm	45 (41–52)	46 (43–50)	44 (41–51)	42 (37–48)	NS
LVDD, mm	51 (48–55)	51 (47–54)	52 (47–55)	51 (48–52)	NS
LVEF, %	55 (45–60)	60 (50–65)	55 (49–61)	55 (45–65)	NS
Peak aortic velocity, m/s	4.2 (3.8–4.8)	2.0 (1.8–2.3)	2.0 (1.7–2.3)	2.0 (1.8–2.3)	< 0.0001
Peak gradient, mm Hg	71 (57–90)	16 (12–21)	15 (12–21)	16 (14–21)	< 0.0001
Mean gradient, mm Hg	47 (40–56)	8 (7–11)	8 (6–11)	10 (9–11)	< 0.0001
AVA, cm^2	0.7 (0.6–0.9)	1.7 (1.6–2.0)	1.8 (1.6–2.0)	1.7 (1.5–2.0)	< 0.0001
AVA index, cm^2/m^2	0.4 (0.3–0.5)	1.0 (0.9–1.2)	1.0 (0.9–1.2)	1.0 (0.9–1.2)	< 0.0001
Cardiac index, L/min/m^2	2.9 (2.6–3.6)	3.0 (2.6–3.6)	3.4 (2.2–4.5)	3.3 (2.5–4.4)	NS
SPAP, mm Hg	42 (37–51)	45 (41–54)	41 (37–47)	41 (38–44)	NS

Abbreviations: AVA, aortic valve area; EF, ejection fraction; LVDD, left ventricle end-diastolic diameter; LVEF, left ventricular ejection fraction; LA, left atrium; SPAP, systolic pulmonary artery pressure.

80.6 years [± 7.0 (46–95)] and mean Logistic EuroSCORE was 24.1% [± 14.0 (3–85)]. A little more than half (45%) of patients were women. The following comorbidities were noted:

Hypertension	58%
Diabetes	27%
CAD	57%
Prior MI	14%
Prior PCI	31%
Prior CABG	23%
AFib	31%
Prior CVA	8%
PVD	26%

Abbreviations: CABG, coronary artery bypass graft; CAD, coronary artery disease; CVA, cerebrovascular accident; MI, myocardial infarction; PCI, percutaneous intervention; PVD, peripheral vascular disease.

The preprocedure parameters were as described as in table below:

AVA (cm^2)	0.64 ± 0.20	(0.2–1.7)
Mean gradient (mm Hg)	49.8 ± 17.8	(15–114)
Peak gradient (mm Hg)	78.3 ± 26.8	(22–169)
% in NYHA class III/IV	86%	
LVEF	51% ± 14	(10–85)

Abbreviations: AVA, aortic valve area; NYHA, New York Heart Association; LVEF, left ventricular ejection fraction.

The procedural results were as follows:

Procedural success	465 (97%)
Mean procedure time	130 ± 49 min
Discharge mean gradient	2.60 ± 4.65 (0–22)
Discharge peak gradient	4.79 ± 8.31 (0–60)
Discharged alive and well with CoreValve	449 (94%)
Regurgitation at discharge	Grade 0 = 37%, Grade 1 = 49%, Grade 2 = 13%, Grade 3 = 1%, Grade 4 = 0%

The mortality results were as follows:

All 30-day mortality	36 (8%)
Procedure related	15 (3%)
Nonprocedure/nonvalve related	18 (4%)
Unknown	3 (< 1%)

The procedural failures were as follows:

Overall procedural failures	13 (3%)
Inability to access vessel	0 (0%)
Inability to navigate vasculature	0 (0%)
Inability to cross native valve	0 (0%)
Misplacement	1 (< 1%)
Aortic root perforation	2 (< 1%)
Aortic dissection	1 (< 1%)
Access vessel bleeding	2 (< 1%)
LV perforation, guidewire	2 (< 1%)
RV perforation, temp pacemaker wire	2 (< 1%)
Difficulty with BAV	1 (< 1%)
Conversion to surgery	2 (< 1%)

(Note: Multiple events in same patients = data not cumulative)
Abbreviations: BAV, balloon aortic valvulopathy; LV, left ventricle; RV, right ventricle.

The procedural complications (0–30 days) were as follows:

MI[a]	3 (< 1%)
Aortic dissection[a]	2 (< 1%)
Coronary impairment	0 (0%)
Acute vascular complications	7 (2%)
Stroke/TIA[a]	8 (2%)
Pacemaker	34 (7%)
Reop for valve failure	1 (< 1%)
Valve dysfunction	0 (0%)
Valve migration	0 (0%)

(Note: Multiple events in same patients = data not cumulative)
Abbreviation: TIA, transient ischemia attack.
[a]Long-term follow-up data is not yet available on registry patients.

DIRECT ACCESS VALVE REPLACEMENT VIA THE TAP—THE EDWARDS LIFESCIENCES EXPERIENCE

Access vessel size, local complication profile, the long and often tortuous vascular tree, as well as the increased stroke risk by retrograde crossing of the highly calcified aortic valve have motivated the author since 2000 to develop the TAP. This third access option (Chap. 6, Access to the Aortic Valves) for TCV implantation was first publicly disclosed by the author in February 2004 at the annual International Society of Endovascular Surgery meeting in Scottsdale, AZ (39). Anecdotally, the presentation took place in the same auditorium where Ulrich Sigwart's presentation inspired Henning-Rud Andersen to invent the valved stent concept 16 years earlier. This third access option was at first validated by a TCV taskforce issuing a position statement supporting the authors' TAP approach as the most promising access at the present time (40) and immediately after the new technique became adopted by clinicians from the surgical (41) and interventional (42) fields as well as by the industry. This process might be quite unique in its way by moving toward fusing two very closely related specialties but of quite diverse training backgrounds and possible leading to a better mutual understanding and collaboration and eventually into a new specialty like the interventional specialist.

A proof of concept study published in 2006 (41) included 30 consecutive patients with mean age 82 years and NYHA of 3.5 over an 8-month period to receive an aortic TCV implantation via the TAP approach. Unfortunately, the study provides little detailed data on inclusion or exclusion criteria of the patient population. Overall, patients with severe AS were selected on the basis of being at high surgical risk defined by a > 11 points logistic EuroSCORE reflected in the mean EuroSCORE of > 27 and presenting an aortic annulus of ≤ 24 mm diameter with equal distribution of calcifications. A Cribier-Edwards device of either 23 (8 patients) or 26 mm (22 patients), both inserted with a 33F delivery system, was used in all cases. In 13 patients, cardiopulmonary support was initiated and all patients underwent rapid pacing at 150/min during BAV and device deployment. Procedural success was present in 29 patients. In one patient, caused by eccentric calcification, the device dislodged retrograde into the left ventricle interfering with the mitral valve. Conversion to SAVR was performed.

Acute results disclosed a reduced peak transvalvular gradient from 76 ± 23 mm Hg to 16 ± 8 mm Hg, a mean gradient lowered from 43 ± 14 mm Hg to 7.5 ± 5 mm Hg, and a jet velocity decreasing from 4.2 ± 0.6 m/s to 1.9 ± 0.5 m/s and no significant changes in the LVEF (52 ± 13% vs 55 ± 12%). Three patients presented trace aortic regurgitation, nine patients 1+, and 2 patients 2+ aortic regurgitation. Of the 14 aortic regurgitations, 5 were of transvalvular and 9 of paravalvular origin. Seven patients had an uneventful recovery. The in-hospital morbidity included two patients undergoing rethoracotomy for hemorrhage-associated complications. A further two patients required cardiopulmonary resuscitation because of complete AV block and because of respiratory dysfunction. None of the patients experienced neurological deficits or stroke as opposed to retrograde implants with stroke rates of 5% to 10%. Mortality reached 10% with two patients dying from nonvalve- or procedure-related origin and one patient expired after biventricular failure at anesthetic induction.

Interim results from the TRAVERCE Feasibility trial of the Edwards SAPIEN™ transcatheter heart valve with the Ascendra transapical delivery system as provided by Edwards Lifesciences, Inc., on May 2008 and presented at the AATS 2008 in San Diego. The purpose of the ongoing prospective multi-center single-arm phase I pilot study is to evaluate the feasibility and safety of the transapical delivery and implantation of the Edwards SAPIEN transcatheter heart valve with Ascendra system. A total of 172 patients are enrolled and interim report data on 135 patients are available with including core lab reviewed and adjudicated data. The primary safety endpoints are death, stroke, valve migration, severe AI, urgent cardiac surgery, or device failure at discharge (< 30 days) and at 6 months. Efficacy endpoints include echocardiographic EOA, NYHA class, and perivalvular leak at discharge (< 30 days) and at 6 months. Inclusion criteria are severe AS with indication for AVR, age > 70 years, additive EuroSCORE mortality risk $\geq$ 9%, EOA $\leq$ 1.2 cm^2, and NYHA class III or IV. Primarily, patients with a native aortic annulus < 19 mm or > 24 mm estimated by echo or patients presenting contraindication for aortic valvuloplasty or TEE were excluded from the study. Additional exclusion criteria were severe chest wall deformity, primary hypertrophic obstructive cardiomyopathy, or history of active endocarditis within last 3 months.

The 135 TAP implantations took place at three different centers with 83 implants at the heart center in Leipzig, Germany, 36 implants performed at Medical University (AKH) Vienna, Austria, and another 16 implants at the University Clinics, Frankfurt, Germany. The baseline demographics of the 135 TAP implants are summarized in the table below.

Age	Mean 81.7 yr $\pm$ 5.1 (63–93)
Gender	Female patients 77%/104
NYHA	3.23 $\pm$ 0.4 (1–4)
Logistic EuroSCORE	26.8 $\pm$ 12.9 (7–59)
Aortic valve area ($n = 100$)	0.55 cm^2 $\pm$ 0.22 (0.24–1.4)
Mean gradient ($n = 108$)	44.76 $\pm$ 14.97 (2.3–80)
Ejection fraction ($n = 111$)	50.75% $\pm$ 15.9% (15–80.6)

Abbreviation: NYHA, New York Heart Association.

The baseline comorbidities are listed in the table below.

Comorbidities	n	%
Systemic hypertension	112	83
Coronary artery disease	64	47.4
Pulmonary disease	48	35.6
Diabetes mellitus	43	31.9
Chronic renal disease	44	32.6
Peripheral vascular disease	35	25.2
Congestive heart failure	30	22.2
Myocardial infarction	27	20.0
Carotid disease	30	22.2
Prior PTCA	25	18.5
Prior coronary artery bypass surgery	19	14.0
Prior stroke	17	12.6

Abbreviation: PTCA, percutaneous transluminal coronary angioplasty.

The total procedural time of 131 implantations was 127.6 ± 82.5 minutes (55–440 minutes). But isolate deployment time measured from balloon aortic valvuloplasty to device deployment ($n = 124$) lasted 8.2 ± 5.6 minutes, with the shortest implant taking 2 minutes and the longest 38 minutes. In 124 (92%) patients, the procedure was performed beating heart (off-pump) and the device was correctly positioned in 126 (93.3%) patients. The reason for conversion to open AVR became necessary in 11 (8%) patients because of malposition ($n = 4$), valve migration ($n = 3$), aortic insufficiency ($n = 5$), ascending aorta dissection ($n = 1$), mitral chordae entanglement ($n = 1$). From baseline to discharge, the AVA increased from 0.55 to 1.46 cm^2, with a mean gradient decreasing from 44.5 ± 15.0 to 7.4 ± 4.5 mm Hg at discharge and 8.3 ± 6.2 at one year (pooled data). The EOA increased from 0.55 ± 0.2 to 1.46 ± 0.5 at discharge and 1.15 ± 0.4 cm^2 at one year respectively. The left ventricular ejection fraction increased from baseline 50.8% ($n = 111$) to 60.4% ($n = 24$). At discharge, 27 (34%) patients had none, 55 (62.5%) had mild (1+), and 6 (6.8%) had mild-moderate (2+). Proportionally, regurgitation increase over the next year to 3 patients (17%) with none, 14 (78%) with 1+, and 3 (17%) with 2+ aortic regurgitation. The intraprocedural complications are listed in the table below.

Complications	$n = 25$ (18.5%)
Vascular—descending aortic dissection	1
Apical bleeding/ventricular injury	8
Arrhythmias requiring intervention	4
Hemodynamic instability requiring intervention	3
Cardiac failure	4
Partial coronary occlusion	3
Coronary occlusion	2

The early deaths are listed in the table below.

Early (< 30 d, no intraprocedural deaths)	$n = 19$ (14.1%)
Cardiac failure	8
Multiple organ failure	2
Respiratory complications	2
Bleeding event	2
Leg ischemia	1
GI complication	1
Embolic event	1
Arrhythmia	1
Sudden death	1
Calcium embolism	1

Abbreviation: GI, gastrointestinal.

The late deaths are listed in the table below.

Late (> 30 d)	$n = 20$ (14.8%)
Respiratory complications	5
Multiorgan failure	3
Cardiac failure	3
Neurological complications	1
Sepsis	1
MI	1
GI complications	1
Autoimmune vasculitis	1
Arrhythmia	1
Sudden death	1
Cerebral bleed	1

Abbreviations: GI, gastrointestinal; MI, myocardial infarction.

The TRAVERCE study experience suggests that the transapical AVR with the Edwards SAPIEN valve is feasible and reasonably safe in high-risk AS patients. No intraprocedural deaths were experienced, no structural valve deterioration up to one year developed, and TCVT valve gradients remain consistent at one year after implant.

Nevertheless, the TAP-related TCVT shows an important complication profile—worsening aortic regurgitation over time, and of 135 enrolled patients only 19 remained at risk at one year. The later results might raise the very justified question if the patients selected for TCVT really benefit from the intervention or if patient selection should be reconsidered in the presence of a growing number of promising medium-term data in the survivors.

TRAVERCE Transapical Trial

At the time the transfemoral transcatheter valve delivery approach was being developed at Percutaneous Valve Technologies, Inc., an alternative delivery method was being performed in animal experiments at Edwards Lifesciences, Inc. Following the Edwards acquisition, the minimally invasive transapical delivery approach through a left thoracotomy incision was further refined in collaboration with North American and European cardiovascular surgeons with initial human trials initiated in late 2004.

The TRAVERCE trial (*TRAnsapical Surgical DeliVEry* of the Cribier-Edwards Aortic Bioprosthesis) was designed as a first in-man pilot study to evaluate the feasibility and safety of the transapical surgical delivery and implantation of the Edwards SAPIEN transcatheter heart valve. The trial was conducted in three European sites. Procedures were performed in cardiac catheterization laboratories or hybrid operating rooms that were in conformance with the necessary hygiene standards for an open procedure with use of the heart-lung machine and floor-mounted fluoroscopy or mobile C-arm machines that were deemed appropriate for possible percutaneous coronary interventions. Following ethics committee approval and health care authority notifications, the phase I study started in December 2004 in Germany. Three patients were enrolled and implanted, all receiving a 23-mm model 9000 valve. All devices were explanted (two at implant and one within 6 hours of implant and replaced with conventional biological valves).

Following modification of the valve with the addition of an outer cloth skirt and change in sizing considerations, the study was restarted in July 2005 with the models 9000 MIS-23 mm and original model 9000-26 mm. In addition, the predilation valvuloplasty procedure was modified to use smaller diameter balloon catheters. One patient was enrolled and an implant was attempted but the device could not be deployed because of issues with the subvalvular mitral apparatus and conventional implantation was done. Additional animal work was undertaken and the first successful transapical implantation was accomplished by Dr. Sam Lichtenstein in St. Paul's Hospital in Vancouver, British Columbia, in October 2005. Successful TRAVERCE study enrollments and implantations resumed again in February 2006. Cloth-covered model 9000 MIS-26 mm was added in May 2006. A total of 24 MIS valves were implanted and then discontinued after the introduction of the model 9000 TFX manufactured with bovine pericardial tissue in July 2006. Enrollment in the TRAVERCE trial was closed in April 2008. A total of 172 patients have been enrolled. The interim data presented are from February 2008 for presentation at the AATS.

The TRAVERCE patient population is very similar to those in the transfemoral trials with the enrollment of symptomatic adult patients who require AVR due to severe (AVA $\leq$ 1.2 cm^2) valvular AS and who are high-risk candidates for routine open heart on-pump cardiac surgery. The primary endpoint is a composite safety event endpoint at 30 days and 6 months that includes cardiac death, bailout surgery, stroke/neurological deficit, valve migration, cardiac perforation/tamponade, device failure, and severe aortic insufficiency. The primary efficacy endpoint was procedural success as well as the evaluation of the hemodynamic parameters EOA and prosthetic valve gradients at discharge, 30 days, 3 to 6 months, and 1 year.

Baseline demographics for the first 135 patients are displayed in Table 6. Patients ranged in age from 63 to 93 with a mean age 81.7 $\pm$ 5.1 years. As in the transfemoral trials, the majority (77%) are female patients. Mean NYHA functional classification is 3.23 $\pm$ 0.4. The predicted operative mortality was calculated using the logistic EuroSCORE with a mean of 26.8 $\pm$ 12.9%. Risk assessment ranged between 7 and 59. STS risk scores were not obtained. For those patients whose EuroSCORE was less than 20%, approval for enrollment was obtained following presentation of the case from the responsible ethics committee. AVA and mean aortic gradient met the inclusion criteria with mean values of 0.55 $\pm$ 0.22 cm^2 and 44.76 $\pm$ 14.97 mm Hg. Ejection fraction was measured at 50.75 $\pm$ 15.9% with a range between 15% and 80.6%.

Implant success in the TRAVERCE study in the first 135 patients was at 92%. Beating heart procedures were performed on 124 patients with 37 patients receiving a 23-mm valve and 87 patients implanted with a 26-mm valve. Mean valve deployment time defined from the time of BAV to the time of valve implantation was 8.2 $\pm$ 5.6 minutes ranging from 2 to 38 minutes. Mean total procedure time was 127.6 $\pm$ 82.5 minutes with procedure time ranging between 55 and 440 minutes. Procedures were performed off-pump in 97 patients (Table 7). Use of the heart-lung machine was at the discretion of the investigator based on the patient's condition. At the beginning of the trial, patients were cannulated femorally and placed on pump as a precautionary measure. As the sites gained more experience a guidewire was placed in the femoral vein and the

TABLE 6   TRAVERCE Baseline Demographics

	Transapical
Age (yr)	*N* = 135
Mean + SD	81.7 yr ± 5.1
Range (min–max)	63–93
< 70 yr	3 (2.2%)
70–79 yr	37 (27.4%)
81– 89 yr	89 (65.9%)
> 90 yr	6 (4.4%)
Gender	*N* = 135
Female	104 (77%)
Male	31 (33%)
NYHA	*N* = 135
Mean + SD	3.23 ± 0.4
Range (min–max)	1–4
Logistic EuroSCORE	*N* = 135
Mean + SD	26.8 ± 12.9%
Range (min–max)	7–59
Aortic Valve Area	*N* = 100
Mean + SD	0.55 ± 0.22 cm^2
Range (min–max)	0.24–1.4
Mean gradient	*N* = 108
Mean + SD	44.76 ± 14.97
Range (min–max)	2.3–80
Ejection fraction	*N* = 111
Mean + SD	50.75 ± 15.9%
Range (min–max)	15–80.6

Abbreviation: NYHA, New York Heart Association.

heart-lung machine primed and on stand-by in the cardiac catheterization laboratory or hybrid operating room. Eleven patients required open conversion to conventional AVR.

As seen in the transfemoral feasibility studies, there is a significant improvement in the hemodynamic parameters. EOAs and mean prosthetic gradients post implantation improve and remains constant over time. Table 8 shows the mean gradient progression and the increase in EOAs over one year. Analyses of these data have been completed by the echocardiographic core laboratory and reflect available echoes of eligible patients at the follow-up interval. The written values reflect pooled data for the 23- and 26-mm valves. These hemodynamic results can be considered to be comparable and in some cases lower than other conventional biological prostheses of the same size.

TABLE 7   TRAVERCE Procedural Outcomes

	Transapical
Deployment time (BAV to valve deployment)	*N* = 124
Mean + SD	8.2 ± 5.6 min
Range	2–38
Total procedure time	*N* = 131
Mean + SD	127.6 ± 82.5 min
Range	55–440
Off pump (*N* = 97)	71.9%
Conversion to open procedure (*N* = 11)	8.1%

Abbreviation: BAV, balloon aortic valvulopathy.

TABLE 8 TRAVERCE Mean Aortic Gradient and EOA

	Baseline	Discharge	3 to 6 months	1 year
Mean aortic gradient (mm Hg)	44.8 ± 15.0	7.5 ± 4.5	8.1 ± 5.4	8.3 ± 6.2
Effective orifice area (cm^2)	0.55 ± 0.2	1.46 ± 0.5	1.34 ± 0.5	1.15 ± 0.4
23 mm $N =$	25	27	12	8
26 mm $N =$	75	57	29	14

Left ventricular function change was controlled by measuring ejection fraction. Again as seen in the transfemoral studies, ejection fraction improved in the transapical group over the course of one year. Pooled results show a baseline value of 50.8% that improved to 52.9% by discharge, then to 57.7% at 3 to 6 months, and is at 60.4% for the 1-year interval. This improvement is shown in Figure 5.

The location and severity of native aortic valve and annulus calcification appears to affect the location and degree of subsequent paravalvular leak and central aortic regurgitation in transcatheter valve replacement. Procedural modifications in the reduction of the size of the valvuloplasty balloon together with a prescribed range of native annular diameter for the 23- and 26-mm valve sizes have in most cases minimized the amount of aortic insufficiency seen following both transfemoral and transapical implantation. Figure 6 displays the aortic regurgitation (both paravalvular and central leak) at discharge, 3 to 6 months, and 1 year from echoes read by the Corelab in TRAVERCE patients. Because of the small number of patients currently available at the one year follow-up, it is not yet possible to determine if the degree of regurgitation has increased or remains stable. For the echoes reviewed in Figure 6, at discharge 33% of patients had no paravalvular or central leak and 60.6% had a trivial or 1+ leak and only 6.4% of patients had a 2+ or mild degree of aortic regurgitation. At the 3- to 6-month interval, 41% of patients presented with no regurgitation and 59% had

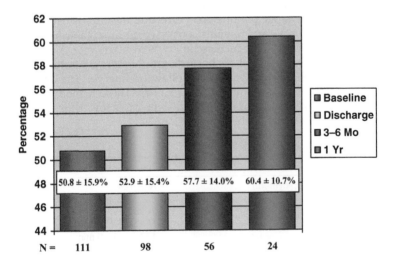

FIGURE 5 TRAVERCE left ventricular ejection fraction.

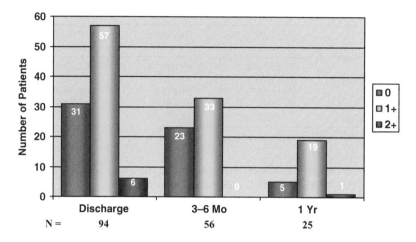

FIGURE 6 TRAVERCE aortic regurgitation.

1+ regurgitation. In the 25 echoes currently available at the one-year follow-up, 20% had no regurgitation, 76% had 1+ regurgitation, and one patient with 2+ regurgitation represents 4%.

There were no intraprocedural deaths during the TRAVERCE trial. At the time of this report, there were 19 (14.1%) early deaths reported and 20 late deaths. Freedom from death at 30 days is 85.3 ± 0.03%, at 6 months 68.9 ± 0.04%, and at 1 year 64.3 ± 0.05%. There has been 100% freedom from prosthetic valve thrombosis and structural valve deterioration. Explants at 30 days reflect those patients who were converted to an open procedure at the index intervention. Only one explant occurred after the 30-day period. Freedom from stroke is 96.1 ± 0.02% at 30 days, 93.2 ± 0.03% at 6 months, and 91.3 ± 0.03% at one year. Freedom from MI at 30 days is 98.5 ± 0.01%, at 6 months 96.5 ± 0.02%, and at 1 year 93.7 ± 0.03%. Freedom from the composite events MACCE is 82.3 ± 0.03% at 30 days, 64.5 ± 0.05% at 6 months, and 59.9 ± 0.05% at 1 year.

REVIVAL II Transapical Trial
Enrollment and follow-up of transapical subjects in the United States under the REVIVAL II IDE Amendment for transapical access feasibility commenced in December 2006. Enrollment was closed in February 2008 and a total of 40 transapical patients have been implanted. The data presented in this section are those presented at the STS in January 2008 on 36 patients.

Patient demographics are expectedly similar to transfemoral REVIVAL II patients and transapical patients in the other studies. The mean age at implant was 83.8 ± 5.3 years (range, 69–93 years). The majority of patients were > 80 years at implant. Prior to the procedure, all patients were in NYHA functional class classes III and IV. Transapical patients had a mean logistic EuroSCORE of 36.5% (range, 6.6–68%) and a mean STS risk calculator score of 12.9 (4–47). Patients who did not meet the specified minimum logistic EuroSCORE and STS risk calculator score had other medical conditions/comorbidities that precluded surgery. At baseline, no significant differences in ejection fraction, AVA, and

TABLE 9 REVIVAL II Transapical and Transfemoral, TRAVERCE High-Risk Conditions

	REVIVAL II TA (N = 34)	REVIVAL II TF (N = 55)	TRAVERCE TA (N = 135)
Porcelain aorta	11 (32.4%)	6 (10.9%)	4 (2.9%)
Radiation of the sternum	7 (6.6%)	4 (7.3%)	0 (0%)
Severe COPD	20 (18.9%)	5 (9.1%)	48 (35.6%)
Chest deformities	4 (3.8%)	3 (5.5%)	1 (0.74%)
Surgical refusal by surgeon	31 (29.2%)	18 (32.7%)	NAV

Abbreviation: COPD, chronic obstructive pulmonary disease.

mean gradient were observed between this cohort and the TRAVERCE transapical cohort. In the REVIVAL II cohort, there are a smaller percentage of female patients (44% vs 77%) and a higher EuroSCORE (36.5% vs 26.8%).

High-risk conditions that were present in the transapical cohort are listed in Table 9 and are compared to available data from the REVIVAL II transfemoral and TRAVERCE transapical data. The REVIVAL II transapical cohort reported 32.4% of patients with a porcelain aorta. It should be noted that except for pulmonary disease these high-risk conditions were not specifically collected in the early feasibility TRAVERCE trial.

Review of the 30-day clinical events in the REVIVAL II transapical cohort shows an early mortality rate of 16.7%. Other early events that were calculated included stroke and valvular thrombosis. Freedom from stroke is reported to be 93.4% and freedom from emergent cardiac surgery is at 97.3%. No valvular thrombosis was reported in any of the patients. Comparable hemodynamic performance improvements are also demonstrated in REVIVAL II transapical patients as can be seen in Figures 7 and 8 at intervals up to 30 days. The valve area increases significantly at 24 hours after implantation and remains constant up to 30 days. Similarly, the mean gradient drops to levels less than 10 mm Hg at 24 hours which is also seen at the 7- and 30-day follow-up.

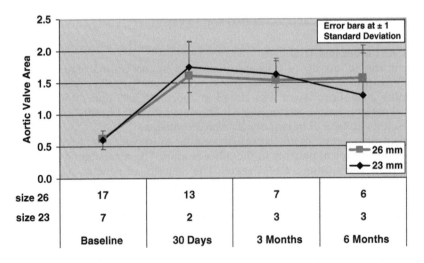

FIGURE 7 REVIVAL II transapical effective orifice area progression.

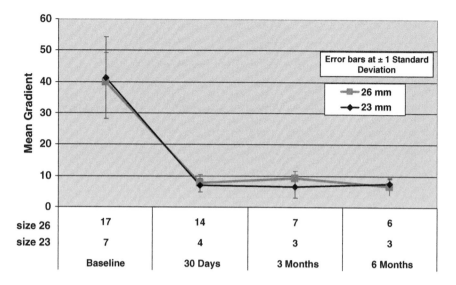

FIGURE 8 REVIVAL II transapical mean gradient progression.

The progression of ejection fraction over the first 30 days is seen in Figure 9. As a time-related event, ventricular remodeling and improvement in ejection fraction progresses over at least one year post implantation. In the chart, it can be concluded that the ejection fraction does not significantly decrease over the first 30 days and shows some improvement at the 30-day interval.

Changes in NYHA functional classification are shown as stepwise improvement over time in the chart labeled in Figure 10. The majority of patients show a one-, two-, or three-step improvement that increases over the

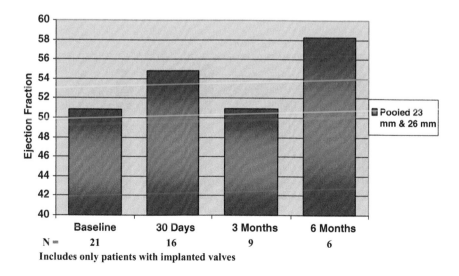

FIGURE 9 REVIVAL II transapical ejection fraction progression.

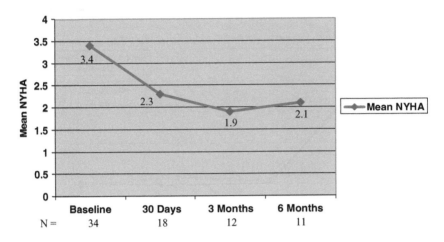

FIGURE 10 REVIVAL II transapical NYHA changes.

first 6 months. Functional improvements were also documented following the administration of quality of life questionnaires at various follow-up intervals in REVIVAL II patients receiving either a transapical or transfemoral implantation. Figure 11 shows the results of the SF-12 Quality of Life questionnaire and Figure 12 shows the results of the KCCQ. Improvements in SF-12 and KCCQ scores were significant at 6 and 12 months when analysis was restricted to patients with complete data at all four time points. The changes were highly statistically significant ($p < 0.01$ for each) in repeated measures ANOVA. In these high-risk patients with critical AS, both general and cardiac specific QOL improved markedly less than six months after treatment with the Edwards SAPIEN transcatheter heart valve using either delivery. General quality of life returned approximately to age-based population norms, and improvements were well maintained at 12 months.

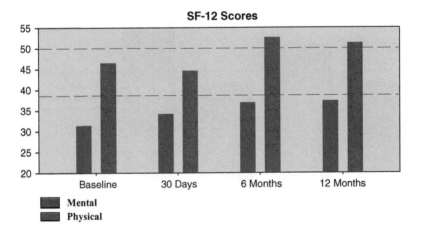

FIGURE 11 REVIVAL II transapical and transfemoral QOL scores SF-12.

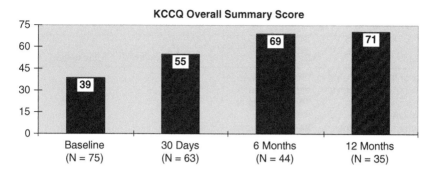

FIGURE 12 REVIVAL II transapical and transfemoral QOL scores KCCQ.

Combined Approach Trial

The PARTNER EU trial is a single-arm prospective multicenter nonrandomized trial of the Edwards SAPIEN transcatheter heart valve for the treatment of severe AS using either a transapical or transfemoral delivery approach. The study is being conducted in the European Union in nine centers in six countries (France, Germany, England, Belgium, Austria, and Netherlands).

The purpose of this trial is to determine the safety and efficacy of the implantable device and the respective Edwards valve delivery accessories in a "real-world" clinical decision-making environment as to best access approach (interventional cardiology and cardiac surgery coinvestigators determine transfemoral vs transapical implantation based upon collaborative review of access characteristics and patient comorbidities). The primary endpoint for this trial is to determine the freedom from death from the index procedure to 30 days and 6 months and NYHA improvement up to 12 months. After providing informed consent, patients were screened for study enrollment. Transapical or transfemoral access for implantation of the study device was determined by a joint decision of the coprincipal investigators after evaluation of anatomical characteristics including the presence and degree of calcification and tortuosity of the vessels of the groin. The main criteria for inclusion were senile degenerative AS with a documented initial AVA of < 0.8 cm^2 (indexed EOA < 0.6 cm^2), mean gradient > 40 mm Hg and/or jet velocity greater than 4.0 m/s, a logistic EuroSCORE ≥ 20 or a STS risk calculator score of ≥ 10. Since there were patients with medical conditions that precluded them from surgery that were not captured within a risk scoring classification, patients with the following conditions were also considered for inclusion into the trial:

1. Porcelain aorta or other precondition that precluded cannulation for cardiopulmonary bypass, cross-clamp application, or surgical access to the mediastinum
2. Surgically unmanageable ascending aortic calcification
3. Radiation treatment of the sternum, chest deformities, or mediastinitis that precluded an open chest procedure
4. Other conditions such as previous CABG surgery or severe pulmonary disease (FEV$_1$ < 1)

TABLE 10   Lists the 9 centers in 6 countries enrolled in the EU PARTNER Trial April 2007–January 2008

Clinical Site	Cardiologist/Cardiac Surgeon	Transfemoral	Transapical	Total
University of Vienna, Austria	Glogar, Wollner	9	10	19
Hôpital Bichat, Paris, France	Vahanian, Nataf	9	9	18
King's College Hospital, London, UK	Thomas, Gamel	7	10	17
West German Heart Center, Essen, Germany	Sack, Thielmann	6	10	16
Hôpital Prive de Massy, France	Lefevre, Donzeau-Gouge	10	5	15
Onze Live Vrouwziekenhuis, Aalst, Belgium	De Bruyne, DeGrieck	8	5	13
Goethe University, Frankfurt, Germany	Schächinger, Wimmer-Greinecker	2	10	12
Charles Nicolle Hospital, Rouen, France	Cribier, Bessou	7	5	12
Thoraxcenter, Rotterdam, The Netherlands	DeJaegre, Kappetein	3	5	8

The participating clinical centers were required to have both interventional cardiology and cardiac surgery departments in-house, imaging equipment in either a cardiac catheterization laboratory or hybrid operating room, and sufficient visualization for percutaneous coronary interventions. Ethics committee approvals were obtained and the trial was registered with the respective ministry of health. Patient enrollment was initiated in April 2007 and completed on January 31, 2008, with a total of 130 patients. A total of 121 of the 130 patients were implanted with the Edwards SAPIEN device by transfemoral ($n = 57$) or transapical ($n = 64$) approach. The enrollment by center and implant approach is provided in Table 10. All sites are actively following their enrolled patients.

A preliminary interim review of the baseline demographics of the PARTNER EU trial shows a mean age 81.5 years with 55% of the enrolled patients being women. AVA during screening was measured to be a mean of 0.47 cm^2 with a mean gradient of 49 ± 15 mm Hg and left ventricular ejection fraction was 54%. NYHA functional classification was reported at 2.93 with 64% of the patients in class III or IV. Logistic EuroSCORE was calculated to be 28 ± 13 and the STS risk assessment score at 12 ± 7. These values are summarized in Table 11. First outcome data presentations are planned for fall 2008.

TABLE 11   PARTNER EU Baseline Demographics

Baseline	
Age	Mean 81.5 yr
Gender	55% female patients
Aortic valve area	0.47 cm^2
Mean gradient	49 ± 15
Ejection fraction	Mean 54%
NYHA functional class	2.93
EuroSCORE	28 ± 13
STS risk assessment	12 ± 7

Transapical and Transfemoral Feasibility Studies Conclusion

More than 1000 patients requiring aortic heart valve replacements have been implanted with the Edwards SAPIEN transcatheter heart valve. Study results suggest that the transcatheter procedure via the transfemoral or transapical approach is feasible and reasonably safe in high-risk AS patients. There have been early procedure-related events that require continued refinement but no structural heart valve deterioration has been reported up to one year post procedure in those patients eligible to that time point. Postprocedural events such as stroke and MI appear comparable to high-risk conventional interventions. Valve gradients and measured EOAs are consistent over time and show considerable improvement and left ventricular function improves.

These unique approaches to AVR do require different patient management and additional physician training. Careful patient selection and screening as well as and collaborative precase planning among medical specialties including interventional cardiology, cardiovascular surgery, anesthesiology, and echocardiography are essential to continue to establish this new technology as a viable alternative to current conventional open heart AVR.

REFERENCES

1. HCPnet. U.S. national statistics. 2005.
2. Iung B, Cachier A, Baron G, et al. Decision-making in elderly patients with severe aortic stenosis: Why are so many denied surgery? Eur Heart J 2005; 26:2714–2720.
3. Edwards Lifesciences SG. Cowen Health Care Conference. Boston, MA: March 2003.
4. Iung B, Baron G, Butchart EG, et al. A prospective survey of patients with valvular heart disease in Europe: The Euro Heart Survey on Valvular Heart Disease. Eur Heart J 2003; 24:1231–1243.
5. Bonow RO, Carabello BA, Chatterjee K, et al. 2008 Focused update incorporated into the ACC/AHA 2006 guidelines for the management of patients with valvular heart disease: A report of the American College of Cardiology/American Heart Association Task Force on Practice Guidelines (Writing Committee to Revise the 1998 Guidelines for the Management of Patients With Valvular Heart Disease) Endorsed by the Society of Cardiovascular Anesthesiologists, Society for Cardiovascular Angiography and Interventions, and Society of Thoracic Surgeons. J Am Coll Cardiol 2008; 52: e1–e142.
6. Huber CH, Göber V, Berdat P, et al. Benefits of cardiac surgery in octogenarians—A postoperative quality of life assessment. Eur J Cardiothorac Surg 2007; 31:1099–1105.
7. Astor BC, Kaczmarek RG, Hefflin B, et al. Mortality after aortic valve replacement: Results from a nationally representative database. Ann Thorac Surg 2000; 70(6):1939–1945.
8. Ambler G, Omar RZ, Royston P, et al. Generic, simple risk stratification model for heart valve surgery. Circulation 2005; 112(2):224–231.
9. Bloomstein LZ, Gielchinsky I, Bernstein AD, et al. Aortic valve replacement in geriatric patients: Determinants of inhospital mortality. Ann Thorac Surg 2001; 71(2):597–600.
10. Chiappini B, Camurri N, Loforte A, et al. Outcome after aortic valve replacement in octogenarians. Ann Thorac Surg 2004; 78(1):85–89.
11. Collart F, Feier H, Kerbaul F, et al. Primary valvular surgery in octogenarians: Perioperative outcome. J Heart Valve Dis 2005; 14(2):238–242, discussion 242.
12. Collart F, Feier H, Kerbaul F, et al. Valvular surgery in octogenarians: Operative risks factors, evaluation of Euroscore and long term results. Eur J Cardiothorac Surg 2005; 27(2):276–280.
13. Craver JM, Puskas JD, Weintraub WW, et al. 601 octogenarians undergoing cardiac surgery: Outcome and comparison with younger age groups. Ann Thorac Surg 1999; 67(4):1104–1110.

14. Edwards FH, Peterson ED, Coombs LP, et al. Prediction of operative mortality after valve replacement surgery. J Am Coll Cardiol 2001; 37(3):885–892, Circulation 2000; 102(19 suppl 3):III70–III74.
15. Rankin JS, Hammill BG, Ferguson TB, et al. Determinants of operative mortality in valvular heart surgery. J Thorac Cardiovasc Surg 2006; 131(3):547–557.
16. Nowicki ER, Birkmeyer NJO, Weintraub RW, et al. Multivariable prediction of in-hospital mortality associated with aortic and mitral valve surgery in Northern New England. Ann Thorac Surg 2004; 77(6):1966–1977.
17. Jamieson WR, Edwards FH, Schwartz M, et al. Risk stratification for cardiac valve replacement. National Cardiac Surgery Database. Database Committee of The Society of Thoracic Surgeons. Ann Thorac Surg 1999; 67(4):943–951.
18. Sundt TM, Bailey MS, Moon MR, et al. Quality of life after aortic valve replacement at the age of >80 year. Circulation 2000; 102:III70–III74.
19. Cosgrove DM III, Sabik JF. Minimally invasive approach for aortic valve operations. Ann Thorac Surg 1996; 62:596.
20. Cohn LH, Adams DH, Couper GS, et al. Minimally invasive cardiac valve surgery improves patient satisfaction while reducing costs of cardiac valve replacement and repair. Ann Surg 1997; 226:421, discussion 427.
21. Yakub MA, Pau KK, Awang Y. Minimally invasive "pocket incision" aortic valve surgery. Ann Thorac Cardiovasc Surg 1999; 5:36.
22. Benetti F, Rizzardi JL, Concetti C, et al. Minimally aortic valve surgery avoiding sternotomy. Eur J Cardiothorac Surg 1999; 16(suppl 2):S84.
23. Minale C, Tomasco B, Di Natale M. A cosmetic access for minimally invasive aortic valve replacement without sternotomy in women. Ital Heart J 2002; 3:473.
24. Cohn LH. Minimally invasive aortic valve surgery: Technical considerations and results with the parasternal approach. J Card Surg 1998; 13:302.
25. Minale C, Reifschneider HJ, Schmitz E, et al. Minimally invasive aortic valve replacement without sternotomy. Experience with the first 50 cases. Eur J Cardiothorac Surg 1998; 14(suppl 1):S126.
26. Lee JW, Lee SK, Choo SJ, et al. Routine minimally invasive aortic valve procedures. Cardiovasc Surg 2000; 8:484.
27. De Amicis V, Ascione R, Iannelli G, et al. Aortic valve replacement through a minimally invasive approach. Tex Heart Inst J 1997; 24:353.
28. Bridgewater B, Steyn RS, Ray S, et al. Minimally invasive aortic valve replacement through a transverse sternotomy: A word of caution. Heart 1998; 79:605.
29. Lutter G, Kuklinski D, Berg G, et al. Percutaneous aortic valve replacement: An experimental study. I. Studies on implantation. J Thorac Cardiovasc Surg 2002; 123(4):768–776.
30. Huber CH, Tozzi P, Corno AF, et al. Do valved stents compromise coronary flow? Eur J Cardiothorac Surg 2004; 25(5):754–759.
31. Cribier A, Eltchaninoff H, Bash A, et al. Percutaneous transcatheter implantation of an aortic valve prosthesis for calcific aortic stenosis: First human case description. Circulation 2002; 106(24):3006–3008.
32. Cribier A, Eltchaninoff H, Tron C, et al. Early experience with percutaneous transcatheter implantation of heart valve prosthesis for the treatment of end-stage inoperable patients with calcific aortic stenosis. J Am Coll Cardiol 2004; 43(4):698–703.
33. Cribier A, Eltchaninoff H, Tron C, et al. Treatment of calcific aortic stenosis with the percutaneous heart valve: Mid-term follow-up from the initial feasibility studies: The French experience [published online ahead of print Feb 9, 2006]. J Am Coll Cardiol 2006; 47(6):1214–1223.
34. Grube E, Laborde JC, Zickmann B, et al. First report on a human percutaneous transluminal implantation of a self-expanding valve prosthesis for interventional treatment of aortic valve stenosis. Catheter Cardiovasc Interv 2005; 66(4):465–469.
35. Webb JG, Pasupati S, Humphries K, et al. Percutaneous transarterial aortic valve replacement in selected high-risk patients with aortic stenosis. Circulation 2007; 116:755–763.

36. Grube E, Laborde JC, Gerckens U, et al. Percutaneous implantation of the CoreValve self-expanding valve prosthesis in high-risk patients with aortic valve disease: The Siegburg first-in-man study [published online ahead of print Oct 2, 2006]. Circulation 2006; 114(15):1616–1624.
37. Grube E, Schuler G, Buellesfeld L, et al. Percutaneous aortic valve replacement for severe aortic stenosis in high-risk patients using the second- and current third-generation self-expanding CoreValve prosthesis: Device success and 30-day clinical outcome. J Am Coll Cardiol 2007; 50(1):69–76.
38. Presented by Maurice Buchbinder at the ACC 2008. The cut-off date is March 15, 2008.
39. Huber CH, Nasratulla M, Augstburger M, et al. Ultrasound navigation through the heart for off-pump aortic valved stent implantation: New tools for new goals. J Endovasc Ther 2004; 11(4):503–510.
40. Vassiliades TA, Block PC, Cohn LH, et al. The clinical development of percutaneous heart valve technology. A position statement of the Society of Thoracic Surgeons (STS), the American Association for Thoracic Surgery (AATS), and the Society for Cardiovascular Angiography and Interventions (SCAI). J Am Coll Cardiol 2005; 45:1554–1560.
41. Walther T, Dewey T, Wimmer-Greinecker G, et al. Transapical approach for sutureless stent-fixed aortic valve implantation: Experimental results [published online ahead of print Apr 5, 2006]. Eur J Cardiothorac Surg 2006; 29(5):703–708.
42. Lichtenstein SV, Cheung A, Ye J, et al. Transapical transcatheter aortic valve implantation in humans: Initial clinical experience [published online ahead of print Jul 31, 2006]. Circulation 2006; 114(6):591–596.

Company Overview

INTRODUCTION TO THE COMPANY SUMMARIES

The following pages have been provided by the companies listed below and shall serve as an overview of clinically used technologies as well as to present future developments and trends in regard of aortic valve procedures. This is not an exhaustive list and data were collected by voluntary response. A total of 24 companies were asked to provide standardized information about business, device development, and clinical or nonclinical data. The following companies were contacted via e-mail: 3F Therapeutics, ABPS, AorTx, ATS Medical, Arbor Medical, **CoreValve**, **Cardious**, DirectFlow, **Edwards Lifesciences**, EndoCor, Endoluminal research Technology, EndoHeart, Heart Leaflet, **JenaValve**, JoTec, LPI repositionable, **Lutter Heart Valve**, Medtronic, **Sadra Medical**, Shelhigh, St. Jude Medical, Sorin, ValveXchange, Ventor.

Six companies provided the requested details (highlighted in bold above). Please note the information was provided by the companies and the author as well as the publisher decline all responsibility about the content.

EDWARDS LIFESCIENCES

Edwards Lifesciences
One Edwards Way
Irvine, CA 92614, USA
Phone: 949-250-2500
Web site: http://www.edwards.com/

Company Profile

Edwards Lifesciences, a leader in advanced cardiovascular disease treatments, is the number one heart valve company in the world and the global leader in acute hemodynamic monitoring. Headquartered in Irvine, CA, Edwards focuses on specific cardiovascular disease states including heart valve disease, peripheral vascular disease, and critical care technologies. The company's global brands, which are sold in approximately 100 countries, include Carpentier-Edwards, Cosgrove-Edwards, FloTrac, Fogarty, LifeStent, PERIMOUNT Magna, and Swan-Ganz. Additional company information can be found at http://www.edwards.com.

Milestones

Since 2002, approximately 500 severe aortic stenosis patients have been treated with the Edwards SAPIEN™ transcatheter heart valve worldwide. Edwards Lifesciences Corporation received CE mark approval for European commercial sales of its Edwards SAPIEN transcatheter aortic heart valve technology with the RetroFlex™ transfemoral delivery system on August 31, 2007.

Studies

Edwards Lifesciences has completed feasibility studies of the Edwards SAPIEN transcatheter heart valve in Europe and in the United States for patients with severe aortic stenosis who were at a high risk for surgery. Additionally, Edwards has begun the PARTNER trial (*Placement of AoRTic TraNscathetER Valves Trial*), a pivotal prospective randomized core lab adjudicated trial for the same patient population. Additional trial information can be found at http://www.clinicaltrials.gov/.

Overview of Characteristics of Technology

Product Information

Stent

Expansion mechanism—balloon expandable valve technology
Material—stainless steel
Dimensions
    Valve size—23 mm and 26 mm
    Profile—22F and 25F

Valve

Edwards SAPIEN transcatheter heart valve
Material—bovine pericardial tissue with Thermafix™ tissue treatment
Configuration—three leaflet aortic tissue valve with uniform leaflet thickness. Obtained through the proprietary Perimapping™ process

The Edwards SAPIEN transcatheter heart valve has leveraged Edwards Lifesciences' more than 40 years of continuous refinement in heart valve technology.

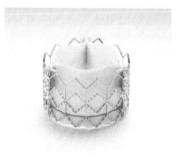

FIGURE 1 Edwards SAPIEN transcatheter heart valve.

Product Information

Delivery Device

Delivery routes—transfemoral and transapical

Expansion devices:
RetroFlex transfemoral valve delivery system
Ascendra™ transapical valve delivery system

Additional data—delivery system also includes the following:
Edwards transcatheter dilator set
Edwards introducer sheath
Edwards balloon catheter (for predilatation)
Edwards crimper
Inflation device

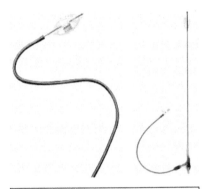

FIGURE 2 Edwards RetroFlex transfemoral delivery system.
FIGURE 3. Edwards Ascendra transapical delivery system.

COREVALVE, INC.
CoreValve, Inc.
1 Jenner 100
Irvine, CA 92618, USA
Tel 949-333-2500
Fax 949-333-2700
E-mail: info@corevalve.com
Acquired by Medtronic Inc, Minneapolis, MN, USA in 2009

Incorporated in 2001, privately owned CoreValve's mission is to reduce the trauma associated with traditional open heart valve replacement surgery and to offer definitive transcatheter aortic valve replacement (TAVR) therapy to patients less suitable or ineligible for surgery. Development programs for **percutaneous transfemoral, subclavian, and transapical** aortic valve replacement systems are in various stages of clinical realization. The company's focus is on percutaneous aortic valve replacement (PAVR) and CoreValve has developed a self-expanding technology for performing TAVR on a beating heart in normal sinus rhythm.

Since inception of the concept, the diameter of the PAVR delivery catheter has been dramatically reduced from 25F to 18F size, and the most recent PAVR *ReValving*™ system procedures have been performed in the catheterization laboratory by the interventional cardiologist under local anesthesia, without the use of surgical cut-down/repair (with preclosing) and without hemodynamic support or artificially accelerating the heart rate during valve placement. These PAVR technique improvements have resulted in a catheterization laboratory procedure that is increasingly similar to complex percutaneous coronary interventions.

Design concept and iterative prototyping took place during 1997 to 2002 and first-generation preclinical, animal, and cadaver work was completed by early 2004. A first in-man feasibility study that enrolled 14 patients with the first-generation 25F PAVR device was conducted between July 12, 2004 (first human implant), and July 2005 at three sites in Germany, Venezuela, and India. A safety and efficacy study that enrolled 65 patients with a second-generation 21F device was conducted between August 2005 and August 2006 at seven sites in Belgium, Canada, Germany, and Netherlands. A safety and efficacy study that enrolled 112 patients with a third-generation 18F device was conducted between October 2006 and June 2007 at nine sites in Canada, Germany, Netherlands, and United Kingdom.

The PAVR safety and efficacy study criteria focused on severe aortic stenosis (AVAI ≤ 0.6 cm^2/m^2) in patients older than 75 years or with logistic EuroSCORE (LE) $\geq 15\%$ or older than 65 years with multiple comorbidities. Study endpoints considered procedural success/morbidity/mortality as well as 30-day and long-term outcomes.

Preliminary analysis (August 8, 2007) of 175 patients enrolled in the combined safety and efficacy studies (21F + 18F) were presented at ACC 2008 (Chicago, IL) by Maurice Buchbinder, MD (San Diego, CA). The combined mean theoretical surgical risk level was LE 24%, with a mean age of 82 years, and mean preprocedural AVA of 0.61 cm^2 and mean gradient 44.3 mm Hg. Approximately one-quarter of patients were deemed totally inoperable and 60% were female patients with 79% of patients in NYHA class III/IV.

Procedural success was 92%, and 91% of patients were discharged with a CoreValve bioprosthesis. The mean gradient was decreased to 7.9 mm Hg and AVA increased to 1.62 cm^2, with 86% of patients in NYHA class I/II. Procedural and procedure-related mortality were <1% and 8% respectively. The total 30-day mortality was 15% and mean follow-up to 12 months (range, 10–32 months) detects a further 16% mortality among these octogenarians, none valve related. At last follow-up, substantially improved quality of life was documented for 85% of surviving patients with mean gradient at 11 mm Hg, ejection fraction of 56%, and 88% in NYHA class I/II. No valve dysfunction or migration was observed either post-procedurally or at long-term follow-up.

After receiving CE mark in mid-2007, the 18F *ReValving* System for PAVR has been the subject of an expanded clinical evaluation at a select number of European sites. The company elected to pursue this strategy to help ensure that interventional cardiologists are well trained, patients are appropriately selected for treatment, and continuing clinical outcomes feedback is obtained during the early stages of expanded use of the technology. CoreValve also established a rigorous training program for physician operators and attending catheterization laboratory personnel. The certification process encompasses both didactic and hands-on proctored clinical requirements. As of summer 2008, approximately 55 sites were actively implanting the device in Austria, Belgium, Denmark, France, Germany, Greece, Italy, Norway, Portugal, Spain, Sweden, Switzerland, Netherlands, and United Kingdom. As of end July 2008, approximately 1500 patients have been treated worldwide with the CoreValve PAVR device. Demographics of the expanded evaluation registry patients are near identical to those of the safety and efficacy studies; however, procedural success is 97% and 30-day mortality is 9%.

During 2007, CoreValve conducted a first in-man feasibility study with its 21F Transapical *ReValving* System. A total of five patients were enrolled at two sites in Germany. A TAVR safety and efficacy study for CE marking purposes was initiated during 2008 (same criteria as mentioned earlier except patients have compromised femoral access). This system implants the identical bioprosthesis design in an antegrade manner by means of a reversed catheter design. The system is advanced over a guidewire, through a small intracostal incision and a transapical puncture of the left ventricle.

The Company plans to initiate a randomized US pivotal trial of the PAVR system, to follow in 2009.

Special Features

- Hourglass frame design voids rotational positioning needs and mitigates coronary jail risk
- Valve design features supraannular valve function and intraannular anchoring
- Self-expansion eliminates risk of valve leaflet damage during delivery
- Self-expansion provides constant force to reduce paravalvular leak risk
- Smallest delivery catheter currently in the clinic (18F with 12Fshaft)
- Proximal repositioning possible during delivery

CoreValve ReValving Bioprosthesis

Frame
- Self-expanding (memory shaped Nitinol)
- Multilevel design incorporates three different areas of radial and hoop strength
  Top: Low radial force area orients the system
  Center: Constrained area to avoid coronaries and featuring supraannular valve leaflets
  Bottom: High radial force for secure intraannular anchoring—avoids recoil—adjusts to annulus size and shape
- Radiopaque

Valve
- Specifically designed for transcatheter use
- Single-layer porcine pericardium
- Trileaflet configuration
- 200 M cycle AWT
- Supraannular valve function unaffected by annulus size or shape within size range
- Intraannular implantation and sealing skirt

CE Marked Sizes
- 26-mm inflow for patient annulus 20–23 mm
- 29-mm inflow for patient annulus 24–27 mm

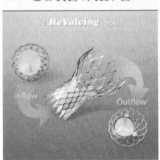

FIGURE 4 Self-expanding multilevel framed bioprosthesis.

PAVR *ReValving* Delivery Catheter

- 18F distal end allows true percutaneous access with preclosing
- 12F stepdown shaft size for enhanced interventional handling characteristics (no need for steerability)
- Over-the-wire (0.035-in compatible)
- Retrograde femoral access
- Integral two-speed handle for controlled loading and delivery of the self-expanding bioprosthesis
- Distal positioning marker
- Self-expansion avoids balloon trauma to bioprosthesis leaflets

Bioprosthesis Loading Process

- Disposable loading system
- Compresses bioprosthesis atraumatically in a consistent manner
- Loads bioprosthesis *into* the distal housing of the delivery catheter

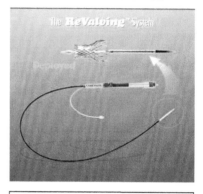

FIGURE 5 CoreValve PAVR delivery catheter.

SADRA MEDICAL, INC.

Sadra Medical, Inc.
1717 Dell Avenue
Campbell, CA 95008, USA
Phone: 408-370-1550
Fax: 408-370-1595
Web site: www.sadramedical.com

Company Profile

Sadra Medical was founded in 2003 by Amr Salahieh and a small group of leading-edge cardiovascular clinicians. The company is pioneering new therapies to minimize the invasiveness of treating aortic valve disease.

Overview

Leveraging the experience from initial approaches to TAVR, the Sadra Lotus™ valve is designed to streamline the procedure; optimize the valve's positioning; and provide a secure, effective bioprosthetic implant. The Lotus valve system consists of the Lotus valve, a bovine tissue trileaflet bioprosthetic aortic valve, and the Lotus delivery catheter, a delivery system for guidance and placement of the Lotus valve. The device is introduced endovascularly via the femoral artery using conventional catheterization techniques. The Lotus delivery catheter is designed to balance flexibility and support to facilitate smooth tracking through potentially challenging diseased anatomy and into the aortic root using a retrograde approach. The valve is intended for placement in the aortic annulus overlying the native aortic valve. The system is engineered to enable placement in a beating heart, and the valve begins to function early in the release process, a key feature designed to minimize systolic ejection forces.

The Lotus valve system is designed to facilitate fine operator control over valve unsheathing, seating, and deployment to aid in precision placement and to help the operator to avoid coronary obstruction and minimize contact with the mitral valve. Prior to releasing the Lotus valve into its final position, the valve may be retracted into the sheath of the delivery system for repositioning and redeployment or removal, as determined necessary by the physician.

Milestones
The company announced the first clinical use of the Lotus valve system in July 2007. Professor Eberhard Grube and Dr. Ralf Müller performed the procedure in the catheterization laboratory at Helios Klinikum, Siegburg.

Studies
Chronic animal studies for replacement of the aortic valve have been conducted in an ovine model to evaluate the short-term healing and seating of the valve. In a series of seven animals, one survived well past a year and two survived beyond 6 months. The valves were positioned and deployed without serious complication. Presacrifice echocardiography indicated that all surviving animals were hemodynamically stable and that the valve was functioning adequately. Gross pathological analysis of the valves, hearts, and other organs indicate that the valves are appropriately seated and healed to the annulus without evidence of excessive pannus ingrowth, valve thrombosis, occlusion of coronary ostia, or embolization. Histological analysis of tissue sections is being conducted by Frederick Schoen, MD, PhD, and Robert Padera, MD, PhD, Department of Pathology at Brigham and Women's Hospital in Boston, MA.

The Lotus valve system is designed to be the first fully repositionable technology to specifically address both the disease etiology of the aortic valve and the unique requirements of a transcatheter aortic valve replacement procedure. In addition to its repositioning and self-centering features that are designed to facilitate optimal positioning of the valve, the device's ability to be resheathed and retrieved prior to final release is designed to provide physicians with more control over the procedure.

Product Information

The Lotus valve is comprised of two principle components—a tri leaflet valve derived from bovine pericardium and a compliant nitinol stent structure designed for support and stabilization of the valve.

- Transcatheter, retrograde delivery
- Self-expanding, self-centering design
- Valve designed to function early during the deployment procedure
- Streamlined proprietary delivery system designed for fine control of valve positioning and repositioning as needed
- Designed to be resheathable and retrievable
- Adaptive™ seal designed to minimize perivalvular leakage

CAUTION: This device is for Investigational Use ONLY. It is not available for sale or commercial distribution. It is not approved for sale or use in the United States.

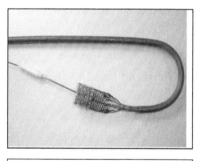

FIGURE 6 Lotus valve system in unsheathed state.

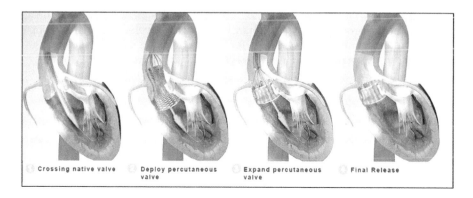

Crossing native valve   Deploy percutaneous valve   Expand percutaneous valve   Final Release

FIGURE 7 TAVR with the Lotus valve system.

JENAVALVE TECHNOLOGY

Disclaimer
The following information contains estimates and forward-looking statements that involve risks and uncertainties. These may include statements regarding future revenues or expenses; earnings and operations; as well as statements regarding demand for the company's solutions and the company's ability to achieve its targets, goals, and initiatives. They are the current beliefs and opinions of certain members of the JenaValve Technology management. The company gives no assurance regarding the achievement of these forward-looking statements, as they are only estimates and the actual outcomes maybe significantly different. Additionally, we expect that these forward-looking statements will change in the normal course of our business. The management specifically disclaims any obligation to update forward-looking statements that we may make in regard to this information.

JenaValve Technology
Nymphenburger Strasse 13
80335 Muenchen, Germany
Tel.: +49 89 55 27 908-0
Fax: +49 89 55 27 908-79
E-mail: info@jenavalve.de

JenaValve and JenaClip are trademarks of JenaValve Technology.

Overview
Transcatheter valve–specific company or division history includes the following:

Data of entrance into transcatheter valve developments: 1995
Prototype completed: Stent: 2007
Start preclinicals: 2007
Beginning of clinical studies: Q4/2008

The company's product idea was first conceived in 1995 by Prof. Dr. med. Hans-Reiner Figulla and PD Dr. med. Dr. disc.pol. Markus Ferrari, both currently at the Clinic of Internal Medicine I of the Friedrich Schiller University, Jena, Germany. Early prototypes of the JenaClip™ were developed in close cooperation with the Fraunhofer Institute for Applied Optics and Precision Engineering (IOF) in Jena, a research and development institute of the Fraunhofer-Gesellschaft. The systems are currently in late preclinical stage and the first clinical trials are in preparation. JenaValve expects its first permanent human implantations by Q4/2008 and CE mark by Q4/2009.

Milestones
The following is a list of key milestones reached:

1995: The "Self-Expandable Heart Valve Prosthesis" patented
1999: Initial stent design (first prototype) completed
First in vitro experiments

2003: Initial catheter design (first prototype) completed in cooperation with the Fraunhofer IOF

Acute animal experiments initiated

2004: First successful acute animal experiments published (*Heart*)

2005: First successful animal (pigs) trials

2006: First financing round completed with Atlas Venture

Dedicated management team established

Transapical catheter design initiated and completed

New transfemoral catheter design initiated

Stent design optimized

2007: Development team completed

Scientific Advisory Board established

First public viewing of JenaValve systems and stent at EuroPCR

Successfully completed acute animal trials (transapical)

Final stent design completed

Secured A-2 financing round with EdRIP (lead investor), Atlas Venture, and NeoMed Management

First temporary human implant

Successful chronic animal trials with a transapical delivering device

Transfemoral catheter design completed

Current milestone calendar

2008: Successful acute animal trial (transfemoral)

Q4/2008: First permanent human implantations

Q4/2009: CE mark

Regulatory Pathways

Studies
- Previous clinical studies: None
- Study overview includes the following:
  Study aim
  Study arms and participating center
  Study endpoints
- Listing of results
- Ongoing clinical studies
- Study overview: Not yet disclosed
  Study aim
  Study arms and participating center
  Study endpoints
- Listing of intermediate results

Planned Clinical Studies
- Study overview: Not yet disclosed
  Study aim
  Study arms and participating center
  Study endpoints

Commercialization: To Be Determined
- Beginning and location of first sales after receiving CE mark
- Sales strategy
- Critical milestones

Intellectual Property Situation

JenaValve is pursuing an active program of patent filing, licensing, and acquisition to generate a portfolio of patents and other intellectual property to protect its JenaClip and delivery system, as well as its pipeline products and methodologies. The company appreciates that patents are not the only form of protection for medical devices and is actively pursuing design, utility model and trademark protection. The company also ensures that all valuable know-how, trade secrets, and special materials are identified and appropriately managed. JenaValve recognizes the importance of competitor monitoring and freedom to operate. It actively searches and analyzes third-party patents for potential risks or obstacles to market, taking appropriate action where and when necessary. The company's patent portfolio comprises 15 patent families that are being actively managed.

The stent per se is protected by many of these patent families, the earliest dating from 1995 onward. The families include granted patents and pending patent applications in Europe, Japan, and the United States and applications pending before the World Intellectual Property Organization. Specific features of the JenaClip are further protected by registered designs in Europe. Features to allow stent location, anchoring, and repositioning are protected by several of the patent families that date from 2000 onward. The delivery system and associated catheter are protected by a number of the patent families dating from 2002 onward, covering the territories of Canada, Europe, and the United States, as well as applications pending before the World Intellectual Property Organization. Further patent applications have been made and are being prosecuted to protect JenaValve's commercial position both from a product development and a defensive point of view. All granted patents are currently in force and pending applications are being actively prosecuted.

JenaValve Technology has designed two integrated aortic valve replacement (AVR) systems, one for the transfemoral approach and the other for the transapical approach. Three state-of-the-art components are used in each system—a catheter delivery unit, the JenaClip—a unique self-expanding Nitinol stent, and a biological valve.

The following patent-protected differentiators enable JenaValve to build safe AVR systems:

- Unique JenaClip design ensures correct positioning
- Repositioning and retrievability possible until final release
- "Clip" mechanism enables firm anchoring of valve onto native aortic valve
- Unrivalled technique for attaching valve on stent

The JenaValve Stent

Trademarked as JenaClip, the company's current stent design, a biocompatible nitinol frame, is the result of more than 30 iterations and is backed by very significant validation tests. Successful animal trials have shown that the exact orthotopic positioning of the stent is the most critical aspect of PAVR. Implantation too deep into the left ventricular outflow tract causes severe aortic insufficiency and implantation too high in the aortic vessel causes occlusion of the coronary arteries. The minimal length of the stent significantly facilitates the passage through the aortic arch, yet robust fixation must be ensured. The ability to position the stent, to check its fit, and the ability to reposition it for optimum effect are crucial features of the recent design.

Unique Features
The construction of the self-expanding nitinol JenaClip relies on anatomical forces rather than simple geometries. It consists of a double-layer system of three clips aligned in two rows, unlike the usual round form. One row is used to affix the valve prostheses onto the stent and another row is used to position the implant exactly and to anchor it into the damaged or dysfunctional native leaflets of the old valve apparatus. This construction fits naturally into the anatomy of the aorta. Thanks to the clipping mechanism, the total length of the JenaClip has been minimized to approximately 30 mm. The passage through the vessels and the aortic arch is as smooth as possible because the catheter is highly flexible. The stent can expand up to 30 mm in diameter, or it can be compressed to 6 mm to fit into a small catheter. The design of the stent together with the expanding properties of nitinol in combination with a unique fixation technology guarantees exact retention (radial force) after implantation. The implant is specified to operate under physiologic blood flow conditions as proved by animal stress testing.

After releasing the stent from the catheter, it expands immediately with its maximal force to a predefined size and adapts to the patient's anatomy. Simultaneously, the biological valve, previously sewed to the stent, starts to function. The native aortic valve leaflets are pressed against the aortic wall and used for fixation in between the JenaClip, similar to a paperclip. This unique feature ensures that the implant does not move downward into the left ventricle. High radial force and its unique concave configuration prevent the implant from moving toward the opposite direction into the aorta. Safe fixation of the new valve is thus assured.

The Catheter Systems
Both the transfemoral catheter system and the transapical catheter system are remarkably easy to maneuver, position, reposition, and deploy. Importantly, they allow complete retrieval of the JenaClip before final release if necessary. The systems are used without any blood flow arrest. The implantation procedure can be carried out without the use of a heart-lung machine. The transfemoral catheter is highly flexible and steerable to pass through the vessels and aortic arch, smoothly guided by a standard guide wire. The transapical catheter is rigid, designed to enable direct access through the apex. The essential features of the catheter systems are as follows:

- User-friendly and ergonomic design
- Easy preimplantation loading
- OTW system: 1:1 torque

- Good visibility of implant due to positioning markers
- Two catheter lengths: 120 cm (transfemoral), 50 cm (transapical)
- Soft tip catheter, bendable to more than 180 degrees for easy and less traumatic crossing of the aortic arch (transfemoral)
- Stiff tip for use like a trocar (transapical)
- Excellent rotational steering for accurate placement of the positioning feelers
- Repositionable and fully retrievable before final release

The Heart Valve Prosthesis

The biological aortic valve is specially designed to connect perfectly to the stent. Thin, yet robust and foldable, the valve is processed and sewed into the stent individually and securely affixed to it. Thanks to the JenaClip design, additional stitch stress is eliminated when the valve is folded. Various valve sizes will be offered as part of the JenaValve product portfolio. They will fit into one catheter size, offering more flexibility and possible cost savings to the hospital. After the physician has decided which size to use, the implant will be loaded into the catheter. All quality requirements and specifications are monitored and verified by the relevant authorities.

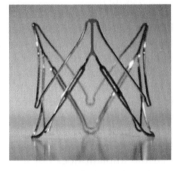

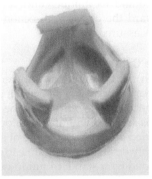

Product Information
Stent
Expansion mechanism
Material (Tech data):
Dimensions (expanded and crimped all sizes)
Radioopacity
Cuff material
Additional data
Valve
Material: Biological
Configuration (number of leaflets, etc)
Thickness
Durability data
Clinical data on surgicalvale implants
Additional data
Crimping Process
Data not disclosed by the company

FIGURE 8 JenaClip stent device.
FIGURE 9 The aortic valve. Previous versions shown, current versions not yet disclosed.

Product Information

Delivery Device

Delivery route(s): Transfemoral and transapical
Material
Dimensions
Expansion device (ex-balloon material, dimensions, etc.)
Handling mechanism
Radioopacity and markers
Additional data

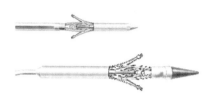

FIGURE 10 The transapical catheter (*above*) and transfemoral catheter (*below*) shown with Jena-Clip. Previous versions shown, current versions not yet disclosed.

CARDIOUS, INC.
Cardious, Inc.
303 Washington Street
Northfield, MN 55057, USA
Phone: 507-663-6170
E-mail: information@cardious.com
Web site: http://cardious.com

AvA™ Aortic Valve Bypass Graft System

Cardious, Inc., was founded to develop and commercialize the AvA aortic valve bypass graft system for use as a minimally invasive beating heart alternative to traditional AVR therapy. The goal of all AVR therapies is to decrease left ventricular load and increase coronary perfusion without producing additional regurgitation. Traditional AVR surgery attains this goal by directly replacing the stenotic aortic valve. In an aortic valve bypass procedure, outflow resistance is reduced by creating a second outflow channel connected to the aorta. By forming a parallel outflow tract, the outflow resistance acting on the ventricle is effectively reduced without replacing the native aortic valve. The native valve is left intact and operational. Since pressure within the large diameter aorta is largely independent of the attachment point of the graft, normal coronary and carotid flow is maintained.

The concept of using an apex to aorta valved conduit to bypass a stenotic aortic valve was first conceived by Nobel laureate Alexis Carrel in 1910 and first performed clinically by Sir John Templeton in 1962. Although Templeton's initial series of human implants proved feasibility of the valved conduit device, the procedure did not gain popularity with surgeons because, precisely at that point in the evolution of surgical techniques, the heart-lung machine was perfected. This led surgeons to select direct aortic valve removal and replacement over Templeton's indirect valve bypass procedure.

Even though direct valve replacement rapidly became the standard, the valved conduit procedure continues to be used in special circumstances by doctors throughout the world. Although there are no commercially available devices approved for aortic valve therapy, there is a substantial body of published literature reporting on the use of surgeon constructed "back table" valved conduit devices used in both "on-pump" and "off-pump" operations. The results document that the procedure provides clinical relief with minimal complications.

The AvA system is the first "apex to aorta" device specifically engineered to ensure a safe and reliable "off-pump" aortic valve procedure. The system includes a pair of custom prosthetic vascular grafts along with a disposable cutting tool. Each textile graft has a polyester-lined titanium housing designed to accept a surgeon-selected, commercially available prosthetic heart valve. The disposable cutting tool is inserted sequentially into each graft to facilitate bloodless attachment of the grafts to heart and aorta. The figure shows a photo of the implants and tool currently in development.

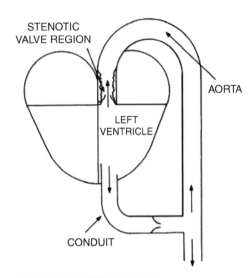

FIGURE 11 Flow schematic.

Implantation Steps
A small incision is made between the ribs at the fifth intercostal space. The aortic graft, with cutting tool inside, is then placed on the descending aorta adventitia and firmly sutured into place. The surgeon activates the cutting tool to excise a circular piece of tissue to form the anastomosis. This is done without any cross or partial clamping of the aorta. The tool (with cut aortic wall securely adhered to it) is removed and the graft is immediately clamped. The surgeon performs a similar technique to insert the apical graft into the ventricle except simultaneous to cutting, the apical graft's rigid connector is advanced into the ventricle thereby

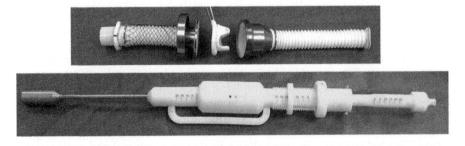

FIGURE 12 AvA aortic valve bypass graft system (shown with surgeon supplied heart valve).

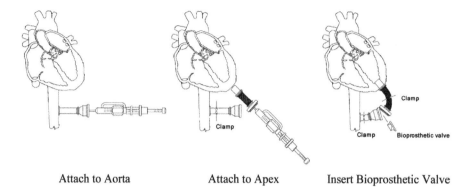

Attach to Aorta   Attach to Apex   Insert Bioprosthetic Valve

FIGURE 13 Minithoracotomy procedure.

allowing a near bloodless insertion. After suturing the graft to the heart wall, the tool is removed and the graft is clamped. The surgeon then selects a bioprosthetic heart valve to insert into the graft housings. No suturing is necessary to install the heart valve. The valve's sewing cuff is used as a sealing gasket. Once inserted, the clamps are removed to create the apex to aorta outflow path.

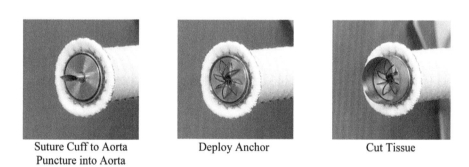

Suture Cuff to Aorta   Deploy Anchor   Cut Tissue
Puncture into Aorta

FIGURE 14 Cutting technique (aortic anastomosis).

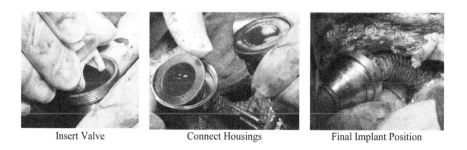

Insert Valve   Connect Housings   Final Implant Position

FIGURE 15 Valve implant technique (animal study).

Potential Benefits to High-Risk Patients

- Long-term implant reliability—allows use of proven traditional bioprosthetic heart valve
- Off-pump—no cardiopulmonary bypass complications
- No aortic clamping or valve excision—reduced emboli generation
- No sternotomy—access through small incision in the fifth intercostal space
- No paravalvular leak
- No conduction system injury
- Line of sight implant management—controlled surgical technique
- Excellent hemodynamics

Milestones

Completed Milestones
- Prototype device developed
- Long-term animal studies underway

Current Milestone Calendar
- Complete long-term animal studies—late 2008
- Initiate human studies—early 2009
- Obtain CE mark approval—2010

Regulatory Pathways
- Europe—CE mark
- US—FDA/PMA

Planned Clinical Studies
- Nonsurgical patients
- Initial study—20 patients/3 sites

Commercialization
- Distributor network

Intellectual Property
- Seven patent applications on file

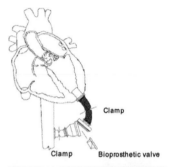

Clamp

Clamp   Bioprosthetic valve

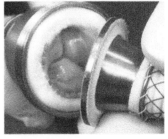

FIGURE 16   AvA implant.
FIGURE 17   Tissue valve inserted into valve housings.

Device Specifications

Implant
- Graft material—polyester
- Graft size—18 mm
- Cuff material—polyester
- Apical connector material—titanium with polyester lining
- Housing material—titanium with polyester lining
- Valve housing size—25 mm (oversized to match valve EOA to graft EOA)

Cutting Tool
- Disposable
- Adjustable puncture and cutting depth
- Hole diameter—18 mm

Valve Compatibility
- 25-mm tissue valve

    Edwards Paramount
    Medtronic Hancock II
    St. Jude Medical Biocor

LUTTER HEART VALVE

Georg Lutter, MD, PhD, and René Quaden, MD
Department of Cardiovascular Surgery, School of Medicine, University of Kiel
Arnold Heller Str. 7, D-24105 Kiel, Germany
Tel: ++49-431-597-4582
Fax: ++49-431-597-4542
E-mail: lutter@kielheart.uni-kiel.de
E-mail: Rene.Quaden@uksh-kiel.de

Overview

In 1993, Dr. Lutter began working on a technology to replace the aortic valve in a surgeon's way: the primary removal of the diseased valve and the consecutive implantation of a valved stent. He started to consider methods to remove the diseased aortic valve before implanting the valved stent. To avoid embolization caused by resected valve fragments, the valve must be isolated from the circulatory system before removal can be initiated. In 2003, Dr. Quaden joined the group and worked with Dr. Lutter on aortic valve resection. Together they developed an aortic valve isolation chamber (AVIC) (Figs. 19, 20) and showed that a high-pressure water stream scalpel and a thulium:YAG laser can be used to resect the aortic valve endovascularly in a nonbeating heart in an animal model and in human preparations. With strong support by Prof. Dr. Jochen Cremer, Head of the Cardiovascular Department, Lutter and Quaden created an international research group with financial support by the German Research Foundation (DFG), the Ministry of Education and Research (BMBF), and the Christian-Albrechts University of Kiel. The Institute of Biomedical Optics (BMO) in Luebeck, the Institute of Microtechnology (IMT) in Braunschweig, the Institute of Anatomy in Kiel, Teccon Engineering in Kiel, STI-Endoscopes in Henstedt-Ulzburg, Erbe-Electromedicine in Tuttlingen, and Wolff-Endoscopes in Knittlingen support this project.

Milestones

Listing of key milestones reached

1. Resection of native and calcified aortic valves in porcine in vitro and in vivo models and in human preparations
2. Development of AVIC

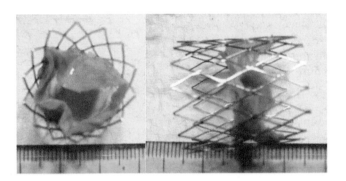

FIGURE 18 A self-expandable nitinol stent for aortic position.

Current milestone calendar

1. Optimal laser source for the resection of calcified valves
2. Optimal AVIC parameters for in vivo use

Studies
Until now, this work has an experimental aim. We are developing optimal parameters for in vivo use. Before starting preclinical and clinical studies, this technology must be proven to be a safe tool.

Commercialization
There is currently no commercial tool available to resect the aortic valve in vivo.

Intellectual Property Situation
IPs are proprietary.

Experimental Aortic Valve Isolation and Resection

AVIC
The reason for isolating the aortic valve is to seal the LVOT just underneath the valve and the ascending aorta in supravalvular position. Therefore, polyethylene balloons have been used: one balloon seals the ascending aorta and another one or two balloons seal the subvalvular area. With selective catheterization, the coronary ostia will be secured.

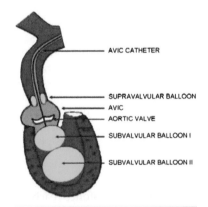

FIGURE 19 Aortic valve isolation chamber (AVIC) scheme.

AVIC Prototype 18/2005

AVIC is an endovascular catheter-based system, using polyethylene balloons and working channels. This prototype is designed for the retrograde approach. The outer diameter is 13 mm with a length of 550 mm. It consists of a stiff proximal part and a flexible distal part to cross the aortic arch. Special sheaths are added at the proximal end to insert the working tools.
The distal balloons can be inflated and deflated independently of one another.

After inflation, the sealing of the resection chamber is proven (**B, C**). The resection is performed with a high-pressure water stream scalpel (**D**) and/or with a thulium:YAG laser.

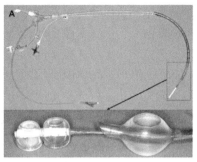

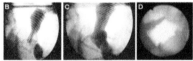

FIGURE 20 (**A**) AVIC prototype 22/2005. (**B**) Installed AVIC in situ (unfilled chamber. (**C**) AVIC in situ (contrast dye-filled chamber). (**D**) Resection of calcified human aortic valve in vitro.

Resection of Human Aortic Valves

The resection of human aortic valves in human anatomical preparations has been performed with a diode-pumped continuous wave thulium:YAG Laser emitting at a wavelength of 2.01 μm with 20 W power-rating (ITL 2000, Lisa Laser Products, Germany). The laser fiber (365 μm) was controlled by a flexible endoscope (7.5F, length 600 mm).

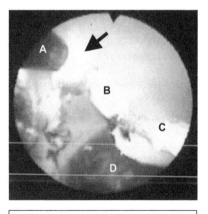

FIGURE 21 Resection sequence with the laser scalpel: (**A**) endo-scopically guided laser fiber, (**B**) right coronary aortic leaflet, (**C**) forceps catheter, (**D**) subvalvular balloon, arrow: laser light.

14 Future Perspectives and Conclusion

ACCESS PORT CLOSURE

Introduction

Access port closure might be one example of future transcatheter valve therapies' (TCVT) evolvements and will contribute to make the transapical direct access valve replacement (DAVR) become a fully percutaneous procedure.

Closure of the access port opening in the left ventricular apex is a key request to further develop the transapical procedure to become a fully percutaneous intervention. Supplementing our work, a three-step experimental approach was initiated to overcome the current surgical access port closure by insertion of a sealing device. In the first step, a muscular ventricular septal defect occluder device was used as a percutaneous plug substitute. In the consecutive follow-up studies, the surgical approach was shifted to an endoscopic access, and finally in the third study step, the closure device was further modified by a pericardial cuff to improve the sealing properties. All the three studies are summarized below.

Transapical Access Port Closure of Left Ventricle with the Use of a Muscular Ventricular Septum Defect Occluder—A Feasibility Study

Introduction

Transcatheter valve techniques as well as endovascular aortic repair (EVAR) procedures require large delivery systems (1–5). Access vessel diameter and quality as well as new access locations limit the use of the available devices. This creates the need for percutaneous closure devices. Most recently, the transapical procedure became one of the preferred access choices for transcatheter aortic valve implantation (6). A restricting characteristic of the procedure is the hemostatic control of the access port in the left ventricular free wall or apex after catheter withdrawal. The closure of the left ventricle access is a challenging procedure. Moreover, there is a consistent risk of air embolism. Currently, bleeding is controlled by a reinforced purse-string suture and the defect is closed surgically after retrieval of the delivery system. Unfortunately, the surgical closure requires a skin incision. A closure device might eliminate the need for direct surgical closure of the access port. Recent developments of sutureless devices for septal defect repairs seem to provide an adequate tool for safe and percutaneous closure of the ventricular access ports.

The following animal studies first verified the suitability of an AMPLATZER Muscular Ventricular Septal Defect Occluder (MVSDO) (7,8) as left ventricular free wall or apex closure device. The second and third experimental studies aimed at limiting the incision size by the use of thoracoscopic visualization and at optimizing the sealing properties by pericardial reinforcement of the occluder device. All experimental work was conducted at the Centre Hospitalier Universitaire Vaudois as part of our transcatheter valve research program.

The following study is partially reproduced with permission from Tozzi et al. Endoscopic off-pump aortic valve replacement: Does the pericardial cuff improve the sutureless closure of left ventricular access? Eur J Cardiothorac Surg 2007; 31(1):22–25.

Materials and Methods

The occluder device is a 12 mm AMPLATZER (AGA Medical Corporation, Golden Valley, MN) made of a nickel–titanium alloy having a predetermined thermal memory shape. The device is made of two interlinked disks sealing the targeted defect by sandwiching the surrounding tissue rim (Fig. 1). A third element, a semirigid guidewire, is secured to the device for driving the deployment. This element is unscrewed once the deployment is completed. The device is mounted into a 30F sheath to simulate the deployment of 25 mm valved stent. The deployment starts in the left ventricle with the release of the endocardial square head. The guidewire is gently pulled back until the square head is in contact with the ventricular wall. The second head is then released by pulling back the sheath, and the guidewire is unscrewed.

In compliance with the European convention on animal care and with permission of the ethics committee of University Hospital CHUV in Lausanne, a porcine experiment was performed. Under general anesthesia, the pigs (55–58 kg) were intubated and mechanically ventilated. Classic ECG monitoring was used. A catheter was inserted into left brachiocephalic vein for drug infusion and

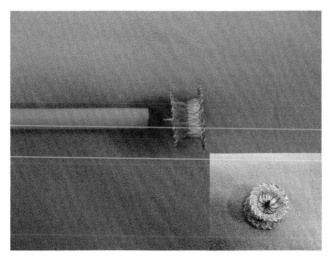

FIGURE 1 Side view and front view (*lower right corner*) of the 12 mm AMPLATZER Occluder made of nickel–titanium alloy and having a predetermined thermal memory shape allowing the device to be crimped into a 12F delivery sheath. The two interlinked circular heads anchor the device by sandwiching the surrounding tissue rim. In this study, the device is mounted into a 30F sheath to simulate the direct access valve replacement of a 25 mm valved stent via the transapical procedure.

another catheter into the left common carotid artery for invasive monitoring and blood sampling including PO_2, PCO_2, $SatO_2$, HT, K, and Na analysis.

The intravascular ultrasound probe (IVUS) (8.5 MHz, Boston Scientific, Sunnyvale, CA) was inserted into left ventricle through a 9F sheath placed in right common carotid artery. This was used to visualize the interior of the LV. The intracardiac echo transducer (ICE) (12.5 MHz, Acuson Corporation, Mountain View, CA) was inserted into the inferior vena cava through a 10F sheath placed in right femoral vein. A 5 cm substernal incision was made and the pericardium opened and suspended for enhanced visualization of the left ventricular apex [Fig. 2(A)]. Intravenous heparin (100 U/kg) was administrated targeting

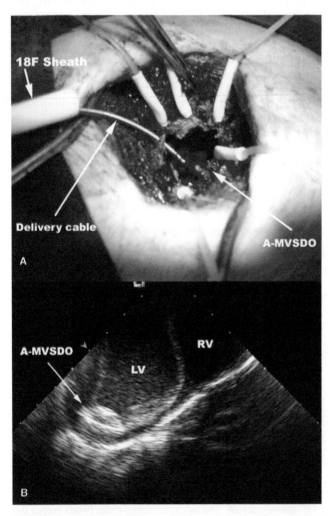

FIGURE 2 **(A)** The MVSDO completely opened and connected with a delivery cable through the substernal incision (18F sheath, external diameter 8 mm). **(B)** Intracardiac echocardiogram showing the MVSDO fully deployed within the prior access port in the LV wall.

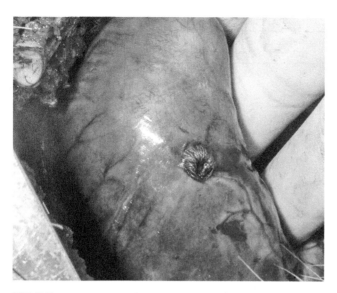

FIGURE 3 Intraoperative finding of a pig's heart. The 30F access port entry of the left ventricular free wall is successfully repaired by the occluding plug.

activated clotting time (ACT) at 200 seconds. The left ventricular apex was punctured for the transapical procedure with a needle and a guidewire, a 9F dilator, and an 18F sheath introduced subsequently into the left ventricular cavity. The 12 mm MVSDO was inserted through the 12F delivery system. Under both echocardiographic and angiographic guidance, the distal MVSDO disk was opened and pulled back out of the left ventricular wall.

Finally, the proximal disc was opened closing the left ventricular puncture hole. The correct location of the MVSDO was confirmed by ICE and angiography [Fig. 2(A) and (B)], and the occluder was detached after safe anchoring within the access port entry (Fig. 3). A pericardial drainage system was placed within the pericardial cavity and the pericardial sac was closed tightly around the transapical puncture site. Time and amount of bleeding were recorded (tank and timer principle). All animals were fully monitored for the next three hours. At the end, an autopsy was performed—particular attention was paid to the position of the occluder and eventual thrombus formation inside the left ventricular cavity.

Methodical Considerations

In all three cases, the MVSDO was successfully released at the desired target location, and all devices did anchor within the left ventricular puncture site. The entire procedure was safely monitored by both intravascular and intracardiac sonographic modalities. Deployment of all three sealing devices was performed precisely and did not require any repositioning.

After deployment, bleeding through the device lasted approximately for two minutes. Hypotension in one animal (58/29 mm Hg) resulted in less blood loss through the device (Table 1).

Single ventricular extrasystoles were common during puncturing and introduction of the sheath. Those resolved spontaneously and did not require

TABLE 1 Perioperative Data from the Feasibility Study in Three Pigs

Pig no.	Age (wk)	Weight (kg)	Bleeding (mL)	Blood pressure	Thrombus on echo	ACT(s)	Autopsy
1 (Male)	8	58	50	59/28/37	Small; between papillary muscles	200	No thrombus; good location good location of occluder
2 (Female)	8	58	650	98/56/68	No	280	No thrombus; good location of occluder
3 (Male)	8	55	800	91/53/65	No	271	Small thrombus at occluder and adjacent wall

medication. The deployment took less than 1 minute and the overall procedure took between 30 and 60 minutes.

During follow-up after implantation of the MVSDO, there were no disturbances in the left ventricular contractility noticed on echocardiographic assessment. The ACT was corrected after satisfactory device placement. In one case, a thrombus formation was suspected on ICE but not confirmed later at autopsy.

Endoscopic Access Port Closure After the Transapical Procedure with a Pericardium Reinforced Percutaneous Closure Device

The second and third follow-up studies are summarized below.

Introduction

As identified from the previous feasibility study (discussed above), the MVSDO device might be used as an anchoring element within the left ventricular free wall or apex plug but the sealing properties of the native occluder device are insufficient. The second aim of the following study is the percutaneous access port closure under thoracoscopic control.

Materials and Methods

To improve the sealing property of the AMPLATZER Ventricular Septal Occluder (discussed above), the ventricular head of the occluder was lined with a 3 cm × 3 cm thin pericardial patch sutured with 6-0 polypropylene (Fig. 4). This pericardial cuff does not affect the pushing/pulling force required to displace the occluder inside the sheath as tested in vitro.

Study design

An acute in vivo evaluation was performed in 12 adult pigs (mean body weight = 55 ± 4.3 kg; range = 43–56 kg) equipped with arterial pressure line in the right carotid artery and ECG. Under general anesthesia, left thoracoscopy was chosen to open the pericardium. One 12 mm port was inserted into the seventh intercostal space for the camera and two 5 mm ports each were inserted into the eleventh and fifth spaces. A pericardial window of 4 cm × 3 cm was then created to improve visualization of the left ventricular apex (Fig. 5). In six animals,

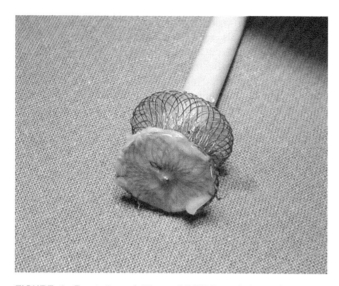

FIGURE 4 Front view of 12 mm MVSDO occluder with the pericardial cuff sutured to the intraventricular device part.

a 3 cm × 3 cm autologous pericardial patch was harvested and sutured onto the ventricular side of the occluder. After heparin injection (100 U/kg), the ICE was inserted into the right femoral vein and advanced into the right atrium under fluoroscopic control. In order to most realistically simulate the transapical procedure (TAP), a 30F sheath was subsequently advanced from the left paraxyphoid area through the left ventricular apex into the left ventricle. Removal of the

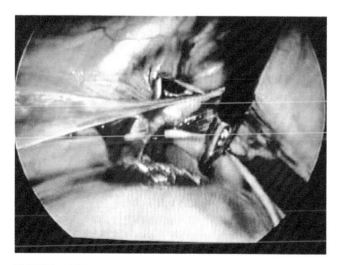

FIGURE 5 Videothoracoscopic view of a pig's heart. The 30F defect of the free wall of the left ventricle has been repaired using the modified MVSDO. The illustration shows the delivery wire still connected to the occluder after full deployment.

sheath was coordinated with insertion and deployment of the occluder system closing the access port. Six animals each were occluded with the standard occluder or with the pericardium reinforced occluder. Observation and data sampling were carried on for three hours, collecting hemodynamic data (heart rate, ECG, blood pressure, Po_2, Pco_2) every 15 minutes. Pericardial bleeding was assessed using the Smart Suction (Cardio Smart LLC, Fribourg, Switzerland), and the blood lost during the procedure was transfused to the animal (9).

Animals were then sacrificed and gross anatomical examination of the heart was carried out at necropsy.

Results

Devices were successfully deployed in all 12 animals in less than one minute. No major arrhythmias were noticed during device insertion and deployment. Blood pressure during the deployment was 50 ± 15 mm Hg. In the native occluder group, bleeding during the deployment was 80 ± 20 mL and after the deployment was 800 ± 20 mL over three hours. In the pericardium reinforced occluder group, bleeding during the deployment was 85 ± 20 mL and was significantly less during the three-hour observational period with bleeding down to 100 ± 5 mL over three hours ($p < 0.001$). Gross anatomical examination demonstrated the correct positioning of the devices. Detailed results are reported in Table 2.

Methodical Considerations

The transapical procedure offers numerous advantages over the remote access retrograde femoral approach and might be considered the next revolution in the cardiac surgery. One of the key steps of the transapical procedure is the closure of the access port. Experienced cardiac surgeons recognize the challenge of safely closing a 30F hole of the left ventricular free wall or apex without extracorporeal support. Moreover, since the procedure aims at substantially reducing the access incision to become a pure percutaneous operation, the closure of the defect seems almost impossible.

The concept of using a two square heads nitinol device to close intracardiac defects has been extensively studied. The 12 mm AMPLATZER Muscular VSD Occluder has a very similar geometry with only an increased distance between

TABLE 2 Hemodynamic Data and Blood Loss During and After Device Deployment[a]

	Baseline		Deployment		Postdeployment	
	Standard	Cuffed	Standard	Cuffed	Standard	Cuffed
Mean arterial pressure	65 ± 5 mm Hg	65 ± 5 mm Hg	48 ± 5 mm Hg	45 ± 5 mm Hg	53 ± 5 mm Hg	55 ± 5 mm Hg
ECG	Sinus rhythm	Sinus rhythm	Ventricular extrasystole	Ventricular extrasystole	Sinus rhythm	Sinus rhythm
Bleeding	n/a	n/a	80 ± 20 mL	85 ± 20 mL	800 ± 20 mL/3 hr	100 ± 5 mL/3 hr
Significance	NS	NS	NS	NS	$P < 0.001$	$P < 0.001$

Abbreviations: n/a, not applicable; NS, not significant.
[a]Two occluders were used: the standard MVSD occluder and the modified device with the pericardial cuff.

the two heads to accommodate for a larger wall thickness up to 7 mm. Figure 3 shows a deployed occluder on the left ventricular wall.

From the initial feasibility study (discussed above) it became clear that the standard muscular VSD occluder can be anchored into the access port defect of the left ventricular free wall or apex but does not provide sufficient sealing to prevent major hemorrhage. The bleeding volume through and around the MVSDO remained important. This observation differs from earlier experiences for closure of right ventricular access ports (8). The difference in the amount of bleeding is caused possibly by higher left ventricular pressure and might explain the lesser bleeding amounts in animals with lower blood pressure.

Transient ventricular extrasystoles (VES) due to the mechanical irritation of the myocardium were noted during penetration of the left ventricular wall. These disturbances vanished after the deployment of the occluder. The occluder did not cause any heart rhythm disturbances in any case after implantation. The suspected thrombus in one of the three pigs of the feasibility study was not confirmed at autopsy.

In summary, a simple modification of the occluder device by lining the intraventricular device head by a 3 cm × 3 cm harvested autologous pericardium allowed dramatic improvement in the device sealing properties as demonstrated by a significant reduction in blood loss from 800 mL in three hours down to 100 mL.

However, before clinical applications, further improvements are necessary. One concern is regarding the ventricular wall thickness: In the present configuration, the occluder does not allow an implantation in a hypertrophic left ventricular wall as both the device heads are too close to each other. Furthermore, a saving bailout strategy in case of device migration needs to be worked out and finally device longevity in this particular anatomic location with very high muscular motion needs to be assessed.

The above studies have demonstrated technical feasibility of endoscopy aided access port closure with a modified ventricular septal device occluder. A device-based access port closure strategy might further enhance the technical superiority of the transapical procedure for direct access valve replacement and allow this approach to become a full percutaneous operation.

FUTURE PERSPECTIVES OF TCVT—AN EXTRAORDINARY JOURNEY

Cardiac surgery and interventional cardiology have jointly embarked onto an extraordinary journey—the journey of transcatheter valve therapies. Treating structural heart disease by catheter-based techniques seems a natural progression shifting maximal invasiveness to scar-free surgical patient care. It is unclear what specialty will ultimately become the primary adopter. Both cardiac surgery as well as interventional cardiology provide excellent conditions to successfully advance in this field. The journey of TCVT realizes the dream of endoluminal repair based on manual skills and "sangfroid," both essential aspects of surgical disciplines. A common denominator describes both specialties well. The Greek word *Kheir* or *Chiro* stands for hand and accurately describes surgical and interventional skills as both being "handwork" and as such closely linked to each other. New developments often create new needs pushing the borders beyond given structures and transcatheter valve therapies might be performed by either specialty but rather will give rise to the interventional specialist or the surgical interventionist but only time will tell us right.

Over the last decade, this new therapy option has become increasingly supported by the clinical implementation. Some might still call it disruptive technology but most have recognized wisely one of the biggest opportunities ever to reconcile both fields to a new surgical interventional discipline. The unprecedented technical acceleration and enthusiastic acceptance by the interventional and surgical community validate the concept of TCVT as does the early clinical data.

What can be expected to come next? The answer lies in the goals this technology should achieve. Industry and most clinicians focus merely on the elderly and high-risk patients. In contrast, our vision is to elevate the transcatheter valve therapies to a state as to replace the current surgical practice of aortic valve replacement by this incision-free technique. At first, the clinical data as well as the various device concepts require consolidation and continuous development. Transcatheter valve therapies are in infancy and enormous progress can be expected in the coming years. Nevertheless, some limitations will remain widely independent from technical progression, for example, the length from insertion site to delivery site defined by the access technique or the diseased vasculature and so forth. The transapical procedure, in contrast, is currently limited only by the required surgical incision and the need for safe access closure. Both the elements can easily be overcome by pure engineering independent of the patient's anatomy or clinical condition.

There can be no doubt that transcatheter valve therapies are facing an extremely promising future, but introduction of a novel technology requires continuous and ongoing efforts set in a limited and controlled clinical surrounding. Early enthusiasm will inevitably encounter drawbacks and unexpected limitations but those will have to be mastered by stepwise adoption.

The position statement issued in May 2008 by the European Association for Cardio-Thoracic Surgery (EACTS) and the European Society of Cardiology (ESC), in collaboration with the European Association of Percutaneous Cardiovascular Interventions (EAPCI) (10), very well opinionated the future progression and level of evidence about transcatheter valve therapies:

> The evidence suggests that this technique is feasible and provides hemodynamic and clinical improvement for up to 2 years in patients with severe symptomatic aortic stenosis at high risk or with contraindications for surgery. Questions remain mainly concerning safety and long-term durability, which have to be assessed. Surgeons and cardiologists working as a team should select candidates, perform the procedure, and assess the results. Today, the use of this technique should be restricted to high-risk patients or those with contraindications for surgery. However, this may be extended to lower risk patients if the initial promise holds to be true after careful evaluation. Conclusion: Transcatheter aortic valve implantation is a promising technique, which may offer an alternative to conventional surgery for high-risk patients with aortic stenosis. Today, careful evaluation is needed to avoid the risk of uncontrolled diffusion.

Undoubtedly, many obstacles remain asking for new answers, but new ingenious approaches merging surgical and interventional advantages and novel technologies will overcome the current shortcomings. Cardiac surgery is evolving in rapid pace toward scar-free surgery, and technological developments are providing the necessary support for the successful embedding into current clinical practice. Operating from within the heart offers tremendous therapeutic benefits to the patients in all risk groups and disease stages.

Direct access valve replacement for the treatment of aortic valve disease joins major advantages of transcatheter valve therapies and surgical approaches and might become the therapy of choice for aortic valve replacement and structural heart disease in the near future.

REFERENCES

1. Bonhoffer P, Budjemline Y, Saliba Z, et al. Transcatheter implantation of a bovine valve in pulmonary position: A lamb study. Circulation 2000; 102:813–816.
2. Criber A, Eltchaninoff H, Bash A, et al. Percutaneous transcatheter implantation of an aortic valve prosthesis for calcific aortic stenosis: First human case description. Circulation 2002; 106:3006–3008.
3. Huber CH, Nasratulla M, Augstburger M, et al. Ultrasound navigation through the heart for off-pump aortic valved stent implantation: New tools for new goals. J Endovasc Ther 2004; 11(4):503–510.
4. Huber CH, Tozzi P, Corno AF, et al. Do valved stents compromise coronary flow? Eur J Cardiothorac Surg 2004; 25:754–759.
5. Zhou JQ, Corno AF, Huber CH, et al. Self-expandable valved stent of large size: Off-bypass implantation in pulmonary position. Eur J Cardiothorac Surg 2003; 24:212–216.
6. Vassiliades TA, Block PC, Cohn LH, et al. The clinical development of percutaneous heart valve technology: A position statement of the Society of Thoracic Surgeons (STS), the American Association for Thoracic Surgery (AATS), and the Society for Cardiovascular Angiography and Interventions (SCAI). J Am Coll Cardiol 2005; 45: 1554–1560.
7. Bacha EA, Cao Q, Starr JP, et al. Perventricular device closure of muscular ventricular septal defects on the beating heart: Technique and results. J Thorac Cardiovasc Surg 2003; 126:1718–1723.
8. Pawelec-Wojtalik M, Antosik P, Wasiatycz G, et al. Use of muscular VSD Amplatzer occluder for closing right ventricular free wall perforation after hybrid procedure. Eur J Cardiothorac Surg 2004; 26:1044–1046.
9. Mueller X, Tevaerai HT, Horisberger J, et al. Smart suction device for less blood trauma: A comparison with Cell Saver. Eur J Cardiothorac Surg 2001; 19(4):507–511.
10. Vahanian A, Alfieri OR, Al-Attar N, et al. Transcatheter valve implantation for patients with aortic stenosis: A position statement from the European Association of Cardio-Thoracic Surgery (EACTS) and the European Society of Cardiology (ESC), in collaboration with the European Association of Percutaneous Cardiovascular Interventions (EAPCI) [published online ahead of print May 12, 2008]. Eur Heart J. 2008; 29(11):1463–1470.

Index

Printed and bound by CPI Group (UK) Ltd, Croydon, CR0 4YY

21/10/2024

01777044-0003